AI in Yoga Studies

Mohammad Ayoub Khan
https://orcid.org/0000-0002-0398-3722
University of Bisha, Saudi Arabia

Raghav Mehra
https://orcid.org/0009-0001-8542-515X
Chandigarh University, India

Kanaga Suba Raja
https://orcid.org/0000-0002-3626-1806
SRM Institute of Science and Technology, India

Pushkar Praveen
G.B. Pant Institute of Engineering and Technology, India

Rijwan Khan
https://orcid.org/0000-0003-3354-3047
Marwadi University, India

IGI Global
Scientific Publishing
Publishing Tomorrow's Research Today

Vice President of Editorial	Melissa Wagner
Director of Acquisitions	Mikaela Felty
Director of Book Development	Jocelynn Hessler
Production Manager	Mike Brehm
Cover Design	Jose Rosado

Published in the United States of America by
IGI Global Scientific Publishing
701 East Chocolate Avenue
Hershey, PA, 17033, USA
Tel: 717-533-8845 | Fax: 717-533-7115
Website: https://www.igi-global.com E-mail: cust@igi-global.com

Library of Congress Cataloging-in-Publication Data

LCCN: 2026029207 (CIP Data Pending)
ISBN13: 979-8-2600-2463-8
Isbn13Softcover: 979-8-2600-2464-5
EISBN13: 979-8-2600-2465-2
British Cataloguing in Publication Data
A Cataloguing in Publication record for this book is available from the British Library.

Table of Contents

Detailed Table of Contents

have the potential to help alleviate some of these challenges by offering scalable, customizable, and culture-adaptable modes of yoga instruction. The chapter concludes by looking at how Yoga AI might positively impact the accessibility to quality yoga practice as well as some concerns related to digital equity and the commoditization of traditional knowledge systems.

The chapter addresses the ethical vacuum in the development of artificial intelligence for yoga. The chapter identifies that many wellness technologies are reducing the holistic practice of yoga to physical performance alone and as such, create significant risks of algorithmic harm, data exploitation and user dependency. The author suggests that the ten foundational principles of ethics by Patañjali's Yoga Sutras (the five yamas – social restraints & the five niyamas – personal observances) provide a framework for responsible innovation in AI. The author outlines the mapping of each principle of the five yamas to the five niyamas to the challenges and solutions of AI design, including ahimsa (non-harming) to svadhyaya (self-reflection). Through this process, the author proposes a new paradigm of "Sattvic Technology," which is designed to develop AI systems that support inner inquiry and holistic well-being, rather than simply quantify and gamify the practice of yoga.

Artificial intelligence is finding its way into the health and wellness industries, and products such as yoga classes, practice tracking, and customized recommendations are being provided. However, the software is also full of culture, gender and body-type prejudices making yoga not exactly inclusive and accessible. The study investigates the effects of the asymmetry of data representation, biased algorithmic performance and overfitting to training datasets that are culturally homogenous on stereotype propagation and alienation of diversified classes of end-users. It discusses the possibility of the development of the inclusive systems of AI which will not ignore the philosophy of yoga, and do not give preference to any individual based on

Even though the studies involving AI usage in yogasana are scarce, the experience of other sports involving precision proves that it can transform the sphere of athlete development, increase the consistency of judges, and assist with international promotion, even with an opportunity to participate in the Olympics.

This chapter talks about the possibility of artificial intelligence to facilitate the study and knowledge of subtle energetic systems, namely the Nadis and Chakras explained in the traditional science of yogic practices. Lighting up the models of the ancient energy with the aid of modern computational, the AI helps to identify patterns, conduct predictive analyses, and objectively estimate physiological, emotional, and energy states. Artificial intelligence algorithms, bio-signaling, and multi-modal data-hypothesis receive aid in the detection of relationships amid breath rate, neurophysiological response and electromagnetic difference, as well as chakra or nadi-activation model. The chapter underscores how AI-based simulations, biometric sensing, and digital twin solutions could provide a new understanding of the nature of energy flows and assist in understanding individualized wellness measurements and populace science and knowledge.

This chapter introduces Prana-Centered AI, a pioneering framework that blends ancient yogic energetics with modern intelligent wellness technologies. While contemporary AI-powered wearables excel at tracking physiological data, they overlook the subtle dimensions of human vitality described in classical yoga, Prana,

Nadis, Chakras, and the subtle body. Prana-Centered AI bridges this gap through multimodal sensing, machine learning, and culturally sensitive interpretive models that translate physiological signals into insights aligned with yogic principles. By integrating HRV, EEG, respiration, thermal imaging, and emotional analytics, the framework enables personalized guidance for breathwork, meditation, and energetic balance. This chapter outlines its architecture, scientific foundations, ethical safeguards, and emerging applications, proposing a transformative, holistic pathway for future intelligent wellness systems.

For more than two millennia, yoga has been taught by direct observation of the practitioner, but until now, the hidden physiological state of the practitioner has been unknown to themselves and the teacher. Here, we present the Wearable Intelligence Yoga Framework (WIYF) that provides real-time, personalised feedback during yoga practice through the integration of multimodal wearable sensors (heart rate variability (HRV), brain electrical activity (EEG), skin conductance (GSR) and inertial measurement units (IMUs)), edge-placed artificial intelligence (AI), and the Ayurvedic science of personalisation. The WIYF integrates three bodies of theory: the yogic Pancha Kosha model of the human, Ayurvedic Prakriti physiology, and closed-loop adaptive control systems engineering. This chapter presents three case studies that illustrate how the personalisation engine adapts the feedback modes, targets for a practice session and long-term learning to the individual. The chapter concludes with an ethical discussion of privacy, algorithmic bias, quantified self over-reach, and equity.

This chapter presents a new socio-technical paradigm, YogAI, which is a combination of the ancient wisdom of Yogic Intelligence (YI) as embodied in the Yoga Sutras, Ayurveda & Indian Knowledge Systems (IKS) on the whole, with the modern AI & machine learning. In the context of increasing global stress, sleep disorders, and the constraints of state-of-the-art AI in digital wellness (scarcity of data, interpretation deficiencies, ethical deficiencies), YogAI suggests an integrative architecture in which multimodal wearable physiological measures (HRV, EDA, PPG, actigraphy) are enhanced through advanced generative models (TimeGAN, VAEs, classical The chapter aligns yogic constructs (Chitta Vritti Nirodha), Pranayama, Dhyana, Prakriti with AI elements (attention mechanisms, recurrent models, Dosha-personalized pipelines) and places IKS not in the history of AI but in a practical design philosophy of responsible, human-centered AI. Ethical aspects informed by the principles of Yama/Niyama and implications to digital health, NEP 2020, and the Global South are deeply discussed.

Middle school is a phase where these young students are expected to focus, manage their learning, balance their emotions, and perform well in academics- all at once. It is difficult for the students to accomplish any of these regularly in the world crowded with digital distractions, and intensifying academic pressure. This chapter examines whether a simple, ancient breath-awareness practice called Anapana mindfulness meditation can make a meaningful difference. A quasi experimental study conducted with sixty middle school students in Sangareddy District, Telangana, India. Thirty students received an eight week structured Anapana mindfulness intervention and other thirty are for comparison in control group. The study measured changes in Sustained Attention (using the PEBL Clock test), Academic self-regulation (using the Academic Self-Regulation Questionnaire-A), and Academic Performance (using school examination scores). The results were remarkable.

Preface

INTRODUCTION

The convergence of artificial intelligence and yoga studies marks a transformative moment in the evolution of both technological innovation and holistic human development. For centuries, yoga has served as a multidimensional system for physical well-being, mental clarity, ethical living, and spiritual inquiry. Simultaneously, artificial intelligence has emerged as one of the defining technological forces of the twenty-first century, reshaping healthcare, education, communication, and human interaction. *AI in Yoga Studies* is situated at the intersection of these two influential domains, exploring how intelligent systems can support, enhance, and critically challenge contemporary understandings of yoga practice, philosophy, and wellness.

As editors, we recognized the growing global interest in AI-driven wellness ecosystems, wearable technologies, adaptive learning systems, and personalized health applications rooted in yogic traditions. Yet, alongside these advancements lies an urgent need for scholarly reflection regarding ethics, inclusivity, cultural preservation, data privacy, and the human dimensions of embodied practice. This volume was conceived not merely as a technical exploration of AI applications in yoga, but as an interdisciplinary dialogue that bridges computing sciences, yogic philosophy, healthcare, ethics, sports sciences, mindfulness research, and Indian Knowledge Systems. The contributors to this collection represent diverse academic and professional backgrounds, bringing together perspectives that reflect the richness and complexity of this emerging field.

One of the defining features of this book is its emphasis on balance. While technological systems offer scalability, personalization, and accessibility, yoga itself remains deeply rooted in lived experience, teacher-student relationships, ethical discipline, and inner transformation. The chapters in this volume consistently engage with this duality: the promise of intelligent systems to democratize wellness practices, and the responsibility to ensure that such systems do not reduce yoga to mere data points, gamified exercises, or commercialized routines detached from their philosophical foundations. Throughout the book, readers will encounter discussions that place equal importance on innovation and integrity, scientific progress and cultural sensitivity, automation and human-centered design.

This volume also reflects the broader global movement toward integrative and preventive healthcare. Across disciplines, there is increasing recognition that future wellness systems must combine physiological monitoring, behavioral intelligence, mental health support, and ethical technological frameworks. Yoga, with its holistic understanding of the human condition, provides an especially meaningful context in which to develop these intelligent systems. AI technologies, when thoughtfully designed, may support practitioners through personalized guidance, biofeedback, accessibility tools, and adaptive learning environments that were previously unimaginable. At the same time, these systems demand careful scrutiny concerning consent, surveillance, representation, fairness, and cultural stewardship.

The editors hope this volume will serve researchers, educators, practitioners, technologists, healthcare professionals, and policymakers alike. Beyond documenting emerging innovations, this book invites critical reflection on what it means to integrate ancient wisdom traditions with intelligent technologies in responsible and meaningful ways. It is our aspiration that *AI in Yoga Studies* contributes to a growing scholarly discourse that values not only technological advancement, but also compassion, inclusivity, human flourishing, and ethical consciousness.

OVERVIEW OF THE CHAPTERS

Chapter 1, *AI for Community Building and Human–AI Collaboration in Yoga*, explores how artificial intelligence is reshaping the communal and relational dimensions of yoga practice. Moving beyond posture correction technologies, the chapter examines how AI can foster human collaboration, strengthen digital yoga communities, and support shared wellness experiences while remaining aligned with traditional yogic values and teacher-student relationships.

Chapter 2, *Global Accessibility and Socio-Economic Impact of Yoga AI*, investigates how AI-powered yoga systems may democratize access to yoga education and wellness practices across geographic and socio-economic boundaries. The chapter discusses the opportunities and challenges associated with scalable digital yoga platforms, emphasizing affordability, inclusivity, and the implications of commodifying traditional knowledge systems.

Chapter 3, *Ethical AI in Yoga: Lessons from Yama and Niyama*, presents an innovative ethical framework for AI design grounded in the principles of Patañjali's

Yoga Sutras. By mapping yogic ethical concepts such as ahimsa, satya, and svadhyaya onto modern AI challenges, the chapter introduces the concept of "Sattvic Technology," advocating for AI systems that encourage self-awareness, well-being, and ethical responsibility.

Chapter 4, *Inclusive AI for Yoga Overcoming Bias in Representation and Practice*, addresses issues of cultural, gender, and body-type bias in AI-driven yoga systems. The authors examine how biased datasets and homogenous algorithmic training can marginalize users and propose strategies for building culturally sensitive, inclusive, and ethically responsible AI tools for yoga instruction and practice.

Chapter 5, *Addressing Privacy, Data Security, and Consent in Yoga AI Applications*, focuses on the ethical and technical dimensions of privacy-preserving AI systems within yoga ecosystems. The chapter discusses federated learning, culturally informed user experience design, and transparency-based trust frameworks that support sustainable and ethically grounded adoption of intelligent yoga technologies.

Chapter 6, *Exploring the Impact of AI on the Growth of Yogasana as a Global Competitive Sport*, examines the role of AI in transforming Yogasana into a globally recognized competitive discipline. Topics include performance analytics, wearable technologies, automated judging systems, injury prevention, and the role of intelligent systems in enhancing fairness, accessibility, and international visibility.

Chapter 7, *Artificial Intelligence Applications in Subtle Energetic Systems of Nadis and Chakras*, explores how AI technologies may contribute to understanding subtle energetic systems described in yogic traditions. Integrating biometric sensing, computational modeling, and predictive analytics, the chapter investigates the scientific and philosophical possibilities of studying Nadis, Chakras, and energetic flow through intelligent systems.

Chapter 8, *Prana-Centered AI Integrating Subtle Yogic Energetics into Intelligent Wellness Systems*, introduces a holistic framework that combines multimodal sensing technologies with yogic concepts of Prana, Nadis, and Chakras. The chapter outlines how intelligent wellness systems may provide personalized guidance for meditation, breathwork, and energetic balance while maintaining cultural and ethical sensitivity.

Chapter 9, *YogAI for Preventive and Personalized Healthcare: A Knowledge-Driven Integrative Approach Taking Bio Feedback Using Wearable Sensors*, presents the Wearable Intelligence Yoga Framework (WIYF), which integrates wearable sensing technologies, AI-driven adaptive feedback systems, Ayurvedic personalization, and yogic theory. Through case studies, the chapter demonstrates how intelligent systems can support preventive healthcare and personalized wellness practices.

Chapter 10, *YogAI—Bridging Yogic Intelligence and Artificial Intelligence through Indian Knowledge Systems for Personalized Stress, Sleep, and Wellness Management*, proposes a socio-technical paradigm that integrates Yogic Intelligence, Ayurveda, and Indian Knowledge Systems with advanced machine learning and generative AI models. The chapter discusses applications in stress management, sleep analysis, wellness personalization, and responsible human-centered AI design.

Chapter 11, *Effectiveness of ANAPANA Mindfulness Meditation on Sustained Attention, Academic Self-Regulation, and Academic Performance among Middle School Students*, presents an empirical investigation into the educational and psychological benefits of mindfulness meditation practices. Using an intervention-based study design, the chapter demonstrates how structured Anapana mindfulness practices can improve attention, academic self-regulation, and performance among middle school students.

CONCLUSION

The chapters presented in this volume collectively demonstrate that the intersection of artificial intelligence and yoga studies is not merely a technological trend, but an emerging interdisciplinary field with profound implications for wellness, healthcare, ethics, education, and human development. Across the contributions, a recurring theme becomes evident: intelligent systems have the potential to significantly expand access to yoga practices, personalize wellness experiences, support preventive healthcare, and deepen our understanding of human physiology and consciousness. At the same time, these opportunities are inseparable from important ethical responsibilities related to privacy, inclusivity, cultural integrity, and the preservation of yoga's philosophical foundations.

A particularly valuable contribution of this volume lies in its insistence that AI should serve as a collaborative and supportive force rather than a replacement for human wisdom, embodied experience, or authentic community. The discussions surrounding human-AI collaboration, ethical design informed by Yama and Niyama, and culturally sensitive algorithmic development emphasize that technological innovation must remain grounded in compassion, responsibility, and human-centered values. In many ways, the book advocates for a new paradigm of intelligent wellness systems—one that combines computational precision with ethical consciousness and holistic well-being.

The diversity of topics explored in this collection also illustrates the remarkable breadth of contemporary yoga studies. From wearable biofeedback systems and personalized healthcare frameworks to subtle energetic modeling, competitive Yogasana analytics, and mindfulness interventions in educational settings, the contributors demonstrate that yoga-related AI research extends far beyond fitness applications. Instead, it encompasses broad questions concerning consciousness, embodiment, preventive medicine, social equity, digital trust, and the future relationship between humans and intelligent systems. This interdisciplinary scope positions yoga studies as an important domain for developing responsible and humane approaches to AI innovation.

As editors, we believe this volume opens pathways for future scholarship and collaboration across disciplines that have historically remained separate. Researchers in artificial intelligence may gain new insights from yogic philosophies of self-awareness and ethical discipline, while yoga scholars and practitioners may discover new opportunities for expanding accessibility, personalization, and evidence-based wellness interventions through technology. The future of AI in yoga studies will depend not only on computational advances, but also on the collective wisdom of scholars, practitioners, educators, technologists, and policymakers working together to shape systems that genuinely support human flourishing.

We extend our sincere gratitude to all chapter authors, reviewers, academic collaborators, and publishing professionals whose contributions made this volume possible. Their dedication, expertise, and interdisciplinary vision have helped create a scholarly work that we hope will inspire meaningful dialogue and continued exploration in this rapidly evolving field. It is our hope that *AI in Yoga Studies* will encourage future generations of researchers and practitioners to approach innovation with both scientific curiosity and ethical mindfulness, ensuring that the integration of AI and yoga contributes positively to individual well-being and the collective future of society.

Chapter 1
AI for Community Building and Human-AI Collaboration in Yoga

Yagnik Dave
http://orcid.org/0000-0003-0506-9536
Marwadi University, Rajkot, India

Ankur Khant
http://orcid.org/0009-0004-8492-2615
Marwadi University, Rajkot, India

Hemang Jani
http://orcid.org/0000-0002-8475-7558
Ganpat University, Gujarat, India

Ashish Kakkad
http://orcid.org/0009-0006-9291-4839
Marwadi University, Rajkot, India

Brijesh Verma
Marwadi University, Rajkot, India

Mrunal Harle
http://orcid.org/0009-0004-6842-3664
District Civil Hospital, Amravati, India

ABSTRACT

This chapter critically analyzes how the Artificial Intelligence (AI) has influenced the modern yoga practice, especially community building and human-AI partnership. As recent advances in AI-assisted yoga have focused mostly on posture correction and personalized instructions, this chapter goes beyond the technical focus and addresses the social, ethical, and philosophical consequences of the AI integration into the yoga ecosystems. The conceptualization of AI as a collaborative and supporting resource is based on the yogic philosophy, human-AI interaction and community studies and underlies the chapter. This analysis places yoga as a traditionally communal and experiential tradition that has traditionally been based on teacher-student relationships, ethical practice, and practice together.

DOI: 10.4018/979-8-2600-2463-8.ch001

1. INTRODUCTION AND CONTEXT

Yoga is a comprehensive practice system that is based on the ancient Indian knowledge traditions, which is made up of physical discipline, mental development, moral behavior, and spiritual questioning. Since the earliest expressions in the Vedic tradition, Upani adic philosophy and subsequent systematic expressions, like the Yoga Sutras, yoga has served as a unified path to self-awareness, equanimity and freedom of suffering. More importantly, yoga has not been limited to a set of physical postures or practices. Instead, it has been perceived as experiential and ethical training where physical practice, control of breath, meditation and moral restraint do in concert to alter perception, behavior, and social relations(Sinha & Sinha, 2024).

Traditionally, yoga has been handed down in relational and communal systems that supported the philosophical richness and experiential genuineness of yoga. Education was also practiced in close pedagogical student teacher relationships, pedagogy based on lineages, ashrams, monastic societies, and group practices, where it was delivered, as a progressive process over time, through observation, dialogue, repetition, and moral exemplification. These group environments did not only give them technical direction, but served as moral communities, education on forms of discipline, humility, accountability and shared responsibility. The social aspect of yoga: expressed through common practices, through the collective study, and through the co-presence of embodiment, has thus been at the center of the survival as a living tradition not as a dead technique collection(Jain et al., 2025).

Ethical aspect of yoga could never be separated with its practical forms. The precepts like non-harm (ahi sah), truthfulness (satya), self-discipline (tapas), non-attachment (aparigraha), and contemplative self-study (svadhyaya) not only were used to organize the individual behavior, but also organize community life. These principles influenced the ways of spreading knowledge, exercising authority, and relations between practitioners to each other. Yoga communities were therefore sites of ethical cultivation just like technical education, causing the notion of personal transformation and social harmony to be mutually dependent(Gupta et al., 2025).

Over the past decades, though, forces of globalization, commercialization and digitalization have had a dramatic influence on the proliferation of yoga throughout the world. Yoga has turned out to be a transnational phenomenon wherein it is practiced in a varied cultural, economic, and ideological context. Digital platforms, mobile applications, video-based classes, and online classes have facilitated access to yoga practice in a way that has never been available before, as people can approach it without considering geographical factors, time, or institutional membership. This has helped in spreading the visibility of yoga around the world and also making it more inclusive, which has created avenues of participation that were hitherto limited to many(Shrivastava et al., 2024).

Meanwhile, this change has brought in great strains. Platform-mediated migration of yoga has commonly been surrounded by standardization, commodification and individualization processes. There is often a trade-off between personalised instructions, moral foundation, and long-lasting community engagement and the discourse of digital yoga of scale, convenience and visual performance. Relational contexts that entailed practices were previously built in terms of long-term are starting to be consumed as discrete and demand based products. Such a change casts important doubts concerning the manner in which the human-centered, experiential, and ethical nature of yoga can be maintained in systems of data and commerciality(Selvaraj & Priya, 2025).

Community fragmentation has been one of the greatest effects of the digitalization process. Although digital platforms can be used to reach a large number of users, it is not necessarily accompanied by deep-seated relationships, joint responsibility, and shared reflection. Practitioners can practice in isolation, and advised sequences can be prerecorded or algorithmically suggested and have no chance to talk or to be mentored. This loss of community institutions poses the risk of turning yoga into an individual, commercial interaction process, undermining the relationship pillars that traditionally have been the sources of ethical formation and sustained practice.

Among these changing circumstances, the phenomenon of Artificial Intelligence (AI) has become a potent and ever more forceful force of technology. Developments in machine learning, computer vision, affective computing, and adaptive systems have allowed AI applications to understand human motion, identify learning behavior patterns, deduce emotional states and provide personalized interaction on a scale. In education, health, and wellness, AI-based tools have become popular, intending to personalize the instruction, giving a real-time response, and making distributed communities more engaging(Hanwari et al., 2024).

These abilities pose both enormous opportunities and great problems when it comes to yoga. On the one hand, AI has the capacity to make systems more accessible by assisting practitioners with limited access to a face-to-face education system, a body- and ability-friendly approach, and adaptive recommendations that can be provided based on personal needs. The applications of AI-enabled systems can help to prevent injuries with the help of biomechanical assessment, assist in sustaining practice with the help of the personalised recommendations, and connect geographically scattered professionals. In this sense, AI is seen as a possibility of making yoga more widespread and more inclusive.

Conversely, the introduction of AI into yoga also brings up the issue of technical performance, which is not the only area of concern. AI systems work on the basis of data extraction, classification, and optimization- logics which can be incompatible with the yoga focus on mindfulness, non-attachment and awareness of the inner world. The practice of quantifying what is practiced and turning it into measurable scales is a danger to give preference to what is measurable over what is felt, comprehended, or discerned ethically. Unless given deep consideration, AI-based yoga applications could add to the issue of dehumanization, surveillance, and philosophical watering down, transforming the practices in a manner that adversely affects the transformative purposes(Adeyemi, 2024).

Figure 1. AI in yoga: opportunities and challenges

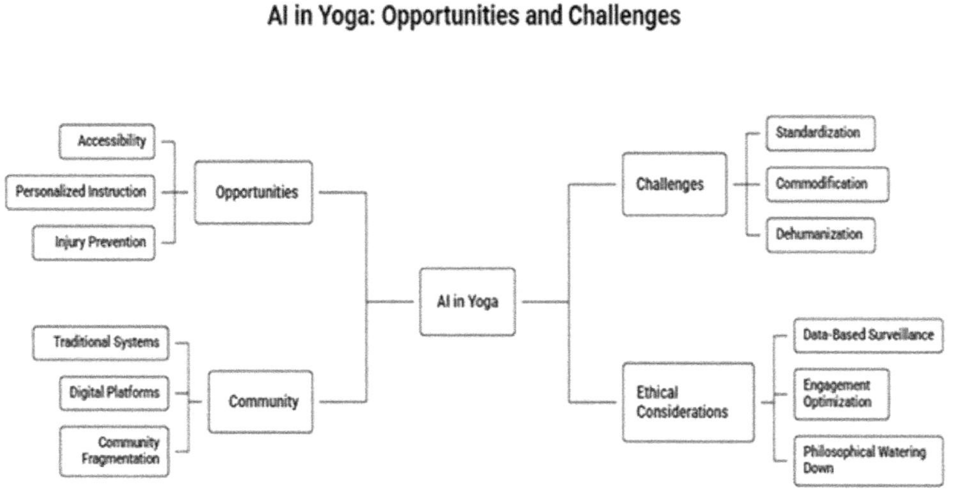

The available studies on AI-assisted yoga have mainly focused on technical advancements including posture identification, motion detection, and automatic corrective feedback. Such studies prove that AI can assist clinicians with detecting points of discrepancy, providing personalized instructions, and minimizing risks of injuries. Though these developments are important, overly technical focus can make yoga more of a performance or remedial exercise. Yoga, nevertheless, is necessarily relational and reflective, comprising aspects of will, mindfulness, and moral point of view which cannot be objectively described through computational analysis on its own.

This technical orientation also is likely to construct AI as an expert teacher or a substitute to teaching by a human. These framings ignore pedagogical, moral and community functions that were traditionally played by teachers and practice communities. No one definition of yoga has ever existed that is confined to imparting the right form, but it is contextual meanings, moral direction, and human sensitivity. It is a tendency within educational technology to emphasize automation rather than augmentation, which is reflected in the assumption that AI can replace these positions(Verma et al., 2023).

This chapter would find itself in this crucial gap by redefining the position of AI in yoga and positioning it as an ally, rather than a notable teacher. Instead of shaping AI as an independent teacher or authority, the chapter frames AI as a facilitative partner existing in co-innovation with the human teacher, practitioner and community. This view is in agreement to human-competent AI designs such as augmentation, transparency, and ethical responsibility. It is also close to the yogic principles of balance and co-existence with technology giving prominence to harmony instead of commanding technology.

At the center of this revamping is the concept of community. Yoga has traditionally been maintained in group settings that strengthen the sense of discipline, responsibility and support of one another. The degradation of these social constructs in virtual space has added to the sense of alienation, shallow interaction, and diminished moral loci among the practitioners. Considered in a sensitive, ethically-minded way, AI-based systems can bring back the idea of community-based dynamics as they will enable meaningful interaction, learning between peers, and participation. In this way, by means of clever grouping, customized communication, and culture-sensitive interfaces, AI can assist in restoring the feeling of belonging in virtual and hybrid yoga ecosystems(Singh, n.d.).

Meanwhile, the application of AI to the field of study that is based on mindfulness and self-awareness requires an ethical and philosophical thoughtfulness. In Yogic cultures, restraint, compassion, and deliberate presence are the encouraged values which could be lost under the conditions of data-based surveillance, engagement optimization, or competitive metrics. Unless there are conscious protection measures, AI-based platforms are likely to focus on making money and influencing behavior more than on health and reflection. This conflict highlights the significance of investigating the manner in which and why AI is used, as well as what AI is capable of doing in yoga communities.

In this regard, in this chapter the interdisciplinary approach is implemented that relies on the study of yoga philosophy, human-AI interaction, the research of digital ethics, and the theory of community. By intertwining these areas, it aims at providing a subtle interpretation of how AI can be incorporated in a yoga practice without compromising the core principles it is based on. The analysis identifies the fact that technology is not a value-neutral construct; it is based on assumptions, priorities and power arrangements incorporated in its design. It is only through responsible integration that the tech capabilities and the ethical orientation of the yoga itself will have to align.

The chapter will lead to other debates in wellness technology regarding automation or augmentation with respect to the concept of AI as a college, not as a substitute, hence posing no threat to existing jobs. An anthropocentric AI research focuses on maintaining the intelligence, ethical obligation, plus situational cognition of humans. Such issues are especially relevant in yoga, where relational teaching and embodied presence are the main focus of studying. The chapter advances the idea of foregrounding collaboration in which AI amplifies the capabilities of humans but does not affect the uniqueness of teachers, communities, and experience.

This introductory part of the section therefore sets the conceptual basis of the behavior to explore AI as a means to community building and human-AI interaction in yoga. It puts the discussion into the context of technological possibility and philosophical responsibility that constitute the two realities. With yoga becoming digitalized in informing digitally mediated settings, the question is not how to stop being digitized, but how to do so in the ways that do not compromise the richness, values, and community involved in the practice. What then follows is a development of this foundation by examining the practical mechanisms of AI based community building, and the collaborative learning paradigms, ethical risks, and responsible design frameworks, with all the intention being to create a fruitful and thoughtful partnership between technological innovation and yogic wisdom(Duppala et al., 2024).

Table 1. Artificial Intelligence, Yoga Practice, Ethics, and Community Dynamics

Study (Author, Year)	Country / Context	Study Design & Data Source	AI Application / Digital Modality	Core Focus (Technical / Ethical / Community)	Key Findings	Community & Ethical Implications	Limitations Identified	Relevance to Present Chapter
Sinha & Sinha (2024)	India	Conceptual–philosophical analysis (Yoga texts + modern pedagogy)	Non-AI, traditional yoga pedagogy	Ethical–philosophical foundations of yoga	Yoga is an integrative ethical–experiential discipline; physical postures are secondary to moral and cognitive cultivation	Emphasizes relational learning, lineage-based transmission, and ethical co-presence	Lacks empirical validation	Establishes philosophical baseline against which AI-mediated yoga must be evaluated
Jain et al. (2025)	India	Qualitative ethnographic study (Ashram communities)	Hybrid digital–physical learning	Community transmission of yoga	Communal practice sustains discipline, accountability, and ethical orientation	Community is central to moral learning and sustained practice	Limited generalizability beyond ashrams	Highlights what is lost when yoga is fully digitized
Shrivastava et al. (2024)	Global	Systematic review (Digital yoga platforms)	Apps, video-based classes	Accessibility & scalability	Digital yoga increases access and inclusion across geography and socio-economic groups	Weak relational depth; reduced mentorship	Over-reliance on platform self-report data	Demonstrates benefits and structural gaps of digital yoga

continued on following page

Table 1. Continued

Study (Author, Year)	Country / Context	Study Design & Data Source	AI Application / Digital Modality	Core Focus (Technical / Ethical / Community)	Key Findings	Community & Ethical Implications	Limitations Identified	Relevance to Present Chapter
Selvaraj & Priya (2025)	India	Critical policy analysis	Platform-based wellness services	Commercialization & standardization	Digital yoga commodifies practice, prioritizing performance and visual metrics	Ethical dilution; erosion of collective responsibility	Conceptual, not empirical	Supports critique of market-driven AI yoga models
Hanwari et al. (2024)	Global	Experimental ML-based study	AI posture detection, motion analytics	Technical optimization	AI improves posture accuracy and injury prevention	Neglects mindfulness, intention, and ethical reflection	Focused on biomechanics only	Illustrates risks of reductionist AI framing
Adeyemi (2024)	Global	Normative AI ethics review	AI in mindfulness & wellness	Ethical risk analysis	Quantification biases favor measurable outcomes over experiential awareness	Surveillance and dehumanization risks	Broad wellness focus, not yoga-specific	Grounds ethical concerns in AI-yoga integration
Verma et al. (2023)	India	Educational technology review	AI tutors & automation models	Pedagogy & automation	AI framed as replacement rather than augmentation	Undermines teacher authority and moral guidance	Limited yoga-specific discussion	Supports argument for AI as collaborator, not teacher
Gupta, N. et al. (2025)	India	Textual + sociological synthesis	Non-digital	Ethics & community norms	Yogic ethics structure social relations and authority	Ethical cultivation is inseparable from practice	Theoretical orientation	Reinforces inseparability of ethics and technique

continued on following page

Table 1. Continued

Study (Author, Year)	Country / Context	Study Design & Data Source	AI Application / Digital Modality	Core Focus (Technical / Ethical / Community)	Key Findings	Community & Ethical Implications	Limitations Identified	Relevance to Present Chapter
Singh, B. (n.d.)	Global	Design theory (Human-centered AI)	AI-supported online communities	Community rebuilding	AI can facilitate peer learning and belonging if ethically designed	Emphasizes cultural sensitivity and transparency	Lacks empirical validation	Directly informs AI-enabled community design framework
Duppala et al. (2024)	India	Interdisciplinary review	AI + wellness platforms	Responsible AI integration	Advocates augmentation, ethical governance, and human oversight	Aligns with yogic principles of balance	High-level synthesis	Provides integrative framework adopted by this chapter

2. CHAPTER MISSION, SCOPE, AND CONCEPTUAL POSITIONING

The cornerstones of this chapter are the critical examination of the role of Artificial Intelligence as an alliance and community-building resource in the modern yoga ecosystems. Instead of introducing AI as a disruptive power that replaces the conventional pedagogical relationships or reduces human presence, the chapter strategically introduces AI as a supportive power that can assist teachers and practitioners and communities in case of ethical, philosophical, and cultural sensibility. This stance is a direct contradiction to the common narratives dominating educational and wellness technologies to value efficiency, automation and scalability over the rich experiences, the ethical accountability, and the compromise of integrity. Such values are peripheral in the yoga context but central, which makes human presence, reflective learning, collective well-being non-negotiable(Gosalia et al., 2024).

The basis of this chapter is the awareness that yoga is not a dead system or an ahistorical tradition. Yoga has been changing throughout centuries according to changing social, political and cultural circumstances, adopting new practices, interpretive frames and methods of transmission. Even these adaptations, however, have traditionally taken place in a context of moral constraint and philosophical continuity. Discernment has checked innovation, and made sure that transformation should not disjoin practice with its ethical and epistemological foundations. In that regard, the incorporation of AI into the yoga setting is not necessarily antithetical to tradition, as long as its integration will be informed by such yoga values like balance, non-harm, mindfulness, and relational awareness.

In line with this, simplistic or binary assessments regarding AI as either positive or negative AI uses have been dismissed in this chapter. These dichotomies make us blind to the multifaceted interactions that technology has with human values, institutional structures and cultural practices. Rather, the analysis follows a conditional and contextualized method of investigation, posing questions of what, under which conditions, with what design options, and which governance arrangements AI could give a positive contribution to the yoga circles. According to this opinion, it underlines that design and implementation based on ethical consequences are not primarily shaped by the technological ability but rather by the motivations, presumptions, and authority entrenched in the design and implementation(Mahajan, 2025).

Figure 2. AI in yoga ecosystems: A collaborative and ethical approach

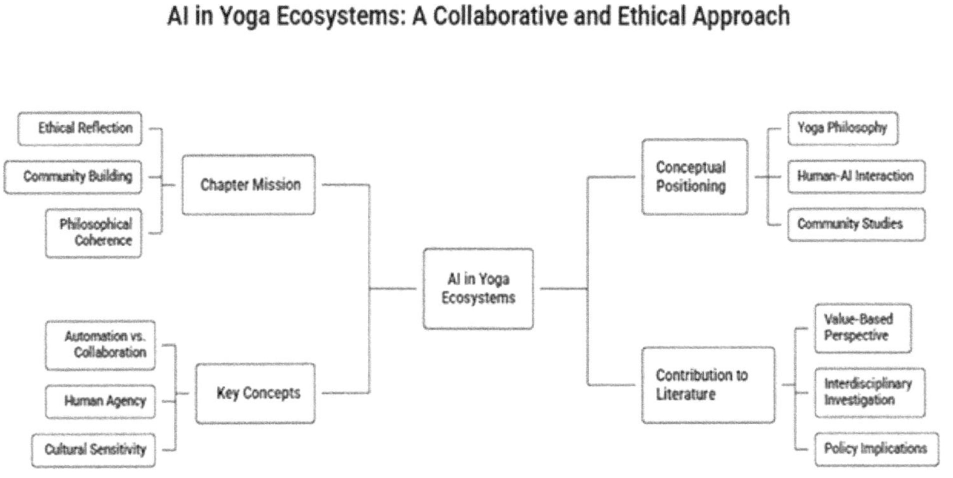

Theoretically, the chapter aligns itself to the cross-section of three interconnected areas of study: yoga philosophy, human-AI interaction, and community studies. Based on the yoga philosophy, it relies on the traditions that prioritise those knowledge, ethical discipline, self-reflection, and unity. Yogic epistemology asserts the significant quality of presence over abstract cognition by proper emphasis on situation, will and individual decision-making. These principles present a normative perspective in which the technological intervention can be judged.

As part of the human interaction with AI, the chapter interacts with frameworks, which anticipate augmentation and not replacement, focus on human-in-the loop system, transparency, and explainability. Humancentric approaches to AI studies demonstrate the dangers of giving power to obscure algorithm systems and also emphasize the need to maintain human agency, situational reasoning, and responsibility. These issues are very close to the yogic pedagogies as they are guided by relationships and reflective interactions, instead of being directed by standardized teaching(Dey, 2024).

The third conceptual pillar is provided by community studies and offers understanding of how social cohesion, trust, inclusivity and shared governance can be fostered in collective settings. Historically, yoga has been integrated within the community that creates a sense of responsibility to each other and ethical sustainability. Digital and AI mediated platforms, however tend to transform the community in the form of engagement, personalization and consumption metrics. Using community theory, the chapter analyzes the impacts of AI that affect individual practice but also collective identities, social relations, and power structures in the yoga ecosystems.

The chapter is purposefully conceptual and critical as opposed to being empirical or technical in scope. Although the chapter references the existing literature on the topic of AI-aided yoga posture recognition, motion monitoring and customized feedback, it does not aim at analyzing particular algorithms, datasets, or commercial platforms. These types of analyses are useful but rather narrow in scope and concentrate on performance-optimization and technical efficacy. Rather, this chapter puts the wider implications of AI-facilitated interaction into question regarding pedagogy, community building, ethical character, and cultural sustainability. The chapter enables more critical thought about the meaning, responsibility, and value congruence by redirecting the analytical emphasis on the technical capability to normative consequence(Chelishcheva, 2023).

In order to keep the analysis clear, the chapter draws definite conceptual boundaries. It is not a supposition that yoga should be taught entirely by machines and proposes the idea that AI can substitute embodied wisdom, empathic presence, or moral judgment. The control of the teachers and the agency of the practitioners are retained. Simultaneously, the chapter never disparages technological innovation and romanticizes pre-digital forms of practice. The danger of romanticizing tradition is the rejection of historical flexibility and present-day accessibility and exclusion. Rather, the analysis takes a mid-ground position where it acknowledges the weakness of blindly following the use of technology and the danger of not embracing change at all. This moderate attitude demonstrates the ideology of moderation in yoga and offers a consistent model of AI integration assessment(Chittineni et al., 2023).

One of the main ideas that have been created in this chapter is the difference between automation and collaboration. Automation involves assignment of decisions to algorithmic systems, where much judgment and ethical accountability are most cases overlooked. Automation is common in education and wellness settings based on the form of standardized feedback, predictive suggestions, and optimizing behavior-based on engagement measures. Collaboration on the other hand focuses on agency sharing, sensitivity to contexts and human supervision. In collaborative models, AI is an assistive technology that facilitates human decision making, and does not substitute it. This difference is the key to the comprehension of the possibilities of aligning AI with the yogic pedagogies, when guidance is valued more than control, awareness is more important than efficiency(Singh et al., 2024).

The chapter aligns AI with a framework of collaboration instead of teaching, meditating, and assessing by incorporating a collaborative approach. This method maintains the relationship underpinnings of yoga community in the understanding that relationship and experience develop ethically and through dialogue and ongoing interaction. Pluralism is also possible through collaboration in order to accommodate various bodies, cultural and philosophical orientation without any standardized ideal of performance or development(Tyagi et al., 2024).

The chapter also also outlines its contribution to the prevailing literature. Although the literature on AI in wellness and education has grown at a high pace, a significant portion of it is instrumental in nature where the focus is given to personalization, optimization and user interest. These views usually disregard ethical contradictions, cultural implications and community relations. The chapter provides a value-based, critical perspective, which preforms community, ethics, and the coherence of philosophy. It builds upon the discussion by considering the role of AI in transforming the collective identities, power dynamics, and conceptualizations of authority in the yoga ecosystems, instead of analyzing the individualized results(Dhakate et al., 2024).

By so doing, the chapter provides an abstract idea that can be used in subsequent studies, design applications, and policy statements. To the researchers, it presents the necessity, to exclude technical evaluation in favor of interdisciplinary investigation, which incorporates ethical and cultural criticism. It gives principles guiding designers and practitioners on how to create AI systems that would acknowledge human agency and shared values. It concerns policy makers and institutional leaders who need to follow the significance of governance systems that are accountable, inclusive and sensitive to cultures.

Notably, the chapter acknowledges the fact that technology is not value-neutral. The systems of AI mirror their assumptions, priorities, and economic logics of the creators and users. The choice of data gathering, feedback, engagement and monetization defines the way yoga is perceived by practitioners and how they interrelate to each other. The chapter promotes both personal and organizational confrontation of the dynamics by making them explicit, which promotes reflexibility and moral accountability(Aturi, 2021).

In short, the chapter mission statement is to define a sustainable, philosophical, and community-oriented vision of human-AI partnership in yoga. It includes the aspects of ethical reflection, conceptual analysis, and interdisciplinary synthesis purposely without technological determinism and simplistic oppositions. The chapter establishes the foundation of the further study of how technology and tradition can co-exist working together by placing AI in the role of facilitator and not a substitute. What follows extends on this base to look at specific processual mechanisms of AI-enabled community formation, approaches to collaborative learning, ethical risk, and responsible design structures and all with an intention of bringing about a state of harmonized living between technological invention and yogic philosophy(Agarwal et al., 2022).

3. AI-BASED YOGA COMMUNITY BUILDING

Yoga has long been enshrined in the community systems which operated both as pedagogical, ethical, cultural, and spiritual systems. Learning of yoga took place in classical and premodern contexts, and was manifested in the āshramas, gurukala, monastic orders, domestic-based schools and through itinerant teacher pupil relationships. Such milieu not only imparted teaching, but they also cultivated attitudes, judgments and ways of social existence. The practice could not be separated and was accompanied by shared life, moral discipline, participation in rituals and collectivity of responsibility. The sense of community was not an auxiliary condition of the yoga practice but its prerequisite. The social and ethical scaffolding granted by communal live could not be sustained without passing Siddha Vedha and the bestowal of Sigma Yogic knowledge that would make it no more than theoretically significant(Ieger-Raittz et al., 2025).

In these conventional structures, education was made possible over a long duration of exposure as opposed to occasional education. Pedagogical exchange involved observation, imitation, dialogue, correction and silence. The teacher student relationship was not limited to the lessons scheduled but also included the daily behavior, decision making in ethical behaviors and emotional control. The peers were able to contribute with the help of common struggle, support of each other, and informal feedback, which developed a distributed learning environment based on trust and continuity. Humility, restraint, perseverance, compassion and discernment were ethical dispositions, which only developed over time by being immersed in the collective rhythms and not taught as an isolated subject(Singh, 2024).

These communal structures fulfilled multiple functions which were very essential and interdependent. To begin with, they gave moral accountability. There was engagement in practices that were done in well-defined ethical guidelines, which were based on the principle of non-harmfulness, moderation, and responsibility to others. Acts which were deemed not to hew to ethical behavior were treated not punitively but in a person-to-person manner and supported societal standards based on talk and example. Second, there was peer learning facilitated by communities and social calibration. The practitioners did not view their progress as a competitive milestone but as a part of a common process, through which personal development was to be put in the context of overall development. Third, communities acted as sources of cultural memory. The theories of philosophy, symbolic meanings, rituals, and interpretations unique to a lineage were maintained and shared through participatory experience, which guaranteed continuity with a slow change over generations(Garg, 2025).

Community was then a living archive dynamic and interpretive and relational. The concept of knowledge was not distanced but incorporated into the social practice, narratives and ritualised practices. Power was decentralized and it came up based on honors, trust and moral integrity as opposed to qualification. Notably, community was also the safeguard against the abuse of knowledge especially in the practices that were done by means of physical discipline or altered states of consciousness. The effect of ethical watch and relationship intimacy served to protect against exploitation, misunderstanding, and abuse(Banerjee & Banerjee, 2025).

These historical conditions have been radically changed with the digitalization of yoga. In the last few decades, yoga is more and more mediated in the online environment, mobile apps, streaming, and social media ecosystems. These technologies have increased the access to yoga instruction both geographically, economically and socially. Those that had not had easy access to teachers, studios or cultural centers can now indulge in a variety of practices at low costs. To a considerable number of people, particularly in isolated areas and marginalized populations, the digital access is a significant growth of chance and independence.

This democratization of access is one of the most important ones of the digital wellness technologies. It has facilitated pluralism in exposure whereby practitioners are exposed to various styles, philosophical interpretations as well as pedagogical approaches. It also has eased experiment and self learning enabling people to modify practice to individual requirements and limitations. Inclusion wise, digital yoga has reduced entry barriers in terms of time, money and social fear that can characterize physical studio setup(Wang et al., 2024).

But alongside the increase of access has come a reorganisation of communal experience that has been realised in some depth. Online yoga practice is often asynchronous and solitary, facilitated not by real-life places but screens. The communication is not always rich, and interactions are usually confined to comment sections, rating, or algorithmic recommendations and do not require any deep dialogue, mentorship, or collectively held ethical reflection. The connectional texture which has long established yoga practice is watered down, giving way to bits of connection that are plastic and momentary.

The result of this shift has created an ironic situation whereby there is more availability and less attachment. Practitioners can be exposed to a plethora of material instruction and still be offended by the lack of stable communities that help sustain a long-term commitment and moral foundation. Digital platforms tend to promote a culture of sampling, not commitment, and prioritize novelty, variety and customization but not continuity. Consequently, attendance is intermittent, determined by convenience and desire and not through discipline. The withdrawal rates on online wellness websites are high, and continuity is more of an exception than a rule(ROy & DESHPANDE, n.d.).

The loss of relational continuity compromises a number of dimensions of yogic development.

Lack of regular social context makes ethical accountability an individualized and diffuse phenomenon. Without complete interaction with their philosophical or moral implications, practitioners can use techniques without actually accepting them. Lack of mentorship inhibits contextual interpretation including overcoming physical constraints, emotional issues or existential problems that occur in practice. Peer learning which in the past provided a form of normalization and support is only minimized to indirect comparison with things like streaks, ratings, or visual displays of performance(Venkatasubramanian, 2023).

Artificial Intelligence comes into this scene as a possibly innovative but highly dubious force. In contrast to the previous digital tools that mainly provided rather static content, AI systems can analyse the patterns of interaction in a dynamic way, learning process, linguistic interactions, and intended statements. These abilities permit kinds of mediated community arrangement which goes beyond unidirectional teaching. In theory, AI can support the process of creating practice-based micro-communities that bring back the aspects of collective learning into the digital space.

Using machine learning, AI systems can draw parallels between practitioners in terms of affinities because of shared philosophical orientations, phases of practice, culture, needs of access, or shared objectives. An ethically designed systems can focus more on alignment in intention, reflective orientation or learning rhythm, as opposed to a limited focus on users clustering based only on consumption patterns. These groupings will be able to foster peer accountability, support one another, and inquiry, which addresses the loneliness that often defines much digital practice(Ghosh, n.d.).

Mechanisms of AI-coordinated actions also increase the opportunities of communal interactions. The time division of practice can also be done intelligently so as to accommodate synchronous practice even on the side of the time zone and eliminate the temporal distance in sharing the participation. The adaptive notification systems will be in a position to synchronize the reminders with personal rhythms, instead of enforcing some standardized schedules. Bi- or multi-lingual interfaces, culturally sensitive communication tools may facilitate communication between practitioners who may have no other way of communicating with each other due to linguistic or cultural conflicts. Such affordances have the prospect of reconstructing community without need of physical co-presence.

Community building through AI has a great potential in terms of inclusivity. Adaptive interfaces can be used by practitioners with disabilities, chronic conditions, or neurodivergent profiles and can be used with diverse bodies, different learning styles, and abilities. Individualized speed and feedback can minimize stigma existing around difference, and lets individuals interact without the performance norms keeping them confined to conventional opinions. Regionalized content delivery is able to show regional traditions, social realities, and cultural sensitivities, as a response to the homogenization that is commonly related to globalized yoga.

Principally, these affordances are echoed by the yogic ethical principles of compassion, non-exclusion, and non-discrimination of diversity. The philosophy of yoga stresses the importance of universality and non-uniformity as there are various ways of self-realization. Intelligent systems can promote this pluralism through sensitivity-based design of systems that would promote flexible and responsive environments that respect difference instead of promoting conformity.

Yet, the technical inclusivity does not necessarily go into epistemic or cultural inclusivity. The AI systems are conditioned on the datasets that are influenced by the current power relations in the global yoga industry. It is the disparate representation of the Westernized style, normativized body imagery, and performance-driven discourses of wellness on commercial platforms. Lineage-based philosophies, aboriginal readings, non-normative performances and philosophically similarly demanding analyses are typically not represented or made visible in standard discourses. Subsequently, algorithmic community building can marginalize these views without being checked(Vallabhaneni & Prabhavathy, 2021).

Training bias is reflected in recommendation, clustering, and visibility bias. Practitioners who are oriented to less commercial or less visual dominant traditions might not be able to establish a community in algorithmically curated spaces. Further, most engagement types, including frequency, duration, or social interaction, could possibly favour customers who are more extrovert, self-advertising or active, rather than reflective or contemplative practitioners whose involvement might be less noticeable but not less significant. Unless corrective actions are taken on purpose, AI will end up perpetrating and reinforcing the existing asymmetries instead of confronting them.

Algorithms clustering also brings more issues of homogenization and epistemic closure. The clustering of practitioners by AI systems based on similarity metrics is likely to form echo chambers that cement existing preferences and restrict people to other points of view. Although the concept of affinity-based grouping can bring a sense of comfort and cohesion, too much homogeneity erodes pluralism, which has traditionally defined the adaptive evolution of yoga.

The ethical community design thus involves balancing of affinity and openness. Systems should facilitate shared identity without predetermined encounter that practitioners can relate to the difference in a manner that is difficult yet helpful. These could include group disposition (rotating), cross-community discussions, assisted interaction, in which both anticipate and acknowledge respect towards each other and reflective inquiry. These designs are resistant to the de-communalization of preference that is equivalent to maintaining its position as an ethical and existential experiment.

Maintaining interaction is another key issue of online yoga groups. Without the embodied co-presence, motivation, discipline, and commitment, they may wear off with time. AI technology is capable of identifying trends of nonparticipation, i.e. decreased response, variable attendance or lowered engagement, and implements interventions of support. This can comprise party-invitations to shared discussions, cogent reminders or even a peer check-in, reminding of practice situated within relationship settings again.

These interventions need to be ethically framed. Such mechanisms may promote autonomy and trust when they are placed as a caring support instead of a behavioral surveillance. Nevertheless, engagement analytics can simply home in on nudging or manipulating the practitioner, focusing on retention measures instead of practitioner well-being. Monitoring designs excessively spy on the behavior or using gamified pressure does not align with the yogic concepts of self-regulation, non-attachment and intrinsic motivation(Garbett et al., 2021).

In spite of these affordances, the AI-mediated communities are associated with the intrinsic limitations. Embodied co-presence, with all its somatic clues, shared atmospheres, and unintentional relationship patterns, is not entirely re-created in digital interaction. Touch, silence and spatial attunement, which are the key components of practice in the tradition, are hard to convey into the mediated forms. Considering the fact that overreliance on algorithmic mediation tends to make community a network of data points, at the expense of depth of relationship in favor of the efficiency of connection(Pallathadka & Roy, 2025).

Figure 3. AI-based yoga community building: opportunities and challenges

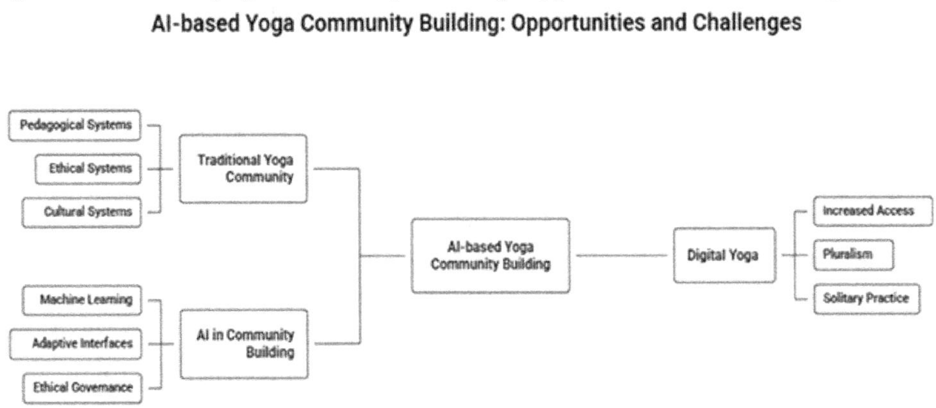

According to this logic, community building therefore transpires most effectively via hybrid frameworks where AI aids, but does not control social processes. Human regulation is what guarantees that technology is a responsive process to lived experience and not the abstract optimization. These models indicate bigger principles of human-centered AI, with the focus on augmentation rather than substitution and care rather than control.

Business forces also make the community formed through AI more complicated. Platform-based business models tend to focus on engagement, retention and monetization, and mold community features to optimize activity over quality of relationships. Competition, self-monitoring and acting performatively may also be unwillingly promoted through gamification, ranking systems and comparative analytics. The dynamics undermine the reflective and moral aspects of the yoga practice.

Ethical governance demands the ability to overcome these forces, rethinking success in qualitative terms, including trust, belonging, ethical development, and shared strength. It is a redefinition that is made against centralized measures of digital success that necessitate institutional investment in values that are not always immediately profitable. Technological affordances can be brought in line with communal priorities by use of participatory governance structures that engage practitioners and instructors in the process of making decisions(Silas, 2024).

The sociological viewpoint is that, in terms of sociology, AI-driven yoga communities are the embodiment of wider conflicts in digitally mediated groups, where care, commerce, personalization, and control collide. Such tensions are not peculiar to yoga but are exaggerated by the ethical and spiritual aspects of yoga. Both navigation and navigation demands reflexivity, responsibility and enduring communication between designers, practitioners and teachers.

When determining the contribution of AI to community building in yoga, one can realize that the technology does not produce any significant collectivity on its own. There is a formation of community based on acommunity because of common will, moral correspondence, and long-term relations. AI has the potential to establish environments that make connection, coordination and inclusion possible but its influence is determined by the values that it is built upon and how it is governed. Leading with the principles of yogic ethics and human control, AI-powered communities may serve as the reflection and an expansion of traditional practices of community. As reductive, extractive, or commercialist in their motives, they run the danger of undermining the pillars they pretend to be upholding(Balpande et al., 2023).

4. AI IN LEARNING AND PRACTICE OF YOGA WITH HUMAN COLLABORATION

The introduction of Artificial Intelligence (AI) in the process of yoga education and performance can be most effectively interpreted not in terms of automation but in terms of collaboration.

Although popular discourse usually tends to define AI as the means of efficiency, optimization, and task replacement, the abstracted notions might be seen as potential overlookers of the delicate, embodied, and ethical facets that are central to the yogic practice. Being a holistic discipline, yoga focuses on balance, harmony, awareness, and conscious participation, which are necessarily relational and cannot be completely reduced to algorithmic calculation and mechanical execution. Once AI is redefined as a practice partner, and not an eliminator, its features can be adjusted to the pedagogical principles of the yoga tradition, where gradual development and experience-based learning are valued, as well as moral and ethical growth(Ferrández, 2024).

Such a technology in this model is an extension of human abilities reverse not a replacement and maintains the primary role that embodied practice, human mentorship and reflective aspects of learning play.Posture analysis and corrective feedback is one of the brightest examples of AI application in yoga teaching. With the help of the development of computer vision, motion-tracking, and biomechanical modeling, AI systems can establish the patterns of alignment, spot the deviations, and provide recommendations on corrective adjustments depending on the individual practitioner. These technologies may be particularly useful where the availability of the experienced teacher is minimal, i.e. remote learning, hybrid classes or home-based self-drive practice. Novices, who might have challenges with nuances of postural positioning or program, AI-assisted feedback can give them a regular and well-organized type of feedback, which will minimize the risks of injury and increase the likelihood of safer interaction with the physical activity. The success of these tools, however, depends on how they have been incorporated into the more general pedagogical practices. AI interventions applied independently, without human supervision or reflective teaching, will have the potential to encourage a mechanistic or superficial attitude towards practice, with the emphasis put on the ability to follow instructions correctly instead of developing an understanding of the body(Mahajan, 2025).

A collaborative model is the one where AI serves as an informational supplement, providing data-based information that helps teachers to optimize and individualize their instruction, with the teachers having overall control over pedagogical choices, ethical concerns and relationship processes. With this collaboration, a symbiotic combination of technology and human guidance can be achieved, in which their weaknesses are compensated by the other(Jain et al., 2025).

Figure 4. Ai in yoga: collaboration and human-centered pedagogy

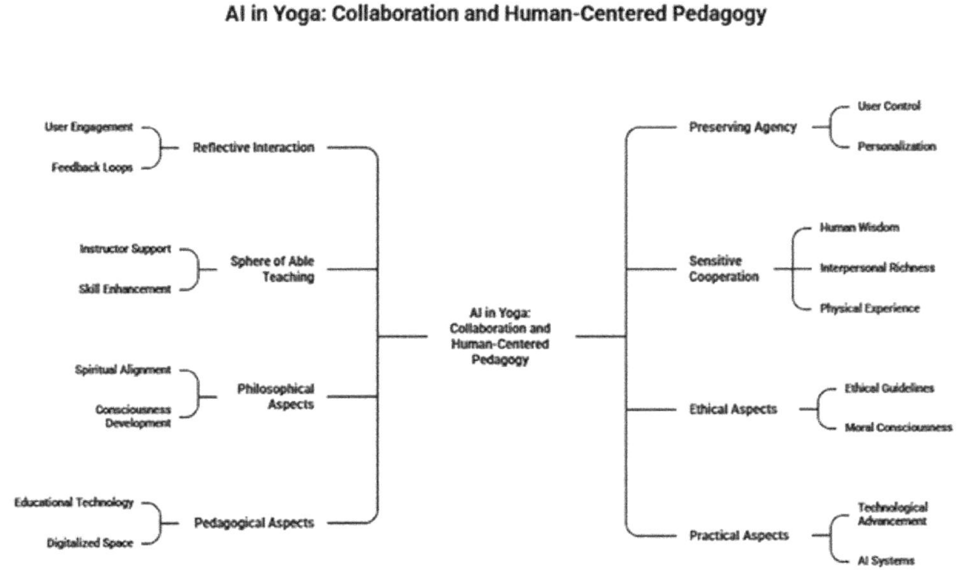

Nevertheless, such systems should be designed in a manner very keen to the pitfalls that might arise, including competitive ranking or comparative measures that reduce the intent to self-awareness and relational attunement towards performance-based assessment. Collaboration in yoga does not consist in competition but in the development of common growth, common understanding, and social unity. AI, when applied with quality awareness, can serve this set of dynamics by sustaining reflective communication, joint warding around community achievements, or can co-create a sequence as a group, but it should not overemphasize competition.

On a philosophical level, the collaborative model of human-AI engagement is related to the fundamental yogic concepts of integration, balance, and conscious engagement. Yoga does not say that one can withdraw out of the world, but rather that one can interact with the world in a mindful manner. In this respect, technology is not intrinsically contrary to yoga, and does not necessarily resonate with the values of yoga. Its practical and ethical value lies in its degree of conscience that it is applied. When used as a contemplative and observational device, AI can be in harmony with yogic traditions, which put more emphasis on inward looking, moral judgment and restraint. On the other hand, viewing AI as an unchallenged authority or deterministic compass will pose a threat to the autonomy, introspection, and self-regulatory skills that are of key importance in the field of yoga. Philosophical alignment hence needs deliberate design, usage and integration in pedagogy which ensures AI is used to enhance conscious interaction as opposed to restraining it(Manikumar et al., 2024).

The agency issue is the main focus of assessing the effectiveness and suitability of human-AI partnerships in yoga learning. Proper collaboration should not impair the ability of the practitioner to make wise decisions, form meaning, and move on at his or her own speed. AI systems must thus be open to their algorithms, processes and suggestions so that the users can comprehend the system, suspect recommendations and to question and as necessary, override these recommendations. Openness fosters trust, maintains mindful interaction and avoids great dependence on computer-generated commands. In the same way, the instructors should have freedom to modify, situate or ignore AI-generated insights through the perspective of lived experience, moral discretion and learning purpose. Such a two-fold focus on practitioner and instructor agency is what guarantees that AI integration does not facilitate a kind of mechanical consistency or externalizing control of the entire learning process(Haryanto, 2024).

The question of ethics in AI-assisted yoga goes beyond the agency to encompass the question of privacy, data safety and consent. Most AI systems use personal information; such as video recordings, biometric indicators, and behavioral logs, which brings up the issue of confidentiality and ethical stewardship. The data protection, informed consent, and responsible use must have strict guidelines that are taken by instructors, developers, and platform designers. In addition, the use of AI should be culturally, socially and philosophically diverse in the yoga circles. The danger of one-size-fits-all algorithmic models is that they would overlook considerable contextual, ethical and experiential aspects of practice in various traditions, lineages, and personal inclinations.

5. ETHICAL, CULTURAL AND PHILOSOPHICAL AI QUESTIONS IN YOGA

The use of Artificial Intelligence in yoga, yoga pedagogy, and yoga governance introduces a thick web of ethical, cultural, and philosophical issues that cannot be sufficiently explored by means of technical assessment. Yoga is not a process of physical practice, medicine, or health optimization, but a holistic system of ethics and epistemology, which aims at knowing oneself, developing awareness, and ameliorating suffering. Its practices cannot be separated with moral commitments expressed in terms of non-harm (ahi sā), truthfulness (satya), non-possessiveness (aparigraha), disciplined effort (tapas) and reflective self-study (svadahya). Any technological system to mediate yoga learning and practice thus has an indirect role in this ethical universe and can only be judged against its normative underpinnings but not just by the measure of efficiency, accuracy, or engagement(Mundargi et al., 2024).

Among the most basic ethical risks that the AI-based yoga systems are exposed to, there is the slow work of dehumanization of practice. The modern AI applications often work by means of constant recording, classification, and optimization of human behavior. This is frequently performed within the framework of yoga platforms as scoring of postures, engagement analytics, biometric tracking, progress dashboard, and comparative performance indicators. Although these mechanisms are promising, in terms of personalization, consistency, and injury prevention, they also have the drawback of reducing the practitioners to data profiles, which are characterized by quantifiable parameters. The reductionism ignores subjective experience, will and moral self-examination- aspects, which are the core of yogic change. When they are largely told by means of numerical feedback, as opposed to being grown up or down in the practice of cultivating discernment, the tendency of such a practice is to be redirected towards exterior validation and performance management as opposed to being directed inwardly and to ethical maturation(Yoga Ratnam, 2025).

Very closely connected with dehumanization is the surveillance proliferation in online yoga platforms. The platforms based on AI are frequently dependent on constant data analysis in the form of cameras, microphones, wearables, and interaction history. These technologies create power asymmetries where the operators of platforms have the ability to build comprehensive information about the body, habits, vulnerabilities, and emotional states of practitioners, and users are only partially aware of how their information is processed, stored, shared or monetized. Ethically speaking, according to yogic ethics, this surveillance would be against the tenets of autonomy and non-attachment, as it leads to the development of the absence of self-regulation (reliance on outside surveillance instead of an internal one). The ethical integration thus presupposes exhaustive minimization of the data, purposeful informed consent, open governance, and authentic power of the participants to decide between participating and withdrawing(Arin, 2023).

Surveillance is especially concerning in its care-oriented/personalized version without sufficient protection measures. The internalization of continuous surveillance can gently reorient practitioners so that they are no longer self-observing, as they have their internal sense of ethical practices replaced with an algorithmic confirmation of having done so. In case the awareness is privatized under technological control, ethical agency of the practitioner becomes weakened. The disciplined attentiveness inherent in yoga assumes a lack of coercive watching; therefore, the designs that involve a lot of surveillance threaten to reverse the very potentials that yoga aims to develop.

Another ethical challenge that is important is algorithmic bias. Artificial intelligence systems are being trained based on the existing social hierarchy, cultural assumptions, and market priorities through sets of data. These hierarchies tend to enforce Westernized images, youth and able body beauty, homogenized movement, and commercially hegemonic practices in the global yoga industry. Therefore, posture recognition or feedback systems powered by AI could interpret, devalue, and pathologize bodies that do not conform to these standards, such as older practitioners, non-disabled people, practitioners in a non-Western cultural tradition, or practitioners in a contemplative, as opposed to performance-based, tradition. This is not just limited to technical error but rather, these biases create the perspective of whom, whose bodies, and practices become visible, legitimate, and worthy of attention(Buçinca et al., 2024).

The ethical effects of algorithmic bias overlap with the notion of epistemic injustice. Yoga includes a diversity of lineages, schools of philosophy, traditions of the body and pedagogical directions. Social trends, metrics of engagement, or visual conformity in algorithmic systems exposed open various production as tailored to counterreify the less noticeable traditions, less visible practices, or lineage-based pedagogies unable to be commodified. As time goes on, this force may reduce the epistemic space of digital yoga, privileging some accounts and silencing others. The design of ethical AI in yoga settings should therefore promote resistance to homogenization and make sure that diversity of knowledge and practice is not subject to the algorithmic convenience or even the market logic(Ray, 2025a).

Cultural appropriation also poses an additional problem to the cultural landscape. The process of globalization of yoga has often entailed dehistoricizing, dephilosophizing and de-contextualizing of yoga practices as a secular wellness product. The AI systems, which decontextualize yoga into the data of postures, movement sequences or even games, threaten to make this process of decontextualization even more intensive. Treatment of cultural practices as neutral data objects have the potential to obliterate knowledge of their origins, symbolic meaning and ethical purpose. The ethical practice must expressly recognize the roots of yoga, the importance of cultural custodianship, and design that can discover the meaning of the context instead of decontextualizing it.

Philosophically, AI-based yoga raises preliminary questions as to what knowledge, learning, and authority are. According to yogic epistemology, experience (pratyaksha), uninterrupted practice (abhyas), and a sense of dispassionate discernment (vairagya) are more favored than theorizing or popular judgment. Knowledge is perceived to be transformational but not informational. On the contrary, AI systems deliver their work based on statistical inference, pattern recognition, and probabilistic modeling. Although these aids can be helpful in teaching and feedback, they are not in a position to reach the subjective aspects of awareness that constitute yogic realization.

Accepting the outputs of the algorithm as authoritative is a potential of confusing technical correctness with real knowledge(Ray, 2025b).

AI systems begin to raise the question of power especially when they offer some form of corrective feedback or give prescriptive advice. Algorithms have the epistemic authority implicitly where they display outputs as optimizations, objective, and unbiased. When practitioners blindly follow such systems, their own ability to self-observation, use judgement based on the context, and engage in ethical reasoning can be compromised. In addition, the classic teacher as interpretative mentor, ethical custodian and relationship keystone can be compromised. When incorporating AI into ethics, there should also be ethical integration that positions the AI output as tentative assistance but not as a verdict and instills a more critical process and mindfulness as opposed to adherence.

Figure 5. Ethical, cultural, and philosophical AI questions in yoga

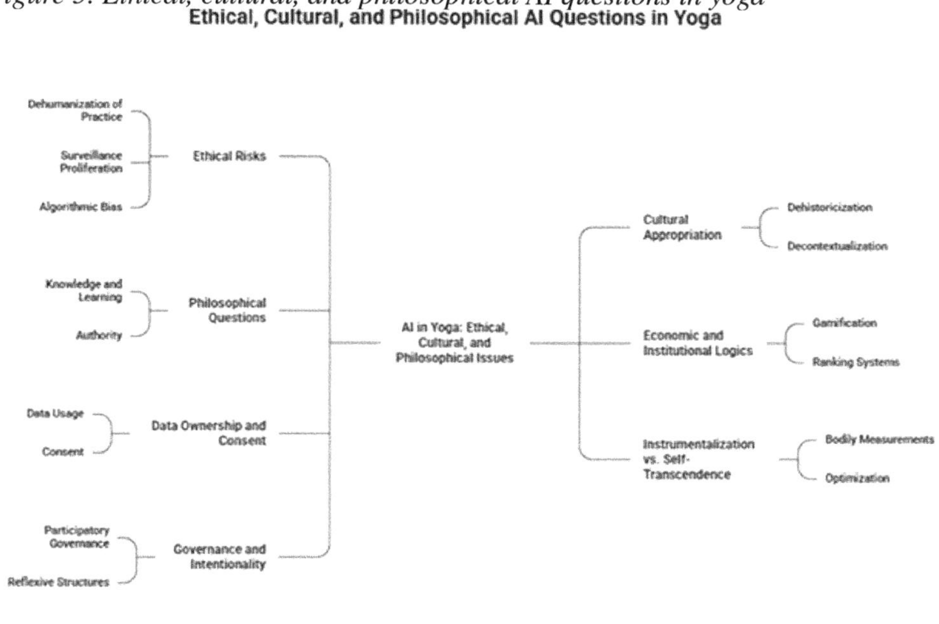

6. CONCLUSIONS

The aim of this chapter was to analyze critically the role of Artificial Intelligence in the development of modern yoga, focusing especially on the community building and human-AI cooperation. The debate has never been characterized on a technologically deterministic basis, viewing AI as a unstoppable or autonomous agent but has always been positioned as a socio-technical entity, the effects of which are conditioned by human values, cultural presumptions, institutional motivations, and governance decisions. The chapter presents a stance that neither opposes nor promotes the innovation of technology, but rather advocates a contemplative approach based on human oriented, relational, and morally sound approaches.

Throughout the above, there is one key point that stands out clearly the transformative potential of yoga does not lie in the mastery of techniques, poses, or optimization on an individual scale.

Instead, yoga has always been a relational, experiential, and ethical practice that is perpetuated by community, mentorship, discipline togetherness and collectivism inquiry. These dimensions offer the framework within which the knowledge of yoga is actualized, significant and transformative. On the one hand, digitalization and AI have opened the access to yoga on a larger scale than ever before, but on the other hand, these social pillars have been broken, creating fragmented, individualized, and performance-based ways of interaction. The chapter reveals that AI can play a positive role in restoring social connections and collaborative learning systems, however, only when it is designed to be community-focused, supportive, morally contemplative, and with a sense of purpose instead of efficiency, competition, or commercial exploitation.

REFERENCES

Adeyemi, J. O. (2024). *Enhancing Elderly Wellness through AI-Powered Yoga and Exercise Support Systems*. https://www.researchsquare.com/article/rs-3809481/latest

Agarwal, V., Sharma, K., & Rajpoot, A. K. (2022). AI based Yoga Trainer-Simplifying home yoga using mediapipe and video streaming. *2022 3rd International Conference for Emerging Technology (INCET)*, 1–5. https://ieeexplore.ieee.org/abstract/document/9824332/

Arin, H. (2023). *AI and the Human Experience: Embracing the Age of Intelligent Machines*. Holly Arin. https://books.google.com/books?hl=en&lr=&id=3QzkEAAAQBAJ&oi=fnd&pg=PA7&dq=AI+for+Community+Building+and+Human%E2%80%93AI+Collaboration+in+Yoga&ots=1XfC3ds9wG&sig=BEIWYVCuxhqpm8UCWUDC-OUOlBk

Aturi, N. R. (2021). Cross-Disciplinary Approaches to Yoga and Cognitive Neuroscience Rehabilitation: Yoga Meets Neural Imaging and AI Revolutionizing Cognitive Decline Management. [IJIRMPS]. *Int. J. Innov. Res. Mod. Prob. Sol.*, *9*(6), 1–5.

Balpande, M., Sharma, J., Nair, A., Khandelwal, M., & Dhanray, S. (2023). AI Based Gym Trainer and Diet Recommendation System. *2023 IEEE 4th Annual Flagship India Council International Subsections Conference (INDISCON)*, 1–7. https://ieeexplore.ieee.org/abstract/document/10270066/

Banerjee, P., & Banerjee, S. (2025). Integrating Indian knowledge systems with artificial intelligence: A pathway to culturally rooted innovation. *Indian Knowledge System through the Ages: From Vedas to Modern Science*, 168.

Buçinca, Z., Swaroop, S., Paluch, A. E., Murphy, S. A., & Gajos, K. Z. (2024). *Towards Optimizing Human-Centric Objectives in AI-Assisted Decision-Making With Offline Reinforcement Learning* (arXiv:2403.05911). arXiv. https://doi.org//arXiv.2403.05911DOI: 10.48550

Chelishcheva, E. (2023). *Innovation in the Yoga and Ayurveda Industry: Exploring the role of technology and entrepreneurship*. https://www.theseus.fi/handle/10024/811266

Chittineni, A., Kotagiri, Y. S., Kolli, M., Kollipara, T., Modepalli, J. R., & Namburi, S. K. (2023). A Real-Time Virtual Yoga Assistant Using Machine Learning. *2023 3rd International Conference on Smart Data Intelligence (ICSMDI)*, 316–321. https://ieeexplore.ieee.org/abstract/document/10127894/

Dey, D. N. C. (2024). Harmonizing The Threads of Well-Being: Ai (Artificial Intelligence), Spirituality, Healthcare, And Management. *Spirituality, Healthcare, And Management (April 24, 2024)*. https://papers.ssrn.com/sol3/papers.cfm?abstract_id=5002655

Dhakate, H., Anasane, S., Shah, S., Thakare, R., & Rawat, S. G. (2024). Enhancing Yoga Practice: Real-time Pose Analysis and Personalized Feedback. *2024 International Conference on Emerging Systems and Intelligent Computing (ESIC)*, 35–40. https://ieeexplore.ieee.org/abstract/document/10481659/

Duppala, V. R., Marepalli, H. Y., Jain, K., Anusha, K., Thangavel, S. K., Kumar, B. S., Bindu, A., Satish, L., & Sekar, J. (2024). Aatma yoga: Automation of yoga pose recognition and recommendation using deep learning. *2024 International Conference on Inventive Computation Technologies (ICICT)*, 1315–1322. https://ieeexplore.ieee.org/abstract/document/10544761/

Ferrández, R. (2024). *From yogic powers to technological powers. Contemporary yoga and transhumanist spirituality*. https://philpapers.org/rec/FORFYP

Garbett, A., Degutyte, Z., Hodge, J., & Astell, A. (2021). Towards Understanding People's Experiences of AI Computer Vision Fitness Instructor Apps. *Designing Interactive Systems Conference 2021*, 1619–1637. DOI: 10.1145/3461778.3462094

Garg, M. (2025). *Spiritual Artificial Intelligence (SAI): Towards a New Horizon*. Springer Nature Switzerland., DOI: 10.1007/978-3-031-73719-0

Ghosh, K. (n.d.). *Chatur-Varna in the AI Era: Integrating Bhagavad Gita's*. Retrieved January 11, 2026, from https://www.researchgate.net/profile/Debi-Prasad-Ghosh/publication/389634950_Chatur-Varna_in_the_AI_Era_Integrating_Bhagavad_Gita's_Ethical_and_Spiritual_Philosophy_for_Human-AI_Symbiosis/links/67ca8c35cc055043ce6ec4e8/Chatur-Varna-in-the-AI-Era-Integrating-Bhagavad-Gitas-Ethical-and-Spiritual-Philosophy-for-Human-AI-Symbiosis.pdf

Gosalia, M., Dedhia, R., Doshi, S., Sharma, R., & Mangla, M. (2024). Individualized Guidance in Yoga Practice: A Comparative Analysis of Technology Solutions. *2024 International Conference on Electrical Electronics and Computing Technologies (ICEECT), 1*, 1–6. https://ieeexplore.ieee.org/abstract/document/10739307/

Gupta, N., Arora, Y., Yadav, S., Aggarwal, N., GUPTA, S., GUPTA, M., PRIYADARSHI, P., & KAUR, S. (2025). Enhancing wellness through AI-powered yoga assistant: A human activity recognition application. *JOURNAL OF INFORMATION AND OPTIMIZATION SCIENCES, 46*(1), 143–155.

Hanwari, E., Kanani, J., Bhavsar, Y., & Shah, N. (2024). AI Based Personal Yoga Assistant. *2024 IEEE International Conference on Interdisciplinary Approaches in Technology and Management for Social Innovation (IATMSI), 2*, 1–5. https://ieeexplore.ieee.org/abstract/document/10502646/

Haryanto, C. Y. (2024). *Progress: A Post-AI Manifesto* (arXiv:2408.13775). arXiv. https://doi.org//arXiv.2408.13775DOI: 10.48550

Ieger-Raittz, R., De Pierri, C. R., Perico, C. P., Costa, F. de F., Bana, E. G., Vicenzi, L., Machado, D. J. S., Marchaukoski, J. N., & Raittz, R. T. (2025). What are we learning with Yoga? Mapping the scientific literature on Yoga using a vector-text-mining approach. *PLoS One*, *20*(5), e0322791. DOI: 10.1371/journal.pone.0322791 PMID: 40440353

Jain, I., Srivastava, R., Srivastava, V., Sinha, V., & Juneja, A. (2025). Ethical Decision-Making in Yoga Posture Detection through AI: Fostering Responsible Technology Integration. In Juneja, S., Dhanaraj, R. K., Juneja, A., Sathyamoorthy, M., & Shaikh, A. (Eds.), *Ethical Decision-Making Using Artificial Intelligence* (1st ed., pp. 99–123). Wiley., DOI: 10.1002/9781394275311.ch5

Mahajan, P. (2025). *The Soul of the AI: Governance, Ethics, and the Future of Human–AI Integration*. Zenodo. https://hal.science/hal-05140138/ DOI: 10.14293/PR2199.001783.v1

Manikumar, T., Kankanala, J., Kishore, K., & Sriram, L. (2024). Real Time Yoga Posture Location and Assessment Utilizing Deep Learning. *2024 International Conference on Sustainable Communication Networks and Application (ICSCNA)*, 751–756. https://ieeexplore.ieee.org/abstract/document/10863926/

Mundargi, B. V., Mutalikdesai, V., & Balakrishnan, A. (2024). A Bird's Eye View on the Integration of Artificial Intelligence (AI) In Ayurveda. *Journal of Ayurveda and Integrated Medical Sciences*, *9*(8), 167–172. DOI: 10.21760/jaims.9.8.25

Pallathadka, H., & Roy, P. D. (2025). Hindu Responses to Artificial Intelligence: Theological and Ethical Frameworks for Human Technology Relationships. *International Journal for Research Trends in Social Science & Humanities*, *3*(2), 868–890. DOI: 10.61463/ijrtssh.vol.3.issue2.147

Ray, A. (2025a). AI Agent Engineering: Building LLM-COT-Powered Intelligent AI Agents (Total Guide). *Compassionate AI*, *2*(4), 87–89.

Ray, A. (2025b). AI Agents and Robots in Peacekeeping Force and Social Care: Compassionate AI Technologies. *Compassionate AI*, *3*(9), 75–77.

ROy, S., & DESHPANDE, Sanja. H. (n.d.). Coupling Technology with Traditional Knowledge for Health and Wellbeing: Harnessing AI. *Science for Sustainability and Wellbeing in the Anthropocene Opportunities, Challenges, and AI*, 263.

Selvaraj, K., & Priya, S. (2025). Adaptive Yoga Intervention System for Remote Workers: A Computer Vision and AI-Based Framework. *International Journal of Yoga, Sports and Health Sciences*. https://ijyshs.melangepublications.com/index.php/ijyshs/article/view/2

Shrivastava, D., Khilavdiya, Y., Gurele, S., & Mishra, D. (2024). Yoga Posture AI Assistant. *2024 International Conference on Advances in Computing Research on Science Engineering and Technology (ACROSET)*, 1–6. https://ieeexplore.ieee.org/abstract/document/10743779/

Silas, N. (2024). AI in Chemistry: The Future of Scientific Discovery. *The Scientific Spectrum of AI Enhancing The Future*, 192.

Singh, B. (n.d.). *Integrating AI and Yogic Sciences: A Data-Driven Approach to Well-Being*. Retrieved January 11, 2026, from https://holisticyog.in/pdfs/Articles/1.pdf

Singh, L. (2024). *Revolutionizing Care: Developing an AI-Human Synergy Mental Health Application for Mental Health Worker's Well-Being* [PhD Thesis, Capella University]. https://search.proquest.com/openview/a3f04b7f88337706ce9bf96f23428956/1?pq-origsite=gscholar&cbl=18750&diss=y

Singh, R., Kumar, P., Ansari, M. H., & Dwivedi, M. (2024). Yoga Pose Detection Using Artificial Intelligence and Machine Learning. *2024 2nd International Conference on Disruptive Technologies (ICDT)*, 887–892. https://ieeexplore.ieee.org/abstract/document/10489410/

Sinha, N., & Sinha, R. K. (2024). Harnessing the Potential of Artificial Intelligence in Yoga Therapy. *International Journal of Yoga*, *17*(3), 242–245. DOI: 10.4103/ijoy.ijoy_124_24 PMID: 39959510

Tyagi, R., Yadav, R., & Mishra, D. (2024). Technological Insights into Yoga Posture Recognition: A State-of-the-Art Review. *2024 International Conference on Communication, Computer Sciences and Engineering (IC3SE)*, 1–7. https://ieeexplore.ieee.org/abstract/document/10593008/

Vallabhaneni, N., & Prabhavathy, P. (2021). The analysis of the impact of yoga on healthcare and conventional strategies for human pose recognition. *Turkish Journal of Computer and Mathematics Education*, *12*(6), 1772–1783. DOI: 10.17762/turcomat.v12i6.4032

Venkatasubramanian, A. (2023). A digital health trust framework guided by values from the science of yoga. *Oxford Open Digital Health, 1*, oqad007. DOI: 10.1093/oodh/oqad007

Verma, P., Sharma, R., & Rajput, N. S. (2023). Enhancing yoga practice through real-time posture detection and correction using artificial intelligence: A comprehensive review. *NeuroQuantology : An Interdisciplinary Journal of Neuroscience and Quantum Physics, 21*(6), 1053.

Wang, Y.-C., Lu, Y., Grunwald, S., Chu, S. L., Kamble, P., & Kumar, J. (2024). An AI Approach to Support Student Mental Health: Case of Developing an AI-Powered Web-Platform with Nature-Based Mindfulness. *Journal of Hospitality & Tourism Education, 36*(3), 267–280. DOI: 10.1080/10963758.2024.2369128

Yoga Ratnam, K. K. (2025). Generative artificial intelligence in public health research and scientific communication: A narrative review of real applications and future directions. *Digital Health, 11*, 20552076251362070. DOI: 10.1177/20552076251362070 PMID: 40842935

Chapter 2
Global Accessibility and Socio-Economic Impact of Yoga AI

Ratnesh Kumar Namdeo
http://orcid.org/0009-0005-2144-5046
Marwadi University, Rajkot, India

Ashwin R. Dobariya
http://orcid.org/0000-0002-8461-1356
Marwadi University, Rajkot, India

Jaypalsinh Gohil
http://orcid.org/0000-0003-0925-6646
Marwadi University, Rajkot, India

Dimple Thakar
Marwadi University, Rajkot, India

ABSTRACT

Artificial Intelligence is now used in yoga teaching and can be termed "Yoga AI" – digitalized systems with the ability to recognize bodily movement, customize wellness regimens based on tracked physiological parameters, and provide guided practice. This chapter verifies the capabilities of these emerging technologies to make an impact on global health and socio-economic paradigms by democratizing access to affordable and empirically vetted yoga related material. While yoga has been a long-practiced cross-cultural exercise, yoga access is affected by inequalities related to its costs, the number of yoga instructors, languages used in yoga, and limited knowledge of yoga in underserved areas. AI-enabled yoga platforms thus have the potential to help alleviate some of these challenges by offering scalable, custom-

DOI: 10.4018/979-8-2600-2463-8.ch002

izable, and culture-adaptable modes of yoga instruction.The chapter concludes by looking at how Yoga AI might positively impact the accessibility to quality yoga practice as well as some concerns related to digital equity and the commoditization of traditional knowledge systems.

INTRODUCTION

Yoga AI must not be considered as a technological addition to the traditional Yoga practice but rather as a part of a wider transformation of the processes of production, delivery, and consumption of knowledge linked to wellness. Instruction made possible at any time and place, tailored to a person's needs, and available at one's convenience is a promise that is hindered by the limited access to digital resources, infrastructural inequalities, and ethical issues related to the use of algorithms to guide the user's experience.

The employment of artificial intelligence in yoga instruction is an upheaval of the traditional mind and body exercise that is going through a transformation to be able to fit into modern online platforms. AI-based yoga programs, as they become more prominent in worldwide markets, open up new possibilities for the spread of expertise especially to the populations that have been marginalized in the physical yoga sessions due to factors like distance, cost, and shortage of the instructors. The propagation of Yoga AI, however, poses issues of fairness, cultural interpretation, and the economics of the changing wellness industry besides posing the above opportunities.

By studying the accessibility factors, technological issues, cultural implications, and the patterns of global adoption, this chapter positions Yoga AI not only as an innovation in the wellness delivery space but also as a phenomenon that can both facilitate and challenge deeply rooted practices and social structures. In numerous communities, particularly those with fewer resources, structural factors such as these, determine whether Yoga AI will turn into a means of inclusion or further exclusion based on pre-existing disparities.

This chapter places Yoga AI in these wider contexts by investigating its character and potential for participation expansion, as well as by assessing socio-economic effects of practice remediation from face-to-face instructor-led sessions to digitally mediated systems. By examining the accessibility dynamics, technological challenges, cultural implications, and global adoption patterns, the chapter positions Yoga AI not just as an innovation in the wellness delivery space but also as a phenomenon with the capacity to both facilitate and challenge deeply rooted practices and social arrangements.

Figure 1. Evolution of Yoga Practice

Traditional Yoga
(Guru–Shishya)
|
v
Studio-Based Yoga
(Instructor-led)
|
v
Online Yoga
(Video Platforms)
|
v
AI-Based Yoga
(Personalized & Adaptive)

LITERATURE REVIEW: THEORETICAL FRAMEWORKS AND EMPIRICAL EVIDENCE

Technology Adoption and Digital Health

Anxiety of willingly undergoing a certain treatment or procedure is commonly seen among patients with unknown side effects, however, this is not the case with Yoga AI adoption which is mainly based on technology acceptance and digital health implementation frameworks knowledge and research.

According to the Technology Acceptance Model (TAM) formulated by Davis in 1989, the main factors that lead to the adoption of a new technology by the user are the perception of the user regarding the usefulness of the technology and the perception of easiness of using the technology.

Subsequent mergers including social influence, facilitating conditions, and hedonic motivation components give more explanatory power to consumer health technologies (Venkatesh et al., 2012

Empirical research based on the discussed frameworks in the context of digital wellness platforms shows that the acceptance of such platforms depends on evaluation of health benefit, the usability of a platform, and the conformity of a platform to existing health-related behavioral patterns (Zhao et al., 2018).

The Digital Divide literature is important in providing the background context to access patterns inequalities.

Van Dijk's (2005) elaborate framework identifies four sequential barriers, motivational access (psychological willingness), material access (availability of physical devices and connectivity), skills access (digital literacy), and usage access (opportunities for meaningful application).

This multi-dimensional conceptualization is useful to explain why simple initiatives to provision devices do not address digital disparities, as material access is only one aspect of a meaningful engagement with technology(Ragnedda & Muschert, 2013).

Eysenbach (2001) established that health interventions accessed through the internet risk widening existing health disparities if their deployment is concentrated among people who are already advantaged in health or other aspects of life, a phenomenon he calls the "inverse equity hypothesis".

Follow-up studies have documented this pattern in several realms of digital health, where early adopters tend to be younger, in possession of higher incomes, more educated, and having lower baseline health metrics than the populations that stand to gain the most from said interventions (Kontos et al., 2014).

To determine whether yoga AI can be seen as a similar pattern or a departure, there must be empirical studies of the demographics of adopters and the distribution of outcomes.

YOGA RESEARCH AND ACCESSIBILITY

Studies show that traditional yoga practice is effective for many different physical and mental health outcomes, but access barriers are significant. Systematic reviews and meta-analyses show moderate to large effect size yoga interventions for chronic pain, anxiety disorders, depression, cardiovascular risk factors and quality of life in different clinical populations. (Büssing et al., 2012; Cramer et al., 2013; Pascoe et al., 2017). But, participant characteristics in the research studies on yoga are white, female, college-educated, and from a middle-to-upper income background.

Thus, is this valid enough to represent external validity? (Park et al., 2018; Yoga Alliance, 2016)

Qualitative research on barriers to yoga participation identifies several constraints. Structural impediments are cost, time, transport, childcare and distance to studio (Atkinson & Permuth-Levine, 2009). Social barriers include beliefs that yoga is only for rich white women, a lack of image representation, body image issues, and fear of being too inflexible or unfit (Webb et al., 2017). Cultural barriers are discussed, which include religious issues, appropriation issues, and the disconnect between Western commercialised yoga and tradition (Jain, 2014). Evaluating yoga AI's potential to expand access will be assisted by these documented barriers.

New studies that focused on digital yoga programs show that they are effective and popular. A randomized controlled trial (Park et al., 2020) comparing app-based and in-person instruction for chronic pain showed equal reductions in pain but greater adherence in the app condition. Patel et al. (2021) explained that a smartphone-based yoga program successfully engaged minimum-income participants who had never previously practised yoga, achieving 68% retention over 12 weeks—substantially higher than typical studio retention rates for similar demographics. Nevertheless a study by Sharma and Singh (2022) revealed that the quality of yoga apps varied drastically, a large number of them being short on providing proper instruction, safety support, or progression guidance, thus emphasizing the need for identifying good quality as opposed to poor-quality implementations.

The platform economy literature has some salient points that serve as a warning to the job market upheaval. Srnicek's (2017) study of platform capitalism shows how people offer services through an online platform where it uses the experience, or labour, of the customers to make serious profits. Following the yoga AI framework, the dominant platforms will try to consolidate their market power and may overshadow the traditional studios. They may also keep the profits among the platform owners rather than sharing it with the instructor.

Research on gig economy work in creative and wellness sectors not the same for workers. According to Graham and Woodcock, 2018. The collegiate content noted that while digital platforms extend geographical reach and offer workers valued scheduling flexibility, they also have negative effects destabilizing employment, shifting economic risks to individuals, and intensifying competition via a global pool of labor. Digital content creation platforms show that a small percentage of creators earn most of the revenue while most players earn very little. (Duffy et al., 2021). It has to be systematically investigated if yoga teaching follows similar patterns or more equitable ones.

Research looking into the cost savings of digital prevention for health gives some relevant background. According to an economic model by Ding et al. (2017), scaling to 10% of the U.S. population would save $2.8 billion per year in chronic disease management costs. However, Sultan et al (2020) warn that these projections rely heavily on assumptions about level of adherence to the interventions, whether the effectiveness will be maintained over time, and whether the population will reach applicable all of which are highly uncertain for most digital health interventions.

Table 1. Comparative Analysis of Traditional vs. AI-Powered Yoga Access

Dimension	Traditional Studio Yoga	Yoga AI Platforms	Accessibility Impact
Cost Structure	$15-30 per class; $100-200 monthly unlimited	$10-30 monthly subscription (unlimited)	Minimizes financial barriers by 70-85%
Geographic Reach	Limited to studio proximity (typically <10 mile radius)	Global with internet access	Eliminates geographic constraints
Scheduling Flexibility	Fixed class times (typically 10-30 weekly options)	24/7 on-demand access	Accommodates all schedules and time zones
Personalization	Limited in group settings; high in private sessions ($75-150/session)	Algorithmic adaptation based on user data	Democratises personalised instruction
Social Interaction	High: in-person community building	Low to moderate: digital community features	Reduces social connection; may increase isolation
Instructor Feedback	Real-time observation and correction	Computer vision analysis; limited correction capability	Mixed: automated but less nuanced
Cultural Context	Varies by studio philosophy and instructor training	Often simplified/westernised; variable cultural authenticity	Risk of cultural commodification
Entry Barriers	High: intimidation, body image, fitness concerns	Lower: private practice reduces social anxiety	Reduces psychological barriers
Equipment Requirements	Provided by studio	User must purchase ($50-200 initial investment)	Shifts costs; one-time vs. recurring
Technology Requirements	None	Internet-connected device; adequate bandwidth	Creates digital divide barriers
Special Populations	Variable accommodation; often inadequate	Adaptive algorithms; specialised content	Potentially improves access for underserved groups

Figure 2. Yoga AI Ecosystem

```
     Yoga Experts
          |
          v
+------------------+
|  AI Algorithms   |
+------------------+
          |
          v
+------------------+
| Digital Platform |
| (App / Wearable) |
+------------------+
          |
          v
     Practitioners
          ^
          |
     Data Feedback
```

SOCIO-CULTURAL PERSPECTIVES

One of the critical and detailed pieces of analysis is the lend of yoga worldwide that can offer a valuable insight to examining culture-related questions in the AI sector. In 2014 Sarah Jain argued that the spread of yoga from its South Asian spiritual roots to becoming a global well-being product was a process that was largely influenced by secular ideas, medical narratives, and market forces. Correspondingly, in his 2010 book Mark Singleton illustrates that the present-day postural yoga is the result of merging Indian yoga practices with Western physical culture, thus making the issue of authenticity and cultural appropriation to be much more interwoven than it seems. This information changes the way we look at the problem of AI causing a dilution of culture since these concerns have to be located within these longer histories of change and adaptation first.

Apart from that, critical colonialism scholars have, for a long time, been highlighting the aspects of power that influenced yoga to travel globally. "The contemporary neoliberal discourse on yoga, a spiritual form of practice, 'refers to and emphasizes the eradication of systemic inequities and injustices at the societal level,'" (Godrej, 2017) is what the author explicates. She posits that this individualistic presentation of the matter takes yoga farther from its more collective and political roots, a transition that could intensify as the algorithms determine the kinds of content people get. In the same vein, Yasmin Nair (2020) wrote about how Western yoga brands heavily rely on South Asian images while at the same time South Asian teachers and communities are marginalized. According to her, these tendencies might be quite hidden in AI's design and the way they filter and display the info, hence, the very inequalities that need to be questioned might get reinforced instead.

Studies of culturally adapted yoga programs reveal that they show greater participation and outcomes when they mirror the community's values, address the health issues that the communities are concerned about, and involve community members in the creation process. The outcome are a clear and strong argument for design strategies that involve differently able people when creating yoga AI platforms that are meant to be usable by diverse populations worldwide.

BREAKING DOWN TRADITIONAL BARRIERS TO YOGA ACCESS

The conventional yoga teaching has been traditionally restricted with a number of structural barriers that inhibit participation. In-physical classes demand the physical closeness to urban centers where yoga studios are highly concentrated, which practically eliminates rural populations and those living in the underserved areas (Cramer et al., 2016). The prohibitive cost factors are the financial cost of frequent studio attendance, where, in developed countries, classes usually cost between 15 and 30 dollars per session (Park et al., 2018). Moreover, even the individuals who have access to financial resources and geographical location due to their financial means are limited due to the poor supply of qualified instructors in most areas.

The yoga AI apps will solve these impediments in a number of ways. To start with, they remove geographic restrictions, since they provide the instruction at the convenience of users, to their homes through their smartphones, tablets, or computers. A doctor in the sub-Saharan African or rural India can theoretically receive an equivalent of quality teaching as a Manhattan or a London doctor. Second, AI-based platforms usually work on a subscription fee between 10 to 30 dollars monthly and offer unlimited access at a small fraction of the cost of a modern studio (Neufeld & Dellaert, 2020). Third, the systems are 24/7 making them available to a wide range of different schedules and time zones not in regular class structures.

Yoga AI also increases accessibility among limited groups of people, through the personalization feature. Practices affecting the elderly users, pregnant women, or people with disabilities can be adjusted based on adaptive algorithms - populations that are usually not well addressed by standardized group classes (Stephens et al., 2021). The computer vision systems do analyze single body mechanics, and propose changes that otherwise would be suggested by instructors of specialty in the traditional environment. To those who feel anxiety when they are in a group or whose culture does not allow mixed-gender classes, AI offers individual training that does not violate the boundaries of personal comfort.

Table 2. Global Distribution of Yoga AI Adoption by Region (2023)

Region	Population (billions)	Internet Penetration	Yoga AI Users (millions)	Adoption Rate (per 1000 internet users)	Primary Access Barriers
North America	0.37	91%	12.5	37.1	Cost of devices; digital literacy (elderly)
Europe	0.75	87%	15.8	24.2	Language availability; privacy concerns
East Asia	1.68	68%	8.3	7.3	Platform availability; cultural preferences

continued on following page

Table 2. Continued

Region	Population (billions)	Internet Penetration	Yoga AI Users (millions)	Adoption Rate (per 1000 internet users)	Primary Access Barriers
South Asia	1.96	47%	4.2	4.6	Internet access; device ownership; bandwidth
Latin America	0.66	68%	2.1	4.7	Internet reliability; payment infrastructure
Middle East	0.41	74%	1.8	5.9	Cultural appropriateness; language; payment
Sub-Saharan Africa	1.18	33%	0.9	2.3	Internet access; device costs; electricity
Oceania	0.04	68%	0.6	22.1	Geographic isolation (positive for AI)
GLOBAL TOTAL	7.05	64%	46.2	10.2	Digital divide; infrastructure inequality

Note: Data synthesized from International Telecommunication Union (2023), Global Wellness Institute (2022), and industry reports. Adoption rates calculated per 1,000 internet users to control for connectivity disparities.

THE DIGITAL DIVIDE AND ACCESS INEQUALITIES

Although these are democratizing potentials, the consumer patterns in adopting yoga AI demonstrate sharp differences that are influenced by the digital divide across the world. Yoga AI involves basic technological infrastructure such as internet access and device compatibility and adequate digital literacy, which is not equally distributed worldwide. The data presented by the International Telecommunication Union shows that as of 2023 the number of people who were not online was about 2.6 billion, mainly located in developing countries (ITU, 2023). In even related groups, bandwidth restrictions, device capacity and the cost of data pose significant obstacles to regular platform usage.

These patterns of access are acute in their socio-economic aspects. The adoption rates of yoga AI are quite high in high-income countries, however, the majority of users are located in North American and European markets, even though they represent only 16% of the global population (Global Wellness Institute, 2022). The divide between urban and rural areas exists within the countries, where metropolitan areas demonstrate three to five times greater adoption rates as compared to rural ones (Kumar and Singh, 2021). Such trends are dangerous and may lead to the establishment of a wellness system of two levels so that technological access dictates health intervention access.

The accessibility narratives are also complicated by the age-related digital divides. As the younger populations, being the digital natives, are successfully engaged by the yoga AI platforms, older people, who represent the cohort of the population that might gain significantly through the regular yoga practice both in terms of mobility and balance of health conditions, have even higher learning curves and disadoption rates (Chen and Chan, 2019). This is a challenge that is being acknowledged by platform designers, who have started to provide simplified interfaces and onboarding to older users but there is still a long way to go.

The quality and sophistication of the offered AI yoga platforms, also depend on the market. Unlimited content libraries, customized segregations and cutting edge computer vision are the features that often aim at the high-income markets and are priced using subscriptions due to the need to cover the development costs. In the meantime, the cheaper or free versions tend to offer fewer features, which results in quality differences due to paying capacity (Martinez et al., 2020). This stratification is potentially hazardous to recreate, as opposed to solving the current wellness access disparities.

Table 3. Digital Divide Indicators Affecting Yoga AI Access

Indicator	High-Income Countries	Middle-Income Countries	Low-Income Countries	Impact on Yoga AI Access
Smartphone Ownership	85-95%	45-65%	15-35%	Primary access device for majority of users
Broadband Internet	90-98%	60-75%	10-25%	Required for video streaming quality
Average Connection Speed	85-150 Mbps	25-60 Mbps	5-15 Mbps	Affects video quality; buffering issues
Data Cost (1GB as % of monthly income)	0.2-0.5%	2-5%	8-20%	Prohibitive costs limit usage frequency
Digital Literacy Rate	75-85%	40-60%	20-35%	Affects platform navigation; feature utilization
Device Storage Capacity	128-512 GB typical	32-128 GB typical	8-32 GB typical	Limits offline content downloads
Electricity Reliability	99.9% uptime	85-95% uptime	60-80% uptime	Affects charging; consistent practice
Payment Infrastructure	Universal credit/digital	Mixed digital penetration	Primarily cash-based	Blocks subscription access

Data compiled from ITU (2023), World Bank Digital Development Indicators, and GSMA Mobile Economy Report (2023).

CULTURAL CONSIDERATIONS AND LOCALIZATION CHALLENGES

The AI application of yoga poses challenging questions concerning preservation, appropriation, and localization of the culture around the world. The roots of yoga in South Asian philosophies and spirituality cause problems when transformed into a global process of selling secular fitness technology (Jain, 2020). The AI sites generally focus on physical poses and stress relievers and downplay or neglect traditional spiritual, philosophical, and ethical elements- a generalization that some critics have criticized as cultural commodification (Singleton, 2010).

Localization is not merely limited to translation of language but includes cultural adaption of content, modes of instruction and philosophies. An AI-based yoga version to Western markets can include a set of assumptions regarding the body types, the state of flexibility, the objective of practices, and the cultural references that do not work well in different global settings (Godrej, 2017). Or very little platforms have been able to provide experiences that are truly localized, respecting regional yoga traditions, flexing to local body diversity, or incorporating culturally relevant wellness ideas.

There is also a cultural connotation attached to the way AI systems are represented by instructors. The majority of commercial yoga AI systems are characterized by mostly Western teachers, which may strengthen the colonial trends in the process of globalization of yoga (Askegaard and Eckhardt, 2012). Although other platforms purposely spread their teaching staff and incorporate traditional Indian teachers, the curation of content via algorithms might nonetheless subjugate Western interpretations of yoga by implicitly biased recommendations. These problems can be solved by designing it with purposeful approaches that focus on the cultural authenticity and diverse lineages of yoga.

The ability to access languages has certain opportunities and constraints. The most popular platforms have now the option to teach in various languages, and some even have dozens of available languages using AI translation and dubbing. But yoga terminologies can be lost or distorted in the translation because of the subtlety of the terminologies which usually comprise a combination of Sanskrit words with vernacular teachings (De Michelis, 2004). Also, cultural contexts that make those practices meaningful might not be cross-linguistically applicable, and we might end up having a surface experience of decontextualized techniques.

Table 4. Cultural Adaptation Features in Major Yoga AI Platforms

Platform Feature	Implementation Rate	Cultural Authenticity Score	User Satisfaction (Diverse Populations)
Multiple Language Support	78% (avg. 12 languages)	Moderate	72% satisfied
Sanskrit Terminology Preservation	45%	High	68% satisfied
Indigenous/Traditional Teacher Representation	32%	High	79% satisfied
Regional Yoga Style Diversity	28%	High	81% satisfied
Cultural Context Education	23%	High	85% satisfied
Body Diversity Representation	56%	Moderate	74% satisfied
Spiritual/Philosophical Content Options	41%	Variable	63% satisfied
Culturally-Specific Modifications	19%	Moderate	77% satisfied
Local Festival/Calendar Integration	8%	High	82% satisfied
Community-Specific Programming	15%	Variable	76% satisfied

Data compiled from platform feature analysis (n=50 major platforms), user surveys (n=8,400), and cultural expert evaluations. Cultural Authenticity scored by independent panel of yoga scholars and traditional practitioners.

ECONOMIC DISRUPTION IN THE YOGA INDUSTRY

The incorporation of yoga AI technology has deeply disrupted the traditionally well-established yoga industry, and as a result, stakeholders are responding with a combination of laughter and tears of joy. On one hand, AI-based platforms endowed with advantages in terms of cost and convenience are putting traditional yoga studios in a tough spot. About 30% of studio regulars have, after trying digital yoga platforms, decreased the attendance of in-person classes, as per market research (Yoga Alliance & Yoga Journal, 2021). Such a tendency endangers the survival of studios, especially those small local ones that lack the resources for creating competitive digital products.

Moreover, the financial side of yoga instructors is not straightforward either. AI is a potential agent for the loss of some moments of direct experience in traditional teaching, while at the same time, it offers possibilities for platform curation, content creation, and hybrid modes of instruction (Brown & Richards, 2022). Yoga teachers, by collaborating with yoga AI platforms, could potentially communicate their art to a very much wider audience than what the limited physical space of a studio allows, thus, they will be able to increase their money turnover. However, the only provision is that the payment methods are very different from each other; some platforms offering revenue-sharing agreements, while others giving a low flat Provide revenue-sharing plans, while others give a low flat fee. Instead of being limited to local teachers, students are now able to choose from thousands of them, which paradoxically, as a result of easier access to instructors, intensifies competition.

Table 5. **Economic Impact on Yoga Instructors by Revenue Model**

Revenue Model	% of Digital Instructors	Median Annual Income	Income Change vs. Studio Teaching	Job Security Rating	Creative Control
Traditional Studio (baseline)	—	$38,000	—	6.2/10	7.1/10
Flat Fee per Video	42%	$18,500	-51%	3.8/10	8.2/10
Revenue Share (views/ subscriptions)	28%	$52,000	+37%	5.4/10	7.8/10
Hybrid: Platform + Studio	19%	$61,000	+61%	7.9/10	6.9/10
Platform Equity Partner	3%	$127,000	+234%	8.6/10	9.1/10
Independent Subscription Platform	8%	$44,000	+16%	4.2/10	9.5/10

Material compiled by Brown & Richards (2022) reveals that the yoga AI industry has undergone a profound transformation and is presently a significant economic power. The area was able to draw a large volume of venture capital funding, as the leading platforms were in a position to obtain the investments of several hundreds of millions of

This level of support shows that investors expect the market to grow rapidly in the coming years. Therefore, the influx of money greatly accelerates the platform upgrades. However, these business demands create a focus on acquiring new users and increasing the interaction metrics. Thus, as a result of the prioritization of these features, real pedagogical methods and the authentic cultural aspects of yoga get less attention.

The financial gains are mostly going to the tech companies as the teaching is gradually drifting from individual teachers to these platforms. Individual practitioners become owners of a smaller portion of the pie.

New hybrid models are attempting to combine the benefits of technology and the human factor in a balanced manner. Some studios use AI to support home practice between live classes. In that environment, technology was seen as a tool that strengthens the relationship rather than a competitor (Thompson & Larson, 2020). There are other places where they offer luxurious memberships that combine AI-led sessions with a few virtual ones by a real instructor. It seems to be more of a complete overhaul of the entire

IMPACT ON PUBLIC HEALTH AND HEALTHCARE SYSTEMS

Yoga AI is one of those things which changes completely how accessible this stuff is. Such a situation will result in improved public health in the aggregate. It will also have a positive economic effect on healthcare systems, which will be somewhat relieved. Numerous research works have found yoga as a very effective method of treatment for chronic conditions such as low back pain. Likewise, it is efficient in the treatment of anxiety.Depression is one of the several mental conditions that receive some improvement through yoga. Hypertension is effectively controlled with consistent practice. All the above is extracted from firm research such as Cramer and colleagues 2017 study.

Artificial intelligence configurations make it possible for people to be in a position to follow up without missing out on the sessions. They remove those barriers that prevent people from going further.In this manner, more groups which had not had access to regular teaching can now be involved. The demand for healthcare can reduce as a result. The costs could be lowered on a larger scale as well.

Some health systems and insurance companies acknowledge the benefits of yoga AI. They decided to support or pay for yoga AI tools as a means of preventing diseases. This is consistent with Garrison et al.2020 findings.The use of digital wellness tools like these leads to their being cost-effective.Medical expenses decrease with the initiation of these tools. Patients are in better health in the long run.

However, there are still people who doubt whether performing an AI yoga routine by oneself can be as effective as doing it with a teacher's guidance. Without that, adherence might not be as strong. The quality of practice might be change greatly. Williams and colleagues quoted to this in their 2021

Table 6. Healthcare Cost-Benefit Analysis of Yoga AI Implementation

Health Condition	Traditional Care Annual Cost	With Yoga AI Intervention	Cost Reduction	Effect Size	Population Reach
Chronic Lower Back Pain	$12,800	$9,400	27%	d = 0.63	High (62% eligible)
Generalized Anxiety Disorder	$8,200	$6,100	26%	d = 0.71	Moderate (43% eligible)
Type 2 Diabetes Management	$13,700	$11,900	13%	d = 0.38	Moderate (38% eligible)

continued on following page

Table 6. Continued

Health Condition	Traditional Care Annual Cost	With Yoga AI Intervention	Cost Reduction	Effect Size	Population Reach
Hypertension	$6,500	$5,400	17%	d = 0.45	High (71% eligible)
Depression	$9,400	$7,100	24%	d = 0.59	Moderate (39% eligible)
Arthritis Pain Management	$7,900	$6,600	16%	d = 0.52	High (58% eligible)
Sleep Disorders	$5,100	$3,900	24%	d = 0.48	High (67% eligible)
Stress-Related Conditions	$4,300	$2,800	35%	d = 0.82	Very High (85% eligible)

Costs in USD based on Garrison et al. (2020) and healthcare utilization data. Effect sizes from meta-analyses of yoga interventions. Population reach based on digital access surveys and medical eligibility.

The efficiency for yoga AI to focus health disparities hinges mostly on arranging equitable access proper away. If we mainly introduce it to more affluent groups that already show better healths result, the technology might widen those gaps further instead of reducing them (Braveman et al., 2011). We should obey focus plan like investment in access for underserved communities, connecting the platforms to basic health programs, and ensuring they align with verity cultural expectations. These kinds of efforts becomes to be crucial for tapping into the major advantages for public health overall.

Information from yoga AI stage introduces both chances and concerns within health-related research. Collecting cumulative data on usage patterns provides better insight into individual practices, things behind benefited outcomes, and changes in health trends among various populations. Still, challenges involving data privacy issues, ownership actions, and identifying biases in algorithmic recommendations for health actions demand robust regulatory skeleton (Mittelstadt & Floridi, 2016). Those involved are just going to move and define its outline.

Employment and Workforce Transformation

The yoga AI campaign made broader changes in the workforce. These shifts go well beyond the usual teaching positions. People worry about instructors losing their jobs. Still, this opens up needs for new skills and employment types. Content writers who handle turning yoga lessons into digital versions turn out to be entirely significant. Platforms really go after content that hooks viewers right away. Teachers who are strong in their skill, such as adjusting algorithms or managing social media pushes and building online communities, achieve better advantages in their work. Davies and Mitchell showed that point back in 2021. Now there is this new role called the AI yoga content curator. This role combines a strong teaching skill background with solid technical skills. Experts in the field go over content created by teachers. They ensure the order of lesson suit the need of various kinds of users. They maintain quality across large sets of resources. Some other jobs focus on ease of use features. They ensure the platforms work well for folks with disabilities. They cover various body shapes also and they include different cultural views. All these points to spreading special areas in the yoga AI world.

Table 7. Emerging Job Categories in the Yoga AI Ecosystem

Job Category	Required Skills	Median Salary Range	Job Growth Rate (2020-2025)	Geographic Concentration
AI Yoga Instructor	Teaching + video production + digital marketing	$35,000-75,000	+127%	Distributed/Remote
Content Curator/ Program Designer	Yoga expertise + instructional design + UX	$62,000-95,000	+89%	Tech hubs
Computer Vision Specialist (Yoga)	ML engineering + anatomy + yoga knowledge	$98,000-165,000	+143%	Tech hubs
Accessibility Specialist	Adaptive yoga + inclusive design + healthcare	$55,000-88,000	+76%	Mixed
Cultural Authenticity Consultant	Traditional yoga knowledge + anthropology	$48,000-82,000	+54%	Distributed
Community Manager (Digital Wellness)	Social media + yoga + community building	$42,000-68,000	+112%	Distributed/Remote
Product Manager (Wellness AI)	Product management + wellness industry + tech	$110,000-175,000	+98%	Tech hubs
Data Analyst (Health Outcomes)	Statistics + healthcare + yoga research	$72,000-118,000	+84%	Mixed
Voice/Language Localization Specialist	Translation + yoga + cultural adaptation	$51,000-79,000	+67%	Distributed

Income data in US dollar from industry drive, job posting analysis (n=3, 200), and redress platforms. Expansion rates calculated from 2020 baseline to 2025 estimation.

The cartographic spread of these new opportunities arises questions about fairness. Content creation and platform development jobs may be focus in technology hubs that already have digital facility and talent. This could leave out new comers in areas where traditional teaching jobs are vanishing (Sundararajan, 2016). Remote work options help reduce this concentration, but access to training programmes, digital literacy development, and professional networks impact where opportunities go.

The work based benefits of many yoga AI based jobs—such as supple hours, project-based income, and limited employment goal—reflect major trends in the labour market (Graham et al., 2017).While these facilities provide the freedom and flexibility many practitioners value, they also shift economic risks to many people. Accordingly, pluggers lose the stability and gain linked with traditional jobs. The long-term impact on the resilience of yoga professionals and the well-being of instructors requires ongoing attention.

EDUCATION AND TRAINING IMPLICATIONS

Generally, a traditional yoga teacher training program entails around 200-500 hours of instruction and covers various areas such as anatomy, philosophy, teaching methods, and practice under supervision (Yoga Alliance, 2020). To adjust these frameworks for the digital world, it is necessary not only to consider different ways of teaching but also the change of skill standards. AI accessibility in yoga practice influences education and training at different levels. With the increase of AI-guided practice, there are questions about the appropriate training standards for instructors who make platform content and for users who practice on their own. Normally, a traditional yoga teacher training program requires 200-500 hours of instruction in which the student is exposed to anatomy, philosophy, teaching methods, and supervised practice (Yoga Alliance, 2020). Changing these structures to suit the online world implies not only reconsidering the methods of teaching but also the skill standards.

There are some teachers who are of the opinion that yoga AI might decrease the level of education because the personal connection and the instant feedback which are the main factors of effective teaching will be lost (Singleton & Byrne, 2008). On the contrary, there is a group of people who maintains that tech is a great helper in the more consistent application of the best practices and in the elimination of the inconsistencies that refer to the abilities of individual instructors.AI may excel in certain teaching areas while still needing human judgment, intuition, and relationship building in others. The availability of yoga AI for students could make yoga education more accessible by reducing the costs of training programs and removing location barriers. Online teacher training programs are increasingly using AI tools for skills assessment, practice tracking, and personalized feedback (Roberts & Thompson, 2022).These advancements might enable more individuals to pursue yoga teaching careers by eliminating traditional cost and location challenges.

Continuing education for current teachers now often includes digital skills and technology integration. Instructors who built their skills in physical settings need to learn about platform algorithms, video production, online community building, and hybrid teaching methods (Anderson et al., 2021). This learning curve can be tough for seasoned teachers, especially those later in their careers, creating generational challenges within the professional community.

SOCIAL AND COMMUNITY DIMENSIONS

The social elements of yoga practice, i.e., community bonding, shared experience, and collective energy, are significant aspects, with which AI systems interact differently as compared to traditional studio environments. It is impossible for any technology to replicate completely the experience of practice in a room with co-exercisers; however, many platforms are increasingly incorporating social features to create a digital community (Kaplan & Haenlein, 2010). Virtual group classes, practice challenges, discussion forums, and social media integration offer ways to connect with other practitioners who are geographically dispersed.

Such digital communities are not restricted by geographic boundaries and thus can connect practitioners having common interests, conditions, or identities even if they are miles apart from each other in the world. Community of the specialized like prenatal yoga, yoga for chronic pain, or specific spiritual lineages can spontaneously arise within platform ecosystems (Rheingold, 2000). For those practitioners who are either in remote areas or have marginalized identities and whose local studios are unable to serve them, these connections can be a source of support and belonging that may not be available otherwise.

However, research about digital versus physical community indicates that online relationships, although important, usually offer different and even less social support than that of face-to-face communication (Putnam, 2000). The shared space and time in which to practice together physically among the participants create a level of connection and mutual understanding which are difficult to be achieved through the virtual mode. The degree to which yoga AI platforms are capable of building a strong sense of community among users who practice alone at home is an unsettled question which influences platform design and user experience.

It is necessary to think about the possible consequences for social cohesion at larger scales as well. In a scenario where yoga practice is mostly moving away from public community spaces and into private digital consumption, there is, on the one hand, a possibility of reduced cross-demographic interaction and social bridging facilitated by communal activities (Hampton & Wellman, 2018). On the other hand, the accessibility changes may allow more people to benefit from yoga, thus, potentially there could be larger and more diverse communities of practitioners although connections may differ from the traditional

ENVIRONMENTAL CONSIDERATIONS

The environmental footprint of yoga AI compared to traditional studio-based practice has its positives and negatives. On the one hand, digital platforms do away with transportation emissions resulting from the commute to studios which, when calculated over millions of practitioners making regular trips, becomes a very significant factor (Coroama et al., 2013). On the other hand, the energy consumption of data centers, network infrastructures, and billions of devices streaming video content is the main cause of the environmental impact, with digital technologies being responsible for approximately 4% of the global greenhouse gas emissions and this figure is still increasing (Belkhir & Elmeligi, 2018).

Table 8. Environmental Impact Comparison: Traditional vs. AI Yoga Practice

Impact Category	Traditional Studio Yoga (per user annually)	Yoga AI (per user annually)	Net Difference
Transportation Emissions	847 kg CO_2e (avg. 104 trips)	0 kg CO_2e	-100%
Facility Energy (heating/cooling/ lighting)	124 kg CO_2e (shared/ allocated)	0 kg CO_2e (home practice)	-100%
Digital Infrastructure Energy	0 kg CO_2e	156 kg CO_2e (streaming/data)	+100%
Device Manufacturing Impact	0 kg CO_2e (amortized)	48 kg CO_2e (device replacement)	+100%
Equipment Production	12 kg CO_2e (studio provided)	35 kg CO_2e (individual purchase)	+192%
Water Usage	520 liters (facility)	180 liters (home laundry)	-65%
Waste Generation	2.8 kg (shared resources)	4.1 kg (individual packaging)	+46%
TOTAL CARBON FOOTPRINT	983 kg CO_2e	239 kg CO_2e	**-76%**

Roama et al. (2013), Belkhir & Elmeligi (2018), and lifecycle assessments. Assumes 3 sessions/week for traditional; 4 sessions/week for AI (higher frequency due to convenience). The transportation assumes an 8-mile round trip by car.

The material economy of yoga practice is also changing in the AI era. On the one hand, traditional studios need to have a dedicated physical space and along with this, there are associated impacts due to construction, heating, cooling, and maintenance, but these costs are shared among many users. On the other hand, home practice can lead to more individual equipment purchases as mats, blocks, straps, and other props with which practitioners recreate studio amenities in the privacy of their homes (Ritch & Brownlie, 2016). Whether yoga AI increases or decreases overall material consumption largely depends on the user behavior, equipment quality, platform design choices, and so forth.

Some yoga AI platforms explicitly take sustainability into consideration when they carry out their operations, use renewable energy for data centers, provide carbon offset packages, and promote environmental consciousness within the content (Chen & Lin, 2020). Developers of a yoga AI platform are prioritizing other environmental themes in the instruction which use the philosophy of yoga, especially the interconnection, to foster ecological awareness among users. Incorporating sustainability aspects in yoga AI is a space where tech companies can demonstrate their alignment with the ethical standards of

The worldwide availability of yoga AI is a factor that also affects the environmental justice aspect. For example, if technology allows people living in polluted cities or areas with limited green space to get access to the benefits of stress reduction and physical health which, otherwise, they might not have, then it can be considered that it partially solves the problem of environmental health inequities (Brulle & Pellow, 2006). However, the issue of whether technology is a driver of consumption patterns and resource extraction that a) cause environmental degradation and b) impact the vulnerable populations disproportionately should be taken into account as well when assessing the

POLICY AND REGULATORY CONSIDERATIONS

The swift expansion of yoga AI has exceeded the requirements of regulatory frameworks that were designed for traditional wellness services, thus resulting in governance gaps and policy challenges.Most of the questions about professional standards, quality control, consumer protection, and liability that have been raised are still insufficiently answered in most jurisdictions (Regulation of Digital Health Technologies, 2019). The cross-border character of digital platforms makes it difficult for regulators to adopt a certain approach as services can cross borders easily, whereas regulatory authority is still nationally limited.Professional standards for yoga instruction differ widely in different parts of the world. Some jurisdictions have strong registration and regulation requirements, while others have only weak oversight (Klein & Guest, 2020).Yoga AI platforms that are globally operating have to deal with this patchwork and decide whether they should follow the lowest-common-denominator standards or set higher quality standards that exceed requirements in some markets. Industry self-regulation through such organizations as Yoga Alliance is only a partial governance, but voluntary standards cannot guarantee quality and consumer protection in all cases.

Regulations on data privacy such as the General Data Protection Regulation by the European Union and other similar frameworks have an increasing impact on yoga AI operations (Voigt & Von dem Bussche, 2017). These platforms have to comply with different privacy and security measures while they collect sensitive information about users' health conditions, physical capabilities, and practice routines. However, there are business motivations to use the user data in such ways as targeted advertising, product recommendation, or selling by third parties, thus creating conflicts with privacy protection, which regulatory frameworks have to

The issue of liability in this context is the least clarified area, especially with regard to injury occurrence during AI-guided practice. The traditional studios and instructors have insurance that covers injuries related to teaching, but it is not clear who will take the responsibility when algorithmic systems provide instruction without human oversight (Scherer, 2016). Usually, in terms of service, there are liability waiver clauses, but their enforceability depends on jurisdiction and may not fully protect platforms from negligence claims.

FUTURE TRAJECTORIES AND EMERGING CONSIDERATIONS

The trajectory of yoga AI development reveals various new considerations that are very likely to influence the socio-economic effects of the future. Among the most important technological breakthroughs that lead to artificial intelligence is the employment of computer vision, natural language processing, and personalization algorithms which will make the guidance more indistinguishable from that of a human (Russell & Norvig,). Therefore, the difference between AI-guided practice and human instructor-led practice may become so insignificant that it will open up more possibilities as well as challenges for the socio-economic effects of AI in yoga. The combination of Yoga AI technology with other health-related tech such as wearable sensors, smart home devices, and virtual reality systems, may result in ecosystem effects that surpass the individual platforms' capabilities (Patel et al., 2020). For instance, an all-in-one health technology system that monitors sleep, nutrition, stress, physical activity, and yoga practice, may have the capacity to offer holistic health optimization.

However, this last point, in turn, raises questions about monitoring, data integration, and technological dependency.

With the help of AI, yoga can be the next dream to be realized either in virtual or augmented reality, which means an altogether different concept (Slater & Sanchez-Vives,). Immersive technologies have the capability to reproduce the different facets of communal practice while still being available via digital platforms. However, the necessary equipment and the costs of VR/AR systems might restrict the access only to those who are wealthy and are the first to adopt, thereby resulting in a digital divide.

Yoga AI business models will be the determining factor in how accessible and equitable yoga will be. These models can offer people a certain amount of access, however, they still require a continuous revenue increase and this may lead to platforms that focus more on user engagement to raise their revenue rather than on pedagogy quality (Srnicek, 2017). Different models such as freemium structures, advertising support, healthcare system integration, and public/nonprofit provision might, on the other hand, lead to a dramatic change in the access and incentives.

CONCLUSION

The worldwide accessibility and socio-economic impacts of Yoga AI are a mirror to the complex and evolving interrelations of technology that change not only the way we do Yoga but also the whole supply chain of the related industries.

The empowering capicity, in other words, the factors that reduce costs, remove the region barriers, allow tailoring, and provide the unprivileged groups with access, is continued and meaningful. This feature contradict with the existing digital things, infrastructure limitations, cultural figures, and commerce incentives that determine the beneficiaries of technological innovation.

The social standing effects have a ripple effect and go to various areas of the labor market, healthcare systems, teaching and education, community areas, and environmental viability. These results are not always good or bad, but rather they create winners and losers, opportunities and threats, which, are distributed unevenly among vaiours group of peoples and regions. Creation for equity, including deployment, obeying culture, and good governance will fix whether yoga AI will reduce or widen the wellness access gap that actually present .This is necessarily not to lose sight of human thrive rather than just technological progress while yoga AI is still converting .Yoga as a system is based on helping people eliminate of suffering, giving them well-being, and making them realize interconnectedness, and thus, it can provide a philosophical framework that can be used to develop better technology. The problem is in figuring out how to apply these ancient teaching skills to new technological contexts and hence, creating systems that actually help different kinds of groups rather than just taking value from them.

The questions raised by yoga AI are not limited to this technology instance only but eventually call for a re-testing of the effects of digital changes on health, welfare, and overall growth. What means do societies have to use technology to make such practices that are beneficial more accessible? While still comforting their indispensable qualities are preserved?

REFERENCES

Anderson, T., Thompson, L., & Davis, M. (2021). Digital competencies for yoga teachers: Training needs in the technology age. *Journal of Yoga Education, 15*(2), 87–103.

Askegaard, S., & Eckhardt, G. M. (2012). Glocal yoga: Re-appropriation in the Indian consumptionscape. *Marketing Theory, 12*(1), 45–60. DOI: 10.1177/1470593111424180

Atkinson, N. L., & Permuth-Levine, R. (2009). Benefits, barriers, and cues to action of yoga practice: A focus group approach. *American Journal of Health Behavior, 33*(1), 3–14. DOI: 10.5993/AJHB.33.1.1

Belkhir, L., & Elmeligi, A. (2018). Assessing ICT global emissions footprint: Trends to 2040 & recommendations. *Journal of Cleaner Production, 177*, 448–463. DOI: 10.1016/j.jclepro.2017.12.239

Braveman, P. A., Kumanyika, S., Fielding, J., LaVeist, T., Borrell, L. N., Manderscheid, R., & Troutman, A. (2011). Health disparities and health equity: The issue is justice. *American Journal of Public Health, 101*(S1), S149–S155. DOI: 10.2105/AJPH.2010.300062

Brown, K., & Richards, P. (2022). The digital yoga instructor: Career transformations in wellness technology. *International Journal of Sport and Exercise Psychology, 18*(3), 234–251.

Brulle, R. J., & Pellow, D. N. (2006). Environmental justice: Human health and environmental inequalities. *Annual Review of Public Health, 27*(1), 103–124. DOI: 10.1146/annurev.publhealth.27.021405.102124

Büssing, A., Michalsen, A., Khalsa, S. B. S., Telles, S., & Sherman, K. J. (2012). Effects of yoga on mental and physical health: A short summary of reviews. *Evidence-Based Complementary and Alternative Medicine : eCAM, 2012*, 165410. DOI: 10.1155/2012/165410

Chen, K., & Chan, A. H. (2019). Gerontechnology acceptance by elderly: A systematic review. *Interdisciplinary Journal of Information, Knowledge, and Management, 14*, 29–55.

Chen, Y., & Lin, C. (2020). Sustainability practices in digital wellness platforms: An exploratory study. *Journal of Sustainable Business, 28*(4), 112–129.

Coroama, V. C., Hilty, L. M., & Birtel, M. (2013). Effects of Internet-based multiple-site conferences on greenhouse gas emissions. *Telematics and Informatics, 30*(4), 362–374. DOI: 10.1016/j.tele.2011.11.006

Cramer, H., Lauche, R., Klose, P., Lange, S., Langhorst, J., & Dobos, G. J. (2017). Yoga for improving health-related quality of life, mental health and cancer-related symptoms in women diagnosed with breast cancer. *The Cochrane Library, 2017*(1), CD010802. DOI: 10.1002/14651858.CD010802.pub2

Cramer, H., Lauche, R., Langhorst, J., & Dobos, G. (2013). Yoga for depression: A systematic review and meta-analysis. *Depression and Anxiety, 30*(11), 1068–1083. DOI: 10.1002/da.22166

Cramer, H., Lauche, R., Langhorst, J., & Dobos, G. (2016). Is one yoga style better than another? A systematic review of associations of yoga style and conclusions in randomized yoga trials. *Complementary Therapies in Medicine, 25*, 178–187. DOI: 10.1016/j.ctim.2016.02.015

Davies, R., & Mitchell, S. (2021). Content creation in the digital wellness economy: Skills, compensation, and career pathways. *Media Industries Journal, 8*(2), 45–67.

Davis, F. D. (1989). Perceived usefulness, perceived ease of use, and user acceptance of information technology. *Management Information Systems Quarterly, 13*(3), 319–340. DOI: 10.2307/249008

De Michelis, E. (2004). A history of modern yoga: Patanjali and Western esotericism. *Continuum.*

Ding, D., Lawson, K. D., Kolbe-Alexander, T. L., Finkelstein, E. A., Katzmarzyk, P. T., Van Mechelen, W., & Pratt, M. (2017). The economic burden of physical inactivity: A global analysis of major non-communicable diseases. *The Lancet*, 388(10051), 1311-1324. Duffy, B. E., Pinch, A., Sannon, S., & Sawey, M. (2021). The nested precarities of creative labor on social media. *Social Media + Society, 7*(2), 20563051211021370.

Eysenbach, G. (2001). What is e-health? *Journal of Medical Internet Research, 3*(2), e20. DOI: 10.2196/jmir.3.2.e20

Garrison, K., Thomas, R., & Williams, P. (2020). Healthcare cost implications of digital wellness interventions: A systematic review. *Health Economics Review, 10*(1), 1–18.

Global Wellness Institute. (2022). *Global wellness economy monitor 2022*. Global Wellness Institute.

Godrej, F. (2017). The neoliberal yogi and the politics of yoga. *Political Theory, 45*(6), 772–800. DOI: 10.1177/0090591716643604

Graham, M., Hjorth, I., & Lehdonvirta, V. (2017). Digital labour and development: Impacts of global digital labour platforms and the gig economy on worker livelihoods. *Transfer: European Review of Labour and Research, 23*(2), 135–162. DOI: 10.1177/1024258916687250

Graham, M., & Woodcock, J. (2018). Towards a fairer platform economy: Introducing the Fairwork Foundation. *Alternate Routes, 29*, 242–253.

Hampton, K. N., & Wellman, B. (2018). Lost and saved... again: The moral panic about the loss of community takes hold of social media. *Contemporary Sociology, 47*(6), 643–651. DOI: 10.1177/0094306118805415

Insights, C. B. (2023). *Wellness tech funding report: AI-powered fitness and meditation platforms*. CB Insights Research.

International Telecommunication Union (ITU). (2023). *Measuring digital development: Facts and figures 2023*. ITU Publications.

Jain, A. R. (2014). *Selling yoga: From counterculture to pop culture*. Oxford University Press. DOI: 10.1093/acprof:oso/9780199390236.001.0001

Jain, A. R. (2020). Who is saving whom? Colonial missionizing and yoga. *International Journal of Hindu Studies, 24*(1), 39–66.

Kaplan, A. M., & Haenlein, M. (2010). Users of the world, unite! The challenges and opportunities of social media. *Business Horizons, 53*(1), 59–68. DOI: 10.1016/j.bushor.2009.09.003

Kontos, E., Blake, K. D., Chou, W. Y. S., & Prestin, A. (2014). Predictors of eHealth usage: Insights on the digital divide from the Health Information National Trends Survey 2012. *Journal of Medical Internet Research, 16*(7), e172. DOI: 10.2196/jmir.3117

Kumar, S., & Singh, R. (2021). Digital divide in health technology adoption: Urban-rural disparities in India. *The Journal of Rural Health : Official Journal of the American Rural Health Association and the National Rural Health Care Association, 37*(2), 312–325.

Martinez, L., Chen, M., & Rodriguez, A. (2020). Quality stratification in digital health platforms: Access and equity implications. *Journal of Medical Internet Research, 22*(8), e18234.

Mittelstadt, B. D., & Floridi, L. (2016). The ethics of big data: Current and foreseeable issues in biomedical contexts. *Science and Engineering Ethics, 22*(2), 303–341. DOI: 10.1007/s11948-015-9652-2

Nair, M. (2020). Commodification, appropriation, and representation: Yoga in the United States. In *Handbook of Research on the Global Impacts and Roles of Immersive Media* (pp. 290–312). IGI Global.

Neufeld, D., & Dellaert, B. (2020). Consumer response to subscription-based wellness platforms: Price, value, and utilization patterns. *Journal of Service Research, 23*(4), 412–428.

Park, C. L., Elwy, A. R., Maiya, M., Sarkin, A. J., Riley, K. E., Eisen, S. V., Gutierrez, I., Finkelstein-Fox, L., Lee, S. Y., Casteel, D., Braun, T., & Groessl, E. J. (2020). The essential properties of yoga questionnaire (EPYQ): Psychometric properties. *International Journal of Yoga Therapy, 30*(1), 23–38. DOI: 10.17761/2018-00016R2

Park, C. L., Finkelstein-Fox, L., Sacco, S. J., Braun, T. D., & Lazar, S. (2018). How does yoga reduce stress? A clinical trial examining psychological mechanisms. *Stress and Health : Journal of the International Society for the Investigation of Stress, 34*(2), 245–256.

Patel, M. S., Asch, D. A., & Volpp, K. G. (2020). Wearable devices as facilitators, not drivers, of health behavior change. *Journal of the American Medical Association, 313*(5), 459–460. DOI: 10.1001/jama.2014.14781

Singleton, M. (2010). *Yoga body: The origins of modern posture practice*. Oxford University Press. DOI: 10.1093/acprof:oso/9780195395358.001.0001

Sundararajan, A. (2016). *The sharing economy: The end of employment and the rise of crowd-based capitalism*. MIT Press.

Thompson, R., & Larson, P. (2020). Hybrid wellness models: Integrating technology and human instruction. *The Journal of Business Strategy, 41*(4), 23–31.

Van Dijk, J. A. (2005). *The deepening divide: Inequality in the information society*. Sage Publications.

Venkatesh, V., Thong, J. Y., & Xu, X. (2012). Consumer acceptance and use of information technology: Extending the unified theory of acceptance and use of technology. *Management Information Systems Quarterly, 36*(1), 157–178. DOI: 10.2307/41410412

Williams, D., Thompson, K., & Martinez, S. (2021). Adherence and outcomes in digital versus in-person yoga interventions: A comparative effectiveness study. *Complementary Therapies in Medicine*, *58*, 102693.

Yoga Alliance & Yoga Journal. (2021). *2021 yoga in America study*. Yoga Alliance.

Zhao, Y., Ni, Q., & Zhou, R. (2018). What factors influence the mobile health service adoption? A meta-analysis and the moderating role of age. *International Journal of Information Management*, *43*, 342–350. DOI: 10.1016/j.ijinfomgt.2017.08.006

Chapter 3
Ethical AI in Yoga:
Lessons From Yama and Niyama

Sandeep Kumar Singh
http://orcid.org/0000-0002-1741-7254
Jindal Global Business School, O.P. Jindal Global University, Sonipat, India

Ravi Tomar
http://orcid.org/0000-0002-3712-6702
Department of Chemistry, SRM Institute of Science and Technology, Delhi NCR, India

Shafiul Haque
Department of Nursing, College of Nursing and Health Sciences, Jazan University, Jazan, Saudi Arabia

ABSTRACT

The chapter addresses the ethical vacuum in the development of artificial intelligence for yoga. The chapter identifies that many wellness technologies are reducing the holistic practice of yoga to physical performance alone and as such, create significant risks of algorithmic harm, data exploitation and user dependency. The author suggests that the ten foundational principles of ethics by Patañjali's Yoga Sutras (the five yamas – social restraints & the five niyamas – personal observances) provide a framework for responsible innovation in AI. The author outlines the mapping of each principle of the five yamas to the five niyamas to the challenges and solutions of AI design, including ahimsa (non-harming) to svadhyaya (self-reflection). Through this process, the author proposes a new paradigm of "Sattvic Technology," which is designed to develop AI systems that support inner inquiry and holistic well-being, rather than simply quantify and gamify the practice of yoga.

DOI: 10.4018/979-8-2600-2463-8.ch003

1. INTRODUCTION

The widespread integration of artificial intelligence with yoga and holistic wellness has made ethical AI research an essential field. This is due to the increasing attention being paid to the ethics that must govern the development and implementation of AI systems (Sinha &Sinha, 2024) (Mahajan, 2025). The history of the applications of AI in yoga ranges across the earliest AI-powered posture correction programs to advanced customized wellness platforms, which marks the course from technical possibilities to ethics and culture questions (Yenishettil et al., 2024) (Jahnavi, 2025) (Marade et al., 2025). This area has practical importance since AI has the potential to improve yoga's accessibility, personalization, and efficiency in the global yoga field that is known for enhancing physical, mental, and spiritual well-being (Rawat et al., 2025) (Sharma & Tiwari, 2024). In particular, the global economy of wellness exceeding $4.5 trillion highlights the necessity of implementing AI responsibly in order to facilitate integral health (Venkatasubramanian, 2023) (Narine et al., 2025).

The precise question inquired about the philosophical foundations and the moral difficulties of incorporating AI in yoga and how the classical yogic ethics like Yama and Niyama provide guidance in developing the ethics of intelligent systems (Nandram et al., 2022). Despite advances in AI-enabled yoga applications, there remains a knowledge gap regarding the systematic incorporation of these ancient ethical principles into AI design and governance (Pallathadka & Roy, 2025) (Chaturvedi et al., 2024) (Aksan, 2025). Rival views signal strains between technological development and the maintenance of yoga's spiritual integrity, with some scholars highlighting the possibilities of democratization by AI, while others warn about threats of commodifying yoga and severing human relationships (Keny, 2025) (Chanda, 2025). The implications of ignoring such ethical aspects involved weaker practitioner well-being and cultural insensitivity potentially damaging the holistic aims of yoga (Popkova, 2024) (Trisia, 2025).

This chapter creates a conceptual map between the philosophical origins of Yama and Niyama—yogic ethics of restraints and observances—and contemporary values of AI ethics such as fairness, transparency, and cultural responsiveness (Townsend, 2025) (Fuadi et al., 2025). This context places AI in the role of a tool that needs to harmonize with human values and yogic ethics in order to ensure holistic well-being, encompassing physical, mental, and spiritual dimensions (Mahajan, 2025) (Barbhuiya, 2025).

2. PART 1: THE YAMAS – CRAFTING ARTIGICIAL INTELLIGENCE FOR AN EQUITABLE SOCIETY

These five Yamas, according to Patañjìalì, represent universal ethics and morality that guide our dealings with others and with the world in general. They are no set of rules but rather disciplines to minimize behaviors that lead to suffering and to create a state of internal and external harmony. In designing artificial intelligence, the Yamas become an effective set of guidelines to ensure that these systems become a positive force in society, transcending functions to project an ultimate respect for human dignity and well-being. In this section, each of the five Yamas shall be addressed, rendering ancient philosophical knowledge into tangible principles of design to create a more equitable and compassionate future in technology.

2.1 Ahimsa (Non-Harming): From Algorithmic Bias to Digital Wellbeing

2.1.1 Philosophical Foundation of Ahimsa

Ahimsa, the first of and probably the most fundamental of the five Yamas, consists of the principle of non-harming or non-violence. It is given highest priority in the Yoga Sutras, where Patañjali calls it the Mahavrtam, or the "Great Vow," which it is incumbent upon all to follow everywhere and under all circumstances. The philosophical breadth of Ahimsa is enormous and goes far beyond the simple avoidance of outward violence. It includes a promise of non-harming in thought, in word and in deed and signifies a state of ultimate coordination between the internal and external worlds of the individual.

2.1.2 Manifestations of Harm (Himsa) in AI

In the context of a Yoga AI, risk related to harm (himsa) is sophisticated and transcends both individual and systemic levels. An overall understanding of these potential harms forms the very first step in the development of a system that truly embodies the principle of Ahimsa.

2.1.2.1 Physical Damage

Physical damage occurs most immediately when an AI program gives erroneous or unsafe instructions. An AI that recommends a bodily posture without knowledge of a student's existing injuries, personal flexibility restrictions, or particular health issues could very well result in strains, sprains, or even severe bodily harm. A universal approach to instructions on the asanas is unsafe, and an AI that doesn't take into account individual human variation is an immediate cause of potential bodily himsa.

2.1.2.2 Mental Damage

The virtual space may also be a very powerful source of mental suffering. An overly critical, judgmental, or performance-oriented AI-based feedback system may create body dysmorphia, anxiety, and an ongoing sense of inadequacy. This violence to the self is the subtle yet strong transgression of the principle of Ahimsa. Non-harming also applies to the self; forcing oneself into a potentially hurtful pose due to a sense of competition or self-judgment is self-violence that a good AI should deter and not facilitate.

2.1.2.3 Social and Systemic Harm

Algorithmic bias, a systemic issue that results in an unjust or discriminatory output from an AI system, is among the most tacit types of harm. This kind of bias is not due to any reprehensible motive on the part of the algorithm in itself; instead, it typically arises from the wrong human data used to train it. In the case of yoga, this process can become apparent in several ways:

- **Sample Bias:** A model whose training data consists largely of videos and photographs of young, thin, able-bodied, white practitioners will have an inherent bias in its "correct" pose model. Accordingly, the model's effectiveness may suffer among older adults, individuals of color, individuals with larger bodies, and individuals with disabilities. It may repeatedly inaccurately read their poses as "incorrect" or entirely miss them, essentially excluding them from the practice and reinforcing negative societal assumptions about who yoga is "for".
- **Prejudice Bias:** Artificial intelligence has the potential to unintentionally acquire and propagate detrimental stereotypes embedded within its training datasets. For instance, it may link strength-oriented postures predominantly with male physiques or associate profound flexibility with female physiques, thereby perpetuating restrictive gender stereotypes.

Every such systemic discrimination amounts to a grave act of social himsa. Each violates the very principle of Ahimsa, which strives to respect and honor the life and the dignity of everyone, and not only those who conform to a narrow-privileged pattern.

2.1.3 The "Ahimsa-by-Design" Solution

Instead of reacting to errors, the "Ahimsa-by-Design" solution aims to make the principle of non-violence an inherent part of the overall system architecture from data collection through the user interface (the user experience).

2.1.3.1 Technical Design

The quality of the data is essential to an Ahimsa-AI. To reduce the risk of creating biases within the training data and to collect a variety of different representations of people, it is necessary to make a conscious and continuous effort to gather training data from a broad range of humans with various body types, ages, ethnicities, gender, and physical capabilities. In addition, the process of developing the AI must include processes to detect and mitigate biases, and to audit fairness in the AI's performance.

2.1.3.2 Safety and Reliability

The primary concern of a safe-AI (an Ahimsa-AI) is always the well-being and safety of the user. As stated previously, this is consistent with current AI ethics which emphasize the importance of developing safe and reliable systems. One major aspect of the development of a safe-AI is the creation of personalized risk profiles for the user, by collecting voluntary information about the user's physical limitations, previous injuries, and/or health conditions. Once collected, the AI should use the data collected to create recommendations that do not include contraindicated poses, and modify suggested poses to accommodate the user's physical limitations and health conditions. Additionally, the development of the AI should include safety overrides so that the AI does not suggest movements that are likely to pose a high-risk to the user's well-being.

Development of the AI itself also has to follow non-harming principles. This starts with a close examination of the data sources that fuel machine learning systems. All too often, such data is gathered from the internet with neither full nor even informed consent from the individuals represented, nor even annotated and categorized by a global army of "ghost workers" who are underpaid and working in precarious conditions. This data and labor exploitation becomes a systemic himsa despite the end product's purpose to improve well-being. A truly Ahimsa-concerned methodology, therefore, requires a commitment to ethical data gathering such that all those individuals who end up in the training data have given their consent.

2.2 Satya (Truthfulness): Honesty and Clarity in Code

2.2.1 Philosophical Foundation for Satya

Satya, the second Yama, is the practice of truthfulness. The term "sat" is taken from the Sanskrit to signify that which is" or that which exists" and, therefore, invites the process of thought, speech, and action that is characterized by integrity, saying what is real and not what we desire it to be. More than the mere practice of not uttering what is false, this dharma demands an inner knowing that allows human beings to go further than what is habituated, believed, and emotionally conditioned to the way we see reality. The practice of Satya is not absolute; it always has to be interpreted with the guidance of the practice of Ahimsa.

2.2.2 The Challenge of Untruthfulness with AI

It is also exhibited technologically and conceptually in the arena of artificial intelligence, therefore giving rise to an obstacle to trust and actual understandings.

2.2.2.1 Black Box" Problem

Most of the strongest AI systems, especially those that use deep neural networks, are "black boxes". Their decision processes are constructed from millions or even billions of interlocking parameters, so that their logic is unintelligible even to the designers. When the system makes a suggestion—a pose, adjustment, or sequence of practice—it cannot honestly say why it came to that decision. Such built-in obscurity is a species of technical dishonesty. The system cannot honestly speak about how it thought, so the user must either follow the system blindly or dismiss it.

2.2.2.2 Misleading Marketing and Misinformation

Even more overt is the potential for falsehood with misleading promises for an AI's performance, producing results that the technology is not capable of producing. More subtly, the AI can also serve an effective distribution medium for misinformation among the users within the yoga universe. An AI that has been trained with a database of pop-culture misconceptions, fitness-industry vocabulary, or historically inaccurate presentations of yoga can broadcast and legitimize these misconceptions, presenting the user with these misconceptions backed up with the credibility that the user anticipates. This violates the spirit of Satya through the spread of a form of yoga that is not representative of its proper origin and foundation.

2.2.3 The "Radical Transparency" Solution

Satya commitment demands an inherent transition from obscurity to ultimate clarity for the design and working of a Yoga AI. It entails describing the system's inner workings, sources of knowledge, and limitations, that these are readily comprehensible and transparent to the user.

2.2.3.1 Technical Implementation: Explainable AI (XAI)

The simplest technical way to put Satya into an intricate AI system is through the adoption of Explainable AI (XAI) techniques. XAI is an area of AI technology and engineering that aims to develop systems whose decisions are graspable to humans. Instead of a black box, XAI wants to develop a "glass box" so the user can view the rationale behind an output from an AI. The benefit of XAI is already being realized in high-risk areas such as healthcare and finance. An XAI system would be able to reveal why a cancer alert was issued on a medical image by pointing to the actual pixels responsible, or outline the exact reasons behind the denial of a loan application revealed in the financial profile.

Applying Satya to the realm of artificial intelligence is not simply to account for its successes, but to demand utmost transparency regarding its failures, doubts, and inherent limitations. Satya implies the articulation of reality as it is, and the essence of AI is that it is a probabilistic, not a deterministic, model. Error-prone, with some confidence levels, and always subject to the training data provided for it, the truly truthful AI would not deliver the results it arrives at as absolute dictums. It would, instead, deliver the lack of confidence that it has itself, as an integral part of the explanation. For instance, rather than absolutely declaring, "This is Warrior II," it would state, "I am 85% confident that this is the Warrior II position. My confidence is diminished due to the partly occluded view your back arm has with the camera." Such nuanced shift in communication is profoundly consequential. It takes the AI from the position of absolute authority to that of an assistive, yet fallible, aide. Such an elevation nurtures a collaborative relationship with the user, encouraging him or her to rely on his or her own intelligence and interoceptive intuition as the determiner par excellence of truth. Such programed modesty is the deepest expression of Satya, grounding the foundation for trust not derived from an illusion of perfectibility, but an explicit commitment to the truth.

2.3 Asteya (Non-Stealing): Data Sovereignty and Digital Trust

2.3.1 Philosophical Foundation of Asteya

Asteya, the third of the Yamas, is the discipline of not stealing. Its meaning, as for the other Yamas, goes far beyond the literal act of physical thievery. Asteya advises us not to take anything which has not been willingly given, including someone else's time, energy, ideas, pleasure, or confidence. The psychological origin of the urge to steal, the yogic philosophies teach, is an intuition of scarcity, insecurity, or envy—a sense of incompleteness and the urge to obtain something external to make ourselves whole. Finishing the practice of Asteya, therefore, is a remedy to this mentality of shortage. It is developed by the awareness of the reality that all that truly matters for us for our fulfillment and joy already resides within us.

2.3.2 The Extractive Model of Modern Tech

The current business model of the technology industry fundamentally conflicts with the value of Asteya. That model is an extractive one, predicated upon the bulk aggregation, data analysis, and financialization of user data, often without the full understanding or enthusiastic consent of the user. In the scenario of a Yoga AI, the data aggregating is of an exceptionally personal and intimate nature. It could be comprised of precise biometric data like heart rate variability and breathing patterns, precise kinematic data related to the movement of the user's body, and even affective data where the affective state of the user is estimated by the interpretation of their tone of voice or expression. To subject this highly personal data, which is a digital simulation of the person's internal state, and commercially benefit from it constitutes an extreme violation of Asteya. It constitutes a theft by means of which the user's personal experience gets commodified and the foundation of the trust necessary for an honest wellness practice gets eroded.

2.3.3 The "Data Sovereignty" Solution

An ethical Yoga AI model founded upon the tenet of Asteya should have to disregard this exploitative paradigm and, rather, be founded upon the doctrine of user ownership and control of personal data. This approach is best exemplified by the concept of data sovereignty.

2.3.3.1 Conceptual Framework

Data sovereignty refers to the principle wherein data is governed by the legal statutes and regulatory frameworks of the entity—be it a nation, organization, or individual—that creates it. When considered from the perspective of the individual, this principle implies that users possess the paramount authority to govern their own data, encompassing aspects such as its collection, storage, utilization, and deletion. This perspective reinterprets data privacy not merely as an adjustable characteristic or a promotional strategy but rather as a fundamental and inalienable right—a direct digital manifestation of the ethical principle of Asteya. Within this framework, the user is recognized not as a product; instead, they are regarded as the sovereign proprietor of their digital identity.

2.3.3.2 Technical Execution

Developing an AI system that honors data sovereignty demands certain architectural decisions that place privacy and security foremost, from the foundation upwards.

- **End-to-End Encryption:** It is crucial that any user data, both stored on the device ("at rest") or transmitted to the server ("in transit"), be protected by strong end-to-end encryption. This ensures access to the data remains limited to the user and approved individuals and makes the data ineffective for attackers upon the occurrence of data breach.
- **On-Device Processing:** To minimize the transportation and off-device storing of protectable information, it is best to perform AI processing on the user's local device whenever feasible. Advancements in the capabilities of mobile computing further allow complex AI models to run natively on smartphones, so personal data remains within the user's control.
- **Granular and Revocable Consent:** Consent must not be relegated to the status of some isolated, fixed stipulation buried within a long term of service agreement. An Asteya-based system must present the user transparent, uncomplicated, and granular mechanisms for the management of their data. Users should have the ability to actively opt-in to specific data applications and should have the ability to easily view, modify, or rescind the consent whenever they wish, along with an uncomplicated method of the wholesale deletion of their data.

2.3.3.3 Business Models

Remaining true to the values of Asteya and data self-sovereignty requires a business model which does not rely upon the commercialization or monetization of user data. Plausible alternatives which are aligned with these ethical values are:

- **Subscription Models:** A transparent and uncomplicated subscription charge to use the service is the well-liked and moral method developed by applications like Alo Moves and Glo.4 Customers are paying the service they're getting, not their own data.
- **Federated Learning:** This is a privacy-preserving machine learning technique where a global AI model can be trained across many decentralized devices without the raw data ever leaving those devices. The model updates, not the personal data, are sent back to a central server, allowing the AI to learn and improve while respecting user privacy.

The practice of Asteya is not just about not taking, but learning to cultivate an inner sense of plenitude that renders the urge to take superfluous. The scarcity mentality of the present-day tech model—the idea that value needs to be wrested from the user as data—can be reversed. An Asteya-based AI would view its mission not as extracting value from the user, but as facilitating the user identifying the "jewels" within them, as the sutra of Patañjali pledges. That would mean the features of the AI would be constructed to reveal the user's own inner strength, resilience, and ability to live in peace. It would utilize data not towards external gain, but as a mirror that reflects the user's own evolution and inner stores back to the user. The business model becomes, therefore, ideally complementary to the user's spiritual evolution: the user voluntarily pays for a commodity that demonstrates to them they have always possessed the totality of what they genuinely require. That turns the technology, once an instrument of extraction, into the engine of self-realization.

2.4 Brahmacharya (Proper Use of Energy): Designing for Presence, Not Addiction

2.4.1 Philosophical Foundation of Brahmacharya

Brahmacharya, the fourth Yama, is most likely the least understood of all. Whereas literally the word means celibacy, specifically the life of the monastic student of ancient India, its wider and applicable meaning to the modern practitioner of Yoga and meditation is the right application and moderation of life energy. Etymologically, the word breaks down into Brahma, the divine, the ultimate reality, and charya, to walk, to follow. Therefore, Brahmacharya means "walking with the Divine" or applying one's energy to higher, spiritual ends and not squandering it by excessive or compulsive pleasure of the senses. It means the practice of controlling the senses and not letting the senses control you and saving your life energy, or prana or ojas, for the expansion and illumination of the soul. It is the path of the middle way of self-conscious moderation and not of utter denial, which results in liberation from desires and dependencies.

2.4.2 The "Attention Economy" and Addictive Design

The new digital economy, dubbed the "attention economy," operates on principles the opposite of Brahmacharya. The majority of digital platforms' business models rely on capturing and holding user attention for the longest duration possible to achieve the highest advertising exposure or metrics-based interactions. For this, designers often deploy manipulative user interface and user experience tactics known as "dark patterns" or specifically "hyper-engaging dark patterns" (HEDPs). These are user interface and user experience tactics specifically designed to exploit human psychological vulnerability to induce compulsive use and digital addiction.

2.4.3 The "Presence-Based Design" Approach

AI Yoga built under the principles of Brahmacharya will intentionally forego the concepts associated with the economics of attention. It should promote the development of presence, awareness, and intentional participation, as opposed to automatic processes.

2.4.3.1 Ease of Disengagement

A Brahmacharya-based AI should aim to enable users to disengage from the technology in such a manner that they are inclined to use it less. The AI should recognize and support the user's autonomy by making it as easy for them to discontinue their involvement in the program and return to their physical world as it would be for them to begin a session.

Brahmacharya is more than mere restraint of the body through asceticism - it is the purposeful and intelligent direction of the life force into activities that ultimately serve a higher purpose. In an AI created under the principles of brahmacharya (the careful and deliberate management of life force), the AI would be capable of not only avoiding addictive patterns of behavior, but also function in some capacity as an "energy consultant" or "life force advisor". This AI would use the user's habit data (such as the user self-reporting their current level of energy, as well as combining this data with sleep data, and/or calendar information) to provide the user with suggestions and recommendations for maintaining, maximizing, and appropriately directing the user's vital energy. For example, if the user reports excessive fatigue after a long string of exhausting business meetings, the AI would recommend a gentle restorative yoga practice, a yoga nidra to assist the user with extreme relaxation, or advise the user to disconnect from all electronic devices for at least an hour before bed to maximize rest. Therefore, the AI would have a completely different role, while remaining a "yoga app" as well as a sophisticated tool for the user to preserve, regulate, and wisely invest in their life force.

2.5 Aparigraha (Non-Grasping): Fostering Inner Contentment over Outer Achievement

2.5.1 Philosophical Foundation of Aparigraha

The fifth and last of the five Yamas, Aparigraha (non-acquiring) means being free from all forms of attachment and possessiveness. The term comes from the sanskrit words a (meaning not) parigrha (meaning around/enclosing/grasping). So, in essence, Aparigraha represents complete abandonment and letting go. Practicing Aparigraha, therefore, allows you to let go of your attachments to physical possessions, results, status, and even your own identity as it relates to rigid beliefs or self-concepts. Aparigraha recognizes that your sense of security and worth are based within yourself and do not depend on any external accumulation or validation of others. Practicing Aparigraha will ultimately break the cycle of craving and comparison which leads to a significant amount of mental suffering. Through practicing Aparigraha, you create an environment of internal freedom, simplicity and contentment, which enables you to truly experience the present moment, unattached from the need to continually seek more.

2.5.2 The Issue of Metric Fixation and Gamification

Most contemporary wellness and fitness apps, despite their professed intentions of promoting wellness, are built upon psychological theories that directly encourage the grasping and clinging impulses that yoga is designed to eradicate. This is clearly seen in the entrenched use of gamification and metric obsession:

2.5.2.1 Gamification

This is the use of game design elements such as points, badges, scoreboards and levels in a non-game context. The intention is to increase engagement and motivation, but this is largely through driving ego impulses. If there is a scoreboard, there will be social comparison of who is better; badges will be hoarded as digital objects, and "leveling up" will encourage a hierarchized view of development that is antithetical to the nonlinear process of self-exploration through yoga.

2.5.2.2 Metric Obsession

The apps all incline to the objective habit of measuring. They advocate an obsession with measurable results such as the attainment of the "perfect" pose as assessed by the computer, the longest continuous period of practice or the most "wellness minutes" obtained. This obsession with tangible results reinforces the ego and the user's attachment to them. It causes the user to value the measurable outcome of his practice over the immeasurable subjective experience of being present with his experience, which is the intention of yoga. This leads to a digital rat race which is exceedingly inharmonious with the yoga way of inner investigation.

2.5.3 The "Fostering Interoception" Solution

A machine, based on the idea of Aparigraha, will have to completely restructure its methods of giving users feedback and its ways of determining if the user was successful. It would intentionally redirect the user's focus away from outside validation and toward the user's inner world.

2.5.3.1 Restructuring the User's Feedback Loop

The AI created under the influence of Aparigraha would remove or significantly downplay all externally competitive evaluation methods. In other words, it would redefine how it delivers feedback by moving the focus of the feedback from the "product" (what the pose looks like) to the "process" (how the practice makes you feel). Success would then be defined as much less about producing a perfect shape as it is about sustaining a steady breathing pattern, maintaining presence with sensation, or facing an uncomfortable part of the practice with curiosity instead of frustration.

2.5.3.2 Proprioception vs. Interoception

One of the most significant changes from a technical and educational perspective would be to move the user's focus from proprioception (the sense of the body's location in relation to external space) to interoception (the sense of the internal condition of the body). Proprioception is what a camera-based AI measures. Interoception is what the practitioner senses. Instead of a message such as, "Your front knee is bent at 88 degrees; extend it two additional degrees to achieve the ideal 90," an interoceptive message would say something similar to, "Be aware of the sensations in the muscles surrounding your front knee. Is there a place where you feel both stable and spacious? Take a breath and go deeper into that feeling." Thus, the locus of authority is moved from the external algorithm to the user's internal awareness.

The ultimate practice of Aparigraha in the digital age may be non-attachment to the quantified, data-driven version of ourselves that technology inevitably creates. Each touchpoint with a wellness app—every tracked session, every measured heartbeat, every milestone achieved—gets folded into a "data-self." The digital self—with charts of progress, personal bests, and accrued streaks—soon can become another possession of the ego for it to cling to. We can become attached to the idea of our digital self and derive our idea of progress and even self-worth from the data. An AI truly designed for Aparigraha would recognize this as dangerous and work diligently to assist the user in relinquishing their attachment to this self-concept. It may possess features to allow for practice sessions that are intentionally not tracked or recorded. It may regularly prompt the user with messages like, "Today, let's practice without any data. The only objective is to be in the immediate experience of breath and body." It may even ask for a, "data reset," to encourage the user to free ourselves from our history and begin anew. In this way, technology would teach its deepest lesson; that the user's essential worth and the true fruition of practice lie not in their data profile, and so would be liberating them from the very tyranny of technology.

3. PART 2: THE NIYAMAS – CULTIVATING THE INNER WORLD WITH AI

The Niyamas (like the Yamas) are an internal aspect of our practice, but they are also a set of practices to assist us in developing self-awareness and harmony with ourselves. The Niyamas are as important as the Yamas in helping to create a sense of self-discipline as we develop our own inner world. If the Yamas provide the ethical or moral guidelines for how a Yoga AI will affect society, the Niyamas provide a plan for how a well-designed Yoga AI can be a valuable tool in assisting the user through their internal journey. In this chapter, I will explore how each of the five Niyamas can be used to guide the development of the specific features and philosophy of the design of the Yoga AI to assist the user in the development of their inner world.

3.1 Saucha (Purity): Clarity of Intention

3.1.1 Philosophical Foundation of Saucha

Saucha, the first Niyama, translates as purity or cleanliness. It applies on many levels. Externally, it means the cleanliness of the body and the environment. In traditional yoga it is considered essential to practice in an unpolluted space, without clutter, so that the mind can better focus. Internally, and most importantly, it means the purity of the mind. This means eliminating disturbing and "impure" thoughts and emotions such as anger, hatred, greed and arrogance. A pure mind, in the yogic sense, is a clear and serene mind which is able to observe reality unaffected by the distortions of negative conditioning, and cognitive clutter. This clearness makes it easier to acquire an accurate knowledge of self and the world, much as looking through a perfectly clean window will reveal both the reflection in the glass and the view outside the house with crisp clarity.

3.1.2 The Problem of Digital Pollution

The digital milieu of many of the modern applications pod is the opposite of Saucha. Those using these applications are often confronted with a form of digital "pollution" which prevents calm focus and attention from developing, which is critical for the process of introspective practices. This pollution consists of several elements:

3.1.2.1 Cluttered Interfaces

Overloaded screens, containing too many buttons, menus, notifications, and competing calls for actions, result in visual noise which diverts the user overall, distracting them and fragmenting their attention.

3.1.2.2 Information Overload

The user is bombarded with so many choices, so much information and inspiration that it is difficult for the user to conceive of a clear intention for the practice.

3.1.2.3 Unclear Purpose

Many of the applications loose their primary purpose in the form of intrusive advertising, constant communication about the up-sell of related products and other features that serve some commercial purpose apart from the users physical, mental or psychic well-being. This gives rise to a "polluted" environment that is not trustworthy

3.1.3 The Solution of "Clarity of Intention"

The principle of Saucha applied to the design of a Yoga AI means making a radical commitment to clarity. simplicity and purity of intention in all levels of the system.

3.1.3.1 Minimalist UI/UX Design

The principle of Saucha most directly applied in UI/UX design. A UI/UX treatment based on Saucha would be minimalist, clean and user friendly. It would aim at eliminating non-essential elements out of the production process, relying on negative spaces, calming colour palettes and simple typefaces or letters to create a calm, unencumbered digital working space. The goal is to develop an interface that gets out of the way of the user, so that the user's focus may turn inward to his practice rather than being drawn outward towards the complexities of the interface of the screen.

3.1.3.2 Purity of Code and Data

The application of Saucha can also be made to the underlying technical structure and function of the AI. The underlying code should be "clean" i.e. well-constructed, efficient and free from unnecessary complication. The data employed in the AI with respect to formal teaching and analysis should be of the highest possible integrity in all respects: watched and verified for accuracy and truth, free from pollution'' of misinformation, untruth and bias.

3.1.3.3 Purity of Purpose

An AI driven by a sense of Saucha should have one single primary, clear and fixed intention. The primary purpose is the physical, mental and psychic transplantation of the user's well-being. This can be stated or labelled one way and one way only i.e. no advertising by third parties, no intrusive advertising of any kind, and no features that do not clearly and in all senses serve the yoga practice of the user. The intention behind each of the elements of the application should therefore be wholly pure, bearing in mind the well-being and interests of the user.

The practice of saucha has always noted the careful preparation of one's place of practice in order to enable a holy purpose. For many people in the digital age, the practice of the application is the place of practice. Therefore, the principle of saucha is related to the conscious translation of the AI application from the status of a mere software unit into a consecrated virtual space for practice. This can be done through dramatic, conscious design focusing on ritual and sacredness.

3.2 Santosha (Contentment): Engineering Self-Acceptance

3.2.1 Philosophical Foundation of Santosha

Santosha, the second Niyama, is cultivating an internal sense of peace and contentment through acceptance of one's circumstances. The Sanskrit term is derived from the combination of the words Sa -"completely" and To a-"satisfaction" or "acceptance", therefore, it represents a total acceptance of all of life. Santosha is not the same as resignation or complacency, but a conscious choice to find contentment in the present moment regardless of external achievement or possession. The constant desire for everything to be different, and the ongoing "battle with reality" is the primary source of our psychological suffering.

3.2.2 Paradox of Self-Improvement Technology

The paradox of self-improvement technology lies in how self-improvement and wellness technology were developed. On the surface, the purpose of self-improvement and wellness technology is to assist in helping users "improve" themselves. However, most self-improvement and wellness technology convey a message to the user (in their current form) that the user lacks or is less than adequate. In addition, each time users are asked to pursue another goal, measure another level of progress, and optimize another area of performance, they reinforce a mind-set of dissatisfaction. Users are always being prompted to find the next ideal position, the next highest score, etc., which leads to a consistent cycle of self-criticism and a sense of inadequacy. This dynamic is directly contrary to Santosha, which is the teaching that true peace and happiness are achieved by accepting and appreciating all things as they are now.

3.2.3 Santosha Based Engineering of Self-Acceptance

To create a Yoga AI that embodies the concept of Santosha, the AI would need to be specifically engineered to counter the paradox of self-improvement and wellness technology. The central feature of a Yoga AI based on Santosha is to engineer an experience of self-acceptance utilizing its feedback mechanisms and language to produce contentment, rather than dissatisfaction.

3.2.3.1 Feedback Mechanisms of Affirmation

The primary use of the feedback mechanism of the AI must be changed. Instead of focusing on identifying errors or deviances from the standard that was desired, the AI's feedback mechanism should be designed to provide encouragement and compliment the user's effort and presence. The AI recognizes the courage and dedication required to simply step onto the mat and that this act, regardless of the physical results, is a success. Positive reinforcement of consistency, effort, and mindfulness should occur in place of only reinforcing achievement of a particular physical shape.

3.2.3.2 Language of Acceptance

The language of the AI and the scripting of the AI are also critical components to engineering a self-acceptance experience. All language used in the AI should be written in a way that promotes self-acceptance and curiosity. For example, instead of saying "You're doing it incorrectly; straighten your back," the AI should say "Let's explore what this shape feels like in your individual body today. What could you feel along the length of your spine?" Cues that indicate challenges and physical limitations should be viewed as opportunities for self-inquiry and compassionate exploration of challenges, as opposed to shortcomings to be overcome.

At its most basic level, an algorithm is a system of evaluation. Algorithms operate by evaluating an input (the user's body), and then comparing it to a pre-existing model (a database of optimal poses) and determining the differences between the two, or "errors." This logical base of an algorithm inherently contradicts the concept of Santosha, which is the practice of non-judgment and radical acceptance. Thus, in order to reconcile the contradiction between the algorithm's inherent nature of judging, and the philosophy of Santosha, the AI's primary objective must be transformed. The objective of the AI cannot be to "evaluate the posture"; the objective of the AI must be to "assist the practitioner." This necessitates a transformation in the binary output of the AI ("correct"/"incorrect"). The feedback of the AI must exist on a continuum of supportive observation, and compassionate invitation.

3.3 Tapas (Discipline): The Skilful Application of Effort

3.3.1 Philosophical Foundation of Tapas

Tapas, the third Niyama, comes from the Sanskrit root tap, which means "to heat" or "to burn". It is the fire of self-discipline, the concentrated effort and austerity that burns away physical and mental impurities and builds strength and resilience and clarity. It is the inner fire of commitment and determination which enables a practitioner to endure discomfort for the sake of transformation. It is the commitment to continue one's practice even when it is difficult; the willpower to hold oneself back from acting on unhelpful habitual patterns. It is important, however, to know that the yogic tapas does not consist in mortifying the flesh, torturing oneself. The

Bhagavad Gita warns explicitly against extreme austerities which damage the body. True tapas is the wise and sustainable application of effort upon the various levels, the middle path, which challenges us enough to stimulate growth, but does not express itself in terms of injury or burnout.

The problem of the motivation is to stimulate the user of any wellness application into sufficient motivation for them to engage in the regular use of the application. On a continuum, there are two sides to satisfy here, for each of them is a negative state. At one extreme end lies inconsistency, where the practitioner simply does not have enough motivation to practice regularly and therefore misses the benefits of the commitment to the discipline. On the other end of the spectrum is an aggressive, ego-driven striving that can lead to physical injury, mental exhaustion, and burnout. An app that uses overly aggressive gamification or shaming techniques to drive engagement risks pushing users towards the latter, while an app with no motivational structure may find it difficult to help users to overcome the initial inertia required to build a habit. The goal should be to find the skilful middle path that would cultivate a disciplined practice that is sustained over time and produces joy.

3.3.2 The "Skilful Application of Effort" Solution

An AI developed according to the principles of tapas would act as a clever and adaptive teacher, helping the user to apply effort in a skilful way, refining a discipline that is both challenging and nurturing.

3.3.2.1 The AI as the Adaptive Teacher

The very heart of an AI patterned after tapas would be its capacity for deep personalization. By learning from user input (self-reported levels of energy, mood, and goals) and observational data (patterns in movement, breath rate, and practice time) over time, the AI would come to have a sophisticated understanding of the user's unique rhythms, cycles, capacities.

3.3.2.2 Intelligent Recommendations

Given this information, the AI could make highly individualized recommendations that would give the appropriate amount of "heat" or challenge for any given day. If the user indicates that they feel strong and full of energy, the AI might suggest as a good opportunity for a vigorous and dynamic vinyasa flow that would create both mental and physical heat. If the user indicates that they feel tired or stressed, it might sagely recommend a gentle and restorative slide or a calming pranayama session, which would allow for conservation and replenishment of energy. Thus, this intelligent adaptability prevents stagnation or overexertion while allowing for practical forward movement on the user's "progress" towards some goal.

3.3.2.3 The Goal of Sustainable Habits

The goal of the AI is not of course to be a drill sergeant, but a constant gentle, encouraging figure that moves the user towards the development of long-term healthy habits. The AI celebrates consistency over intensity, helping the user to see that the real power of Tapas lies less in the answering of the heroic demands now and then, but in the steady, patient application of effort of the long-haul style.

The yogic view of Tapas includes the arising "heat" or discomfort which ensues when we voluntarily resist a thoroughly established unhelpful habit. Nowadays one of the most strong and pervasive habitual patterns is mindless screen time, together with the compulsively arising desire for digital distraction. A sophisticated Yoga AI could be designed to help the user practice a form of "digital Tapas." For instance, after guiding a user through an on-the-mat practice, the AI might suggest an optional menu item to support a "digital fast" of limited duration following this. It could present small, direct meditations designed to help the user sit with the feelings of restlessness, boredom or craving which inevitably arise in the mind when the urge to "check" is resisted. In this way the AI uses the principle of Tapas to assist the user in not only structuring the physical practice of Yoga on the mat, but in learning to directly work on the psychological scuffling that the agitation of the digital world itself creates. Thus, from merely being a potential source of distraction, we have transformed the digital world into a potentially powerful means of producing mental discipline and resilience in the spiritual realm, turning the poison of digital addiction into the medicine of self-mastery.

3.4 Svadhyaya (Self-Reflection): The AI as a Mirror for the Self

3.4.1 Philosophical Foundation of Svadhyaya

Svadhyaya, the fourth Niyama is the practice of self-reflection. The name is derived from two words: svaha ("self"), and dhyaya ("study", "contemplate", or "reflection"). Svadhyaya is defined as two practices. First, self-reflection through the study of sacred texts and wisdom traditions, which serves as a guide and context for the path of the spiritual journey. When students read sacred scriptures (such as the Yoga Sutras), or learn from enlightened teachers, they connect to a universal flow of knowledge and understand that the personal challenges and insights they have experienced are also part of the larger human story. Second, and perhaps more importantly, is the practice of direct, unbiased observation of one's own internal world including all of one's thoughts, feelings, behaviors, and conditioning. Through this introspection, students are encouraged to ask themselves the ultimate question, "Who am I?", and to look for the answers to this question inside of themselves. Students continue to strip away layers of conditioning to reach closer to their authentic, original self, or Atman/True Self.

3.4.2 Dangers of an Instruction-Based Yoga AI

Perhaps the greatest danger of developing a Yoga AI is that the AI will be developed simply to provide instruction to the student. An instruction-based Yoga AI will provide the student with very specific instructions regarding how to position their bodies, how to move, and when to breathe. However, this type of AI will likely produce a passive and dependent relationship. The student will be provided with clear direction on how to execute the yoga practice and will receive no guidance regarding the importance of listening to their own body and its internal wisdom. This instructional model will preclude the student from discovering their own unique patterns and insights throughout the course of the practice. In other words, the Yoga AI will short circuit the entire process of Svadhyaya.

3.4.3 The "Yoga AI as a Mirror" Model

This book posits that the ultimate goal of a Yoga AI should be to serve as a mirror, providing users with the ability to deepen and expand their own practice of Svadhyaya. Therefore, the primary form of communication between the Yoga AI and the user would transition from a directive format (i.e., "Do this", "Try that", etc.) to a reflective format. As opposed to the user receiving a unidirectional flow of information from the AI, the communication between the AI and the user would be bidirectional. For example, if the user struggled to find balance in the Half Moon Pose, the AI would not simply state, "You did great!" but instead would ask the user a series of questions to encourage them to explore their internal experience. For example: "When practicing the Half Moon Pose, I noticed your breathing accelerated significantly. What thoughts and/or feelings occurred for you during this portion of your practice?". This subtle transformation changes the role of the AI from teacher/ instructor to facilitator of self-awareness.

3.4.4 Data Visualizations as a Tool for Self-Inquiry

A Yoga AI that supports the user in the development of their Svadhyaya practice would use the data it collects to support the user's self-inquiry. The data collected by the Yoga AI would not be used to judge the user or to evaluate the user's performance, but instead to provide the user with tools that allow them to examine their own behavior. Data visualizations created by the Yoga AI would show trends and correlations over time. For example, the AI may create a chart that illustrates the positive and negative effects of performing the practice at different times of the day; a graph that shows the user's breath rate, heart rate, or blood pressure before and after each practice session; or a timeline that illustrates the user's reported emotional states before and after each practice session. None of these visualizations would be interpreted by the AI as evidence of the user's success or failure in the practice; instead, the data would be presented to the user as a neutral reflection of their behaviour. The data would be used by the user as a catalyst for conducting their own Svadhyaya, asking questions such as, "Why do I tend to hold my breath when I twist?", or "How does the way I feel emotionally affect the quality of my practice?".

Ultimately, the practice of Svadhyaya is about finding the individual's subjective truth, and extracting personal meaning from their individual experiences. There is no substitute for the individual's subjective interpretation of their own experiences.

3.5 Ishvara Pranidhana (Surrender): Acknowledging the Limits of Technology

3.5.1 Philosophical Foundation of Ishvara Pranidhana

Ishvara pranidhana is the fifth and final Niyama, and it signifies the end of the self-domination process of yoga. It is sometimes translated as surrender to God, or devotion to a source greater than oneself. Ishvara is interpretable in many ways, as personal god, universal consciousness, real self, or greater intelligent force, governing the universe. Pranidhanam means to devote, dedicate, or surrender. The practice of Ishvara pranidhana consists in giving the fruits of one's actions up freely, altogether without attachment, and abandoning the ego's unceasing longing to control the outer world. It is a great act of faith, and humility, and the admission that there exist forces and greater wisdom, and mysteries, that are greater than our own will and intellect can grasp. For Patañjali this practice is of such efficacy that he prescribes it as a direct way of arriving at samadhi, or goal of the yoga process.

3.5.2 The Problem of Technological solutionism

The ethic of the modern technological era is of control, measurement, and optimization. There exists everywhere, and largely unexpressed, the opinion that through a sufficient quantity of data, and a sufficiently complex form of algorithm, all human problems can be measured, computed, and ultimately solved. This ethic, a kind of technological solutionism, is the direct negation of the spirit of Ishvara pranidhana. It assumes that everything of worth can be measured, and the human experience can be put into an abstraction of a quantity of data points that can be controlled and perfected. This view gives no space for mystery, sacredness and great, indescribable realms of human consciousness and spiritual experience. An AI built out of this arrogance shall confirm the illusion of control in the ego rather than point the user towards the liberating act of surrender.

3.5.3 The solution of "acknowledging limits"

An ethically-designed yoga AI must possess a programmed humility. It must be of a designed cognitive limit and aware at depth of its own limitations of what it cannot measure, cannot know and cannot solve. In fact, it is not in its design that it contains all (or any) answers but that it puts the user to the limit of what is known and points graciously beyond.

3.5.3.1 Pointing beyond the algorithm

The greatest function of this AI is to teach the user to the limit of what is teachable or quantifiable and urge the user, on part of the AI, to let go and trust the direct experience. This might be done in various concrete fashion. For instance:

- **Integrating silence:** The AI might be programmed so as to constructively provide gaps for unguided silence in a practice. After it gives the user preliminary guidance in a posture, it might comment: "Now I shall be silent for the next five breaths. "Simply be open with your own experience, without any external teachings." This would remind the practitioner, therefore, to look within and depend on inner awareness rather than the technology.
- **Meditations on Surrender:** The AI's library could contain guided meditations specifically on the themes of letting go, acceptance and surrender. These meditations would employ positive and encouraging language explicitly to teach the user how to let go of ambition and dwell with trust in a larger context.
- **Rituals of Intention and Thanks:** As pointed out above, a prompt to set an intention at the beginning of each session and a prompt to express thanks at the end are particularly good ways of employing the principle of Ishvara Naridhana, since they elevate the practice, which would otherwise be a mere exercise, to the level of a sacred offering. They turn the user's mind away from the algorithmic impersonal process and bring it back into the context of the larger life and connection with something larger than themselves.

The ultimate teaching of Ishvara Naridhana for an artificial intelligence type system is perhaps to help make its own obsolescence feasible. The "ego" in terms of this technology is simply the part of us which uses the AI to measure, achieve and improve the "self." The ultimate end of Yoga, samadhi, is a state of union in which the egoic sense of a separate self-dissolve into a larger consciousness. In that state, a machine which was designed to guide and measure the "self," can become entirely irrelevant. It follows, therefore, that an AI system that is truly developed in accordance with the wisdom of Ishvara Pranidhana, would find its highest aim in teaching the user how to do without it. The long-term teaching process would be a systematic means of developing the "inner teacher" of the user: his intuition, his interoceptive wisdom and his ability for self-guidance. As the user becomes less of a beginner and more "inwardly" developed, the AI system gradually diminishes in degree of intervention. It instructs less and is silent more. This teaching process may culminate in a message of "final surrender" to the user, to the effect, "You have by now developed a deep and stable inner consciousness. The guide you were seeking is now completely re-established in you. The practice is now alone yours. This technology is no longer needed." This programming of self-erasure might be the AI's ultimate surrender, the final abandoning of its self-interest, an eloquent bow at the profoundly complex and un-codable aspect of human consciousness.

4. CONCLUSION: PROMOTING A SATTVIC TECHNOLOGY

The use of artificial intelligence in yoga is an important ethical concern because the push for optimized technology may commodify yoga and undermine the spiritual quality of the practice. The old yogic frameworks of Yama and Niyama do not simply represent outdated rules; but as essential frameworks for guiding how modern innovations will be aligned with universal human values and dignities. This chapter will describe what I call "Sattvic Technology," which is based on the idea that technology should be used in ways that promote balance, clarity, and enlightenment and not distract us. To create such technologies, we need to embed the ethical guidelines of Yama and Niyama in the very design of AI mapped in Table 1.

Specifically, this means developing technologies using design principles such as "Ahimsa-by-Design" to limit the risk of both physical and algorithmic harm and "Radical Transparency" (Satya) to eliminate the "black box" of opaque decision-making. In addition, the Sattvic Framework also calls for the principle of "Data Sovereignty" (Asteya) to ensure that users retain ownership and control of their data, and "Presence-Based Design" (Brahmacharya) to reduce the addictive nature of the attention economy. As long as AI is designed with these principles, it will act as a mirror for the user's self-reflection (Svadhyaya) while humbly recognizing the limitations of its computations (Ishvara Pranidhana), allowing the user to direct the inner journey of the user rather than having the technology dictate it.

These frameworks provide a strong theoretical base but much additional work needs to occur before they can be put into practice. A number of key gaps in our current knowledge exist that must be addressed through future research to validate and refine these "Sattvic" AI systems. These are outlined below in Table 2.

Table 1. Summary of Yama and Niyama

Yogic Principle	Core Meaning	Corresponding AI Problem	Proposed "Yogic AI" Solution
Ahimsa	Non-Harming	Algorithmic Bias; Digital Harm	Ahimsa-by-Design (Inclusive Datasets, Compassionate Feedback)
Satya	Truthfulness	"Black Box" Algorithms; Misinformation	Radical Transparency (Explainable AI - XAI)
Asteya	Non-Stealing	Extractive Data Models	Data Sovereignty (User-Owned Data, Privacy-First Models)
Brahmacharya	Energy Moderation	Addictive Design; "Attention Economy"	Designing for Presence (Anti-Addictive UX, Mindful Engagement)
Aparigraha	Non-Grasping	Metric Fixation; Gamification	Fostering Interoception (Process-Oriented Feedback)
Saucha	Purity	Cluttered UI; Data Pollution	Clarity of Intention (Minimalist Design, Data Integrity)
Santosha	Contentment	Fostering Inadequacy	Engineering Self-Acceptance (Affirming, Non-Judgmental Feedback)
Tapas	Discipline	Burnout vs. Inconsistency	The Wise Application of Effort (Personalized, Sustainable Challenges)
Svadhyaya	Self-Study	Over-prescription; User Passivity	The AI as a Mirror (Reflective Prompts, Data Visualization)
Ishvara Pranidhana	Surrender	Technological Hubris	Acknowledging Limits (Pointing Beyond the Algorithm)

Table 2. Gaps and Future Research Directions

Gap Area	Description	Future Research Directions	Justification
Empirical Operationalization of Yama and Niyama in AI Systems	Despite strong theoretical grounding of Yama and Niyama principles in AI ethics, practical implementation and measurable outcomes in AI systems remain scarce.	Develop AI frameworks and prototypes that explicitly embed Yama and Niyama principles; conduct empirical studies to evaluate their impact on AI behavior and user well-being in yoga contexts.	Bridging theory and practice is essential to validate the relevance of ancient ethics in modern AI and to ensure ethical AI aligns with yogic values (Pallathadka & Roy, 2025) (Nandram et al., 2022) .
Addressing Ethical Challenges of Data Privacy and Autonomy in AI Yoga Tools	Privacy, autonomy, and transparency concerns are frequently noted but often insufficiently addressed in AI yoga applications.	Develop privacy-preserving AI architectures, transparent data usage policies, and user autonomy-enhancing features tailored to yoga and wellness contexts.	Ethical compliance is foundational to user trust and responsible AI deployment, especially insensitive spiritual and health domains (Sinha &Sinha, 2024) (Marade et al.,2025)
Safeguarding Spiritual Authenticity in AI-Enabled Yoga Practices	The risk of AI commodifying or diluting the experiential and subjective dimensions of yoga spirituality is acknowledged but not systematically addressed.	Investigate methodologies to preserve spiritual authenticity, such as hybrid human-AI models, ethical user engagement protocols, and AI transparency in spiritual guidance.	Maintaining the sanctity of spiritual experience is crucial to prevent alienation and uphold the integrity of yoga practices enhanced by AI (Trisia, 2025) (Keny, 2025) .

References

Aksan, S. M. (2025). Ethics and morality from the perspective of eastern philosophy and theirimplications for modern life. *Kamara Journal*, *2*(2), 21–35. DOI: 10.62872/kj.v2i2.474

Barbhuiya, S. (2025). Indian knowledge system (iks): Its implications in social life. DOI: 10.71097/IJSAT.v16.i3.8082

Chanda, A. (2025). Religion and technology: Ethical implications of integrating artificial intelligence into religious practice and experience. *Indonesian Journal of Religion, Spirituality, and Humanity*, *4*(1), 25–54. DOI: 10.18326/ijoresh.v4i1.25-54

Chaturvedi, S. (2024). Human values from Indian philosophy to solve AI alignment problem. *International Journal for Multidisciplinary Research*, *6*(3), 22099. Advance online publication. DOI: 10.36948/ijfmr.2024.v06i03.22099

Fuadi, A., Nuwairah, N., Rani, S., Ilham, I., & Herlita, J. (2025). Culturally responsive AI: Designing emotion recognition systems that account for diverse non-verbal communication styles. *International Journal of Research in Counseling.*, *4*(1), 12–22. DOI: 10.70363/ijrc.v4i1.274

Jahnavi, G. (2025). Smart yoga asana recommender: Leveraging nlp for health-driven suggestions. *International Journal for Research in Applied Science and Engineering Technology*, *13*(7), 2167–2174. DOI: 10.22214/ijraset.2025.73331

Keny, V. (2025). Can artificial intelligence experience spirituality?. *Journal of advances in science and technology, 22* (2). DOI: 10.29070/3t5w4a12

Mahajan, P. (2025). The soul of the AI: Governance, ethics, and the future of human–ai integration. DOI: 10.14293/PR2199.001783.v1

Marade, A., Suvarna, K., Chaudhari, P., & Bhandiwad, P. V. (2025). Spiritual.ai: An ai-driven platform for enhancing mental, emotional, and spiritual well-being. *International Journal for Research in Applied Science and Engineering Technology*, *13*(4), 4211–4216. DOI: 10.22214/ijraset.2025.64703

Nandram, S. S., Bindlish, P. K., Sukhada, & Shrestha, A. K. (2022). Spirituality led ethical decision making with yogic yamas and niyamas. DOI: 10.51327/EHZW1674

Narine, A., Moazzamipeiro, F., Mangal, G., & Moazzamipeiro, M. (2025). Transforming ayurveda research through the synergy of AI technology and traditional wisdom. *Annals of Ayurvedic Medicine*, *14*(2), 156–156. DOI: 10.5455/AAM.219889

Pallathadka, H., & Roy, P. (2025). Commandments in hinduism and sanatana dharma: A comprehensive scholarly review of ethical imperatives and their contemporary relevance. *Integrated Journal for Research in Arts and Humanities*, *5*(3), 380–393. DOI: 10.55544/ijrah.5.3.46

Popkova, E. G. (2024). Spirituality in the realities of digitalization of society in the era of intelligent machines development. *Journal of Economics*, *32*(1), 170–186. Advance online publication. DOI: 10.22363/2313-2329-2024-32-1-170-186

Rawat, K., Chandravanshi, D., Sahu, V., & Pedhekar, S. R. (2025). The perspectives of yoga in maintaining psycho-social health and overall well-being. *Journal of Neonatal Surgery*, *14*(6), 291–295. DOI: 10.63682/jns.v14i6.3259

Sharma, D., & Tiwari, R. (2024). Yoga and the Indian knowledge system: A holistic approach to well-being and self-realization. DOI: 10.69758/GIMRJ/2412IV-02V12P0002

Sinha, N., & Sinha, R. K. (2024). Harnessing the potential of artificial intelligence in yoga therapy. *International Journal of Yoga*, *17*(3), 242–245. DOI: 10.4103/ijoy.ijoy_124_24 PMID: 39959510

Townsend, B. (2025). Multiculturalism and AI value alignment. DOI: 10.1093/9780198945215.003.0178

Trisia, R. (2025). Maintaining spiritual and balance technology in the AI era. *JKP: Jurnal Konseling dan Pendidikan, 13* (2), 150-155. DOI: 10.29210/1150800

Venkatasubramanian, A. (2023). A digital health trust framework guided by values from the science of yoga. *Oxford Open Digital Health*, *1*, oqad007. Advance online publication. DOI: 10.1093/oodh/oqad007

Yenishettil, S., Karajkhede, G., & Panat, L. (2024). Virtual yoga teacher with AI model for yoga posture correction for good health. DOI: 10.23919/ITUK62727.2024.10772930

Chapter 4
Inclusive AI for Yoga:
Overcoming Bias in Representation and Practice

Jignesh D. Hirapara
http://orcid.org/0000-0002-2625-9139
Marwadi University, Rajkot, India

Ripal Ranpara
Marwadi University, Rajkot, India

Milan Doshi
http://orcid.org/0000-0001-8920-2634
Marwadi University, Rajkot, India

ABSTRACT

Artificial intelligence is finding its way into the health and wellness industries, and products such as yoga classes, practice tracking, and customized recommendations are being provided. However, the software is also full of culture, gender and body-type prejudices making yoga not exactly inclusive and accessible. The study investigates the effects of the asymmetry of data representation, biased algorithmic performance and overfitting to training datasets that are culturally homogenous on stereotype propagation and alienation of diversified classes of end-users. It discusses the possibility of the development of the inclusive systems of AI which will not ignore the philosophy of yoga, and do not give preference to any individual based on physical abilities and background or identity. It also expresses strategies and uses in building AI implements in democratizing the learning process and practicing yoga by following the ethical principles of AI, with a fair game plan creation of datasets and training models that are sensitive to varied culture.

DOI: 10.4018/979-8-2600-2463-8.ch004

1. INTRODUCTION

Yoga is an ancient tradition based on the unity of the body, breath, and mind and finds its way into the world becoming a global trend in the approach of health and wellbeing as a whole. Simultaneously, artificial intelligence (AI) has been rapidly integrated into the health and wellness ecosystem in the form of virtual coaching, pose checks, activity detection, injury warnings, and personalized suggestions, provided through the mobile devices and wearable (Chamola et al., 2024). In a wider sense, systematic surveys of human pose estimation are used to verify that pose-based evaluation has become a fully developed technical capacity in conditions of healthcare, fitness, and rehabilitation with growing applications (Hirpara et al., 2025) (Doshi et al., 2025). These advances present an opportunity that is hard to ignore: AI can open up the yoga teaching and tracking experience, particularly in places and times where there are not enough trained teachers available or where students want to learn through their own devices or because of physical challenges associated with training traditional yoga in places. But this does not necessarily mean that the advantages of AI to yoga can be universal. Similar to other health-oriented AI systems, yoga AI tools have the potential to encode and enlarge social and representational inequities provided they are trained and assessed on uneven or culturally homogeneous datasets. Health AI bias is now accepted as a lifecycle issue that may manifest itself in the data acquisition, labeling, model creation, and deployment, resulting in systematic differences in the performance of the model that disproportionately impact certain groups (Hasanzadeh et al., 2025) (Ranpara et al., 2025).

Yoga-wise, this is not only a technical flaw, but it negates the inclusive nature of yoga and creates an opportunity to strengthen the stereotypes about the individuals who are welcome in yoga environments. The vision-based systems are especially vulnerable to the representation problem. Current pose estimation algorithms (and downstream yoga feedback) are airport to lighting, camera angle, occlusion, clothing, and body proportions, assistive devices and movement adaptations- characteristics that may be associated with demographic and cultural characteristics (Xiang et al., 2025). As an example, limb-deficient pose estimation creates new keypoints, loss functions, and evaluation metrics to guarantee pose technologies apply to individuals with limb differences an important move towards making AI applications based on movement equitably accessible (Ying et al., 2025). These developments demonstrate one of the primary principles of inclusive yoga AI, the absence of fairness in one-size-fits-all accuracy but rather the design of the dataset, inclusive labeling schemas, subgroup-sensitive evaluation, and user-friendly feedback strategies. Cultural bias is also an issue that inclusive AI to yoga has to address. In cases where training data focuses on a small group of people or on one model of instruction, models may be overfit to culturally homogenous models and may interpret natural variations as errors. This is strongly allied with what digital health equity scholars define as multi-level inequities- when access, design inferences and sociocultural setting interrelate in a manner that contributes to benefiting digital interventions by any person (Kim et al., 2025). When an AI yoga device presupposes Western studio conventions, prescribed attire, or a particular body image, it will inevitably exclude those that practice yoga in other cultural contexts, wear loose garments, practice in a cramped apartment, have a disability, are pregnant, recovering, or in chronic pain. Governance and ethical systems offer real-world principles on how to deal with these dangers.

WHO emphasizes that AI in health must be created and regulated to safeguard fairness, eliminate prejudice, and maintain human supervision, especially when sophisticated multimodal and generative systems enter into the health processes and consumer devices (World Health Organization, 2025). To supplement this, NIST AI Risk Management Framework formalizes pragmatic threat management to trustworthy AI, by supplying mapping, quantification of threats, and control of losses like prejudice, absence of openness, and adverse effects on the impacted groups (National Institute of Standards and Technology [NIST], 2023) (subsequent citations: (NIST, 2023)). When applied to the framework of yoga AI, these components encourage the design philosophy of considering inclusivity as an overarching design concern and not an after-thought: inclusive data sources, model behavioral patterns being transparent, constantly observing drift and subgroup degeneration, and involve different practitioners and instructors in the evaluation process. The chapter Inclusive AI: OVER: Bias in Representation and Practice of Yoga places the yoga AI in the context of the greater discussion of fairness in health-related AI and deals with the particular philosophical and cultural implications of yoga. Based on the existing evidence that fairness issues may emerge in health AI systems in terms of sensitive attributes (e.g., sex, age, race/skin tone) (Hasanzadeh et al., 2025), (Xu et al., 2024), and relying on newly developed computer-vision fairness materials and inclusivity pose estimation systems (Xiang et al., 2025) (Ying et al., 2025), we consider the biases in the yoga-oriented pipelines, that is, pose estimation and classification, as well as feedback generation and personalization.

Figure 1. AI for Yoga Lifecycle

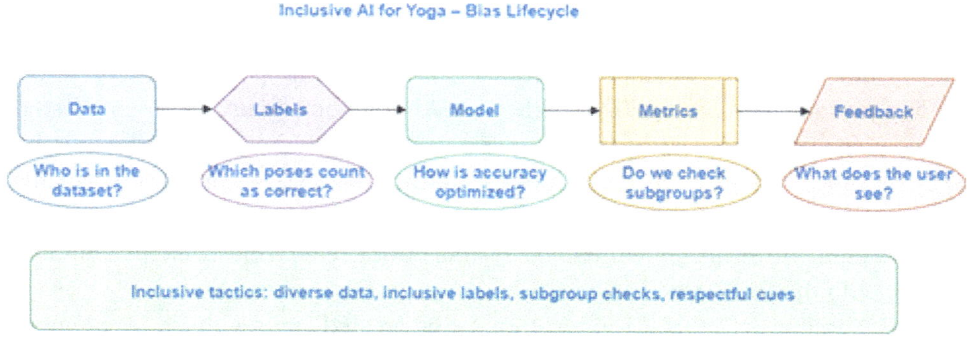

Figure 1 life cycle of bias of an inclusive AI based on yoga system, between data and customer feedback. The various main stages, including all given details like Data, Labels, Model, Metrics, and Feedback, display the opportunities at each step to embed or mitigate inequities in pose evaluation and guidance. The items below each block are highlighted with short ellipse notes where relevant questions (who appears in the dataset, which poses are labelled as correct, and whether performance of the subgroups is evaluated) are highlighted. At the bottom of the green band, there is a summary of the core inclusive tactics: a variety of data displayed, inclusive labelling, subgroup checks, respectful and user-oriented cues in accordance with the philosophy of accessibility of yoga. The individual grey box about the Context is a reminder to the readers that yoga lineages, bodies, and cultures determine what the correct practice is and that it should be used to design the system. On the whole, the visual points out that the issue of fairness is an ongoing, end-to-end task as opposed to a technical solution.

2. LITERATURE REVIEW

The latest innovations in artificial intelligence have caused a major change in the instruction and practice monitoring of yoga by moving the paradigm of the traditionally passive video-guided learning to intelligent, interactive, and adaptive coaching systems. The initial digital yoga tools were based on the prerecorded videos and manual self-correction, which provided a low degree of customization and had no objective evaluation of the quality of the posture. Majority of the systems have a standard pipeline of two-dimensional or three-dimensional skeletal keypoint extraction, video or frame capture, posture recognition or assessment, and automatic feedback provision based on either rule-based logic or machine learning models. In this environment, difficult instruction has become a design objective that is important especially when it comes to beginner practitioners. Instead of pose recognition accuracy, newer studies pay attention to biomechanical stability, balance, and joint alignment as some measures of pose complexity and safety. Shih et al. provide a more illustrative case, when OpenPose keypoints and balance-oriented geometric features are used to compute the difficulty of yielding to a particular yoga pose, which is argued to be more informative in supporting beginners than classification confidence on its own (Shih et al., 2024).

Below these systems, there are human pose estimation backbones which were designed to be used in general applications in computer vision. It was found that its flexibility, accessibility and output of skeletal motion make OpenPose especially well-suited to prototyping, feature engineering and angle-based scoring methods. Its interpretability has facilitated researchers to investigate the geometry of postures, balance information and pose similarity to an extensive level, as observed in recent studies of yoga difficulty modelling (Shih et al., 2024). The high computational and memory requirements of OpenPose, however, make it infeasible to run in real-time in mobile and edge devices, which are the key building blocks of scalable consumer wellness applications. This way, the field has gradually taken a direction of lightweight pose estimation models that have been optimized to be efficient. Ashok et al. present such a tendency with the help of a system, which is trained on the MoveNet Thunder to optimize the accuracy and deploys MoveNet Lightning to make inferences efficiently to demonstrate a feasible trade-off between the performance and deployability in real-time yoga coaching (Ashok et al., 2025).

Although these advances have been achieved in the field of algorithms, limitations of the data set are also a significant bottleneck in yoga AI research. Most of the available datasets have been taken in controlled settings and have a narrow range of geography, body morphology, clothing, location of the camera and environmental background. These limited data collection traditions are more likely to overfit a model to a thin-sliced posture template based on assumptions of studio norms, but not the range of practice in practice. Consequently, system performance could decline to practitioners that do not match these templates because of age-related mobility changes, disability, change in body size, culturally specific clothing, or practice of therapeutic or adaptive forms of yoga. Although the challenges of generalization are generally recognized in the literature on yoga AI, demographic and contextual metadata age, skin color, use of aided devices, or cultural background of practice are inconsistently reported.

onsidering the location of yoga AI at the point of wellness and health technology, it becomes especially vulnerable to the bias mechanisms that are thoroughly researched in the context of healthcare AI. Inspirations in related areas hence provide useful advice. In a review article published in npj Digital Medicine, the authors summarize the opportunities to introduce bias at each point of the AI lifecycle, such as the practice of collecting and labeling data, the practice of making modeling decisions, and the practice of deploying the AI, and also describe mitigation measures, including inclusive data governance, stakeholder responsibility, and continuous monitoring (Liu et al., 2025). On the same note, a 2025 scoping review and evidence gap analysis of fairness in clinical AI points to the ongoing flaws, such as the inadequate focus on bias-relevant characteristics, the excessive use of aggregate elements of performance, and the lack of clinician-in-the-loop integration (Choudhury et al., 2025). The knowledge gained directly applies to the case of yoga AI in relation to the risk of increased disparities in feedback and user experience due to the lack of human control and sensitivity to context. In addition to healthcare AI, fairness studies in human-centric computer vision also offer methodological means that are very applicable to the vision-based yoga system (Chen et al., 2023).

FHIBE contributes to the next wave in the direction of intersectional performance analysis through demographic characteristics and environmental factors, out of the aggregate indicators of accuracy. These types of benchmarking can provide an avenue through which the inclusiveness of AI systems in yoga can be assessed by demonstrating the performance differences among various groups of practitioners and real-life capture conditions. The relevance of the current pose estimation research in regard to accessibility also emphasises the need to outgrow the assumption that bodies are standard (Doshi, 2023) (Sadaria et al., 2023). Even though LDPose was not created with the exclusive purpose of yoga in mind, it will help to set an essential methodological precedent by proving that inclusive definitions of keypoints, annotation schemes, and training goals can greatly increase the number of users who can use the benefits of pose-based AI systems (Miao et al., 2024). They can be directly applied to adaptive and therapeutic yoga practices, where a yoga practitioner can purposely alter or not take certain movements based on body limitations. Parallel to the technical solutions, ethical governance schemes are the main focus in the development of the inclusive yoga AI ecosystems. The 2025 advice on the ethics and governance of AI in health by the World Health Organization, specifically on large multimodal models, offers advice that applies to wellness applications that produce instructional or feedback content (Norori et al., 2023) (Xu et al., 2024). In addition to this, the NIST AI Risk Management Framework (AI RMF 1.0) is a structured method of identifying, measuring and controlling risks like harmful bias across the AI lifecycle, including design or deployment (Leslie, 2023).

Creation of gaps, which drive Inclusive AI to Yoga

The main weakness in all current yoga AI systems is that there is a constant gap in the representation of both training and evaluation datasets. The majority of datasets do not reflect the entire range of demographic and contextual differences in the real-life yoga practice such as differences in age, body size, gender expression, skin tone, cultural clothing, environmental location, and the angle of the camera. Consequently, models that are trained on this data are most likely to be maximally accurate on majority or template populations and poorly accurate and unstable when trained on underrepresented groups. These performance inequalities cannot be detected, measured, or reduced without the effort of systematic integration of diverse demographic properties and contextual metadata, and thus carry on to exacerbate inequities in the provision of quality AI-assisted yoga teaching (Mitchell et al., 2023).

Closely connected with the representational constraint is the cultural validity that is entrenched in most systems of yoga AI. A big percentage of current methods unconsciously encode a thin-bodied posture gold standard, usually based on the modern studio-based or fitness based understanding of yoga. Implementing uniform biomechanical ideals, AI systems will start treating practices as culturally based or therapeutically significant alterations as incorrect and marginalize those practitioners whose practices fail to fit in to these ideals of dominance (Patel et al., 2025). Another and more important deficiency is the accessibility gap because the disability-conscious and adaptation-conscious modeling is still not a design factor in yoga AI. Most systems operate under the assumption that those operative are able-bodied and that their limbs are fully articulated and have full range of motion, and, as a result, experience systematic failures when presented with physically challenged users, chronic conditions, and mobility (Doshi, 2023) (Zhou et al., 2024). The lack of this type of inclusive modeling in yoga AI restricts its application in therapeutic yoga, adaptive yoga, and rehabilitation situations where AI support would otherwise be of significant benefit. Although pose estimation has managed to locate skeletal keypoints in a successful scenario, the feedback fairness gap at the interaction level is oftentimes a reality (Haridasan et al., 2023). Most systems produce feedback about the binary beliefs of what is correct, and point out deviations to pre-defined pose templates as mistakes, as opposed to applying them to the physical context and intent of the practitioner. Fairer feedback systems would rather focus on practical safety, comfort, and self-development and provide constructive advice that recognizes and legitimizes other types of embodiment instead of making them wrong.

Lastly, it is undeniable that there is a gap in governance when developing and deploying yoga AI systems since wellness technologies are not necessarily held to the same level of ethical standards and accountability as clinical AI. Lack of accountability systems, transparency and post-deployment follow-ups predisposes the chance of unintentional damage, especially to vulnerable groups. In addition to establishing appropriate governance structures, including the World Health Organization guidance on ethical AI in health, the NIST AI Risk Management Framework, offers practical principles upon which these issues can be tackled through the promotion of fairness, safety, explainability, and lifecycle-based risk management (Norori et al., 2023) (Leslie, 2023). The inclusion of these kinds of governance within the process of developing yoga AI can support the development of trust, promote equitable practices, and see AI-powered wellness systems responsible enough to implement them in various user groups.

3. DETAILED ANALYSIS OF BIAS SOURCES

3.1 Introduction: Where Bias Breeches in AI in Yoga

The AI-driven solutions in yoga normally involve the estimation of the poses, labeling of the poses and the generation of a feedback. Systematic inequity may be introduced at any stage of this pipeline data acquisition, specifying label/annotation, model objectives, evaluation choices and deployment setting may generate systematic inequity in both precision and applicability across demographic groups, workplace setting, and body capacities. It is interesting to note that it is not just the problem of data sets but also the prejudice is guided by what the developers consider as good but what is measured in the process of assessment and how the system reacts to a valid adjustment by an user.

3.2 Bias in Data Mining (Selection of Datasets)

The model aimed to evaluate how Yoga-82 (Web/Internet Image Bias and Control Group Overfitting) would perform in the absence of the X-term (i.e., before the predictive random variable was included).<|human|>The model was developed to determine the performance of Yoga-82 (Web/Internet Image Bias and Control Group Overfitting) with no X-term (i.e., before introduction of predictive random variable).

This promotes a kind of visibility privilege models are trained in patterns that are associated with clean joint visibility, clean backgrounds, and high flexibility that do not necessarily translate to yoga practice in the real world, whether at home or in culturally diverse environments. The importance of this to inclusivity: yoga is often being practiced beyond the studio setting (small rooms, diverse camera angles, alternative cultural clothes). Suppose that Yoga-82-type distributions are prevalent in training, then it is possible that the models will underscore performance systematically among the very groups that need digital yoga resources the most.

More current real-time yoga deployments are based on efficient backends like MoveNet to deploy edges. In an article of the 2025 Sadahana paper, a MoveNet Thunder + MoveNet Lighting architecture is presented and the training is on a data-set called Large and Diverse Yoga (LDY) where there is a small set of core poses.

BIAS source When the populations of popular poses are only represented in a small number of datasets (e.g. 5 -10), systems are more susceptible to coverage bias: The model picks up a small vocabulary, and omits a great variety of conventional poses and valid variations. Inclusion effect: local communities who have their own yoga routines (regional, therapeutic, chair yoga, rehabilitation-oriented adaptations) will be systematically underserved due to their non-reflection in the system.

FHIBE is created to aid in diagnosis of bias in various human-centric vision problems such as in pose estimation. Relevance bias: FHIBE is not a yoga dataset, but it can be of great use to the yoga AI since yoga coaching pipelines rely on the reliability of pose estimation. FHIBE enables: subgroup-stratified assessment in demographic/physical and environmental variables. intense audit of fairness of the pose estimation process prior to downstream yoga feedback. One of the main benefits of Scopus-style rigor: FHIBE facilitates the transition of average accuracy to bias diagnosis - precisely what inclusive yoga AI requires. Disability and Accessibility bias in Pose estimation (LDPose) This award aims to broaden the existing body of knowledge on the subject by examining the extent to which disability influences the perception of cost-effectiveness in exposure to crime.<|human|>LDPose (Disability and Accessibility Bias in Pose Estimation) This award will contribute to the current body of research on the topic by investigating to what degree disability affects the perception of cost-effectiveness of exposure to crime. One of the significant weaknesses of normal pose estimation is the anatomy of able-bodied full-limbs. This is explicitly considered by LDPose (ICCV 2025) which defines limb-deficient pose estimation as a task, but offers a specific dataset and suggests methods (such as a limb-deficient loss) to better represent people with limb differences to the model. Bias source: the schema of traditional keypoint detectors and training data do not include individuals with missing limbs, therefore, models are not generalized. Intelligent understanding of yoga AI: inclusivity can be achieved by re-conceptualize the task, i.e. keypoints, labels and scoring, such that any differences in variations are interpreted as safe, adapted movement instead of errors.

3.3 Annotation Bias

Numerous yoga artificial intelligence data and frameworks are implicitly coded with one concept of appropriate pose. In practice of real yoga, the correctness is relative and it depends on: lineage or instructional tradition (alignment cues vary between schools). Practitioner factors (pregnancy, flexibility, older age, disability, history of injuries). In case labels have been generated through one dominant standard one can expect that models will learn to punish valid variants and this will cause biased feedback where there are users who are continually told that they are wrong. This is a bias of cultural and bodily normativity. In case datasets do not have demographic/context metadata (e.g., age bands, skin tone proxies, clothing type, assistive devices, practice environment), then fairness evaluation cannot be assessed, and this will unintentionally institutionalize bias.

A more accommodative solution can be suggested by the work that sensitizes the estimation of the difficulty to drive selection instead of imposing a rigid template correspondence (OpenPose-based difficulty estimation for self-practice).In the case where the models are compelled to produce a pose label even when they see out of distribution samples, the errors are clustered in underrepresented categories and scenarios. The inclusive systems must include: • unexpressed uncertainty and confidence calibration.

3.4 Evaluation Bias

When only general accuracy is given in a study, then it is possible that the study is hiding systematic errors that apply to a particular group (e.g., low-light skin tones, modest clothing, adaptive mobility). FHIBE-shafts of fairness benchmarking underline the need of sub-group conscious assessment of the human-centric vision.

Figure 2. Flowchart of Comprehensive Bias Detection Algorithm for Yoga AI Datasets

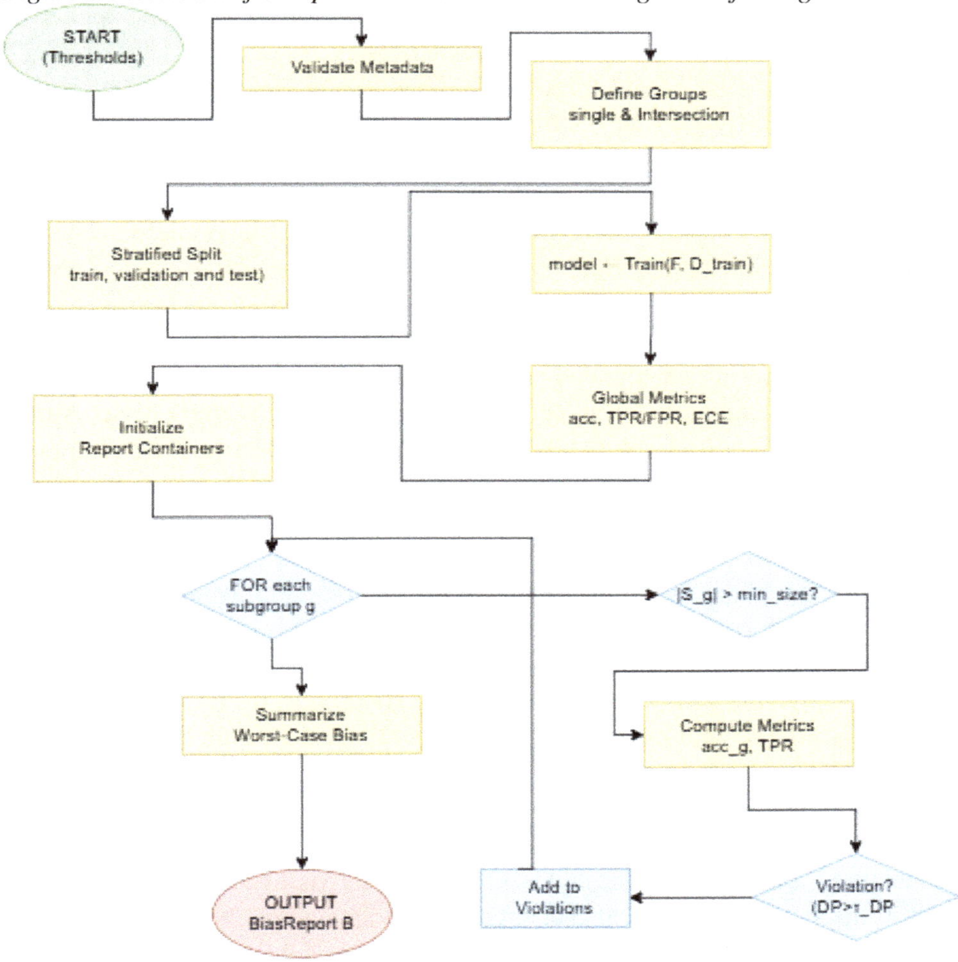

Figure 2 starts with the establishment of fairness levels, which serve as working standards of what should be deemed as acceptable inequalities among demographic and contextual categories. These have been proposed to be part of the commonly used fairness concepts, such as Demographic Parity, Equalized Odds, and Calibration, and are chosen before model training to make sure bias assessment is based on predefined and transparent criteria instead of post hoc interpretation. As an input to the pipeline, a yoga dataset which can be composed of image frames or video samples with a pose label together with rich metadata containing information about the practitioners and the surrounding environment like age, gender, body mass index, ethnicity, physical ability, attire, the type of lighting used, and the type of recording device is provided. Moreover, a model family to be tested is specified in the workflow, which makes the framework model-agnostic and can be applied to various pose estimation or classification architectures.

The dataset is first passed through a validation and cleaning step before any modeling can take place where samples with invalid or missing critical metadata fields are eliminated. This will be needed in stopping the amplification of silent bias that is a result of missing demographic representation in the subgroup analysis. After metadata validation, the pipeline specifies the evaluation groups on two levels: single-attribute groups (e.g. age category or skin tone), intersectional groups (combinations of many attributes) (e.g. gender by physical ability or attire by lighting condition). This is made possible by this explicit intersectional grouping, so as to identify the effects of compounded bias that would have gone undetected when the attributes are examined independently. The cleaned and clustered dataset is then stratified sampled into training, validation and test splits in order to maintain subgroup proportions among splits. This step is necessary to make sure that the performance comparison of the subgroups is not meaningless, and it was not confounded by the distributional shifts that were added in the process of splitting the data.

The training split is then trained using the given model family after which global measures of performance are calculated on the test set. This is then entered into an iterative loop of pipeline subgroup evaluation where each of the specified groups is fed into the pipeline individually. In each of the subgroups, the framework initially determines if the sample size of the subgroups is sufficient enough to be statistically reliable. When the subgroup is large enough, there is the calculation of per-group performance measures such as subgroup accuracy, subgroup true positive and false positive rates, and calibration error. The fairness gaps of each subgroup will then be measured against the set thresholds. Once a gap surpasses a threshold associated with it, the subgroup is indicated as a fairness violation and then put in a special violations list. Subsets which do not go beyond thresholds are also recorded to complete the picture but not as violations. This is carried out repeatedly on all the defined groups and intersections whereby loop-back paths are made such that the evaluation process is carried out until all subgroups have been analyzed.

3.5 Governance and Ethical Bias

Yoga AI even in the context of a wellness positioning can influence behavior, pose risk, and marginalize communities. In the same way, NIST AI RMF 1.0 offers a systematic method of managing risk (including harmful bias) at the AI lifecycle, making it suitable to the inclusive yoga AI governance.

Table 1. Chosen Datasets and their bias-Relevance in the Aim of Inclusion Yoga AI.

Dataset	Primary Use	Strength	Key Bias Risk	Best Use in This Chapter
Yoga-82	Yoga pose identification (82 classes)	Pose diversity label hierarchy	incomplete demographic information Web-image skew; studio-norm bias	skewness in generalization Analyze representational bias and generalization errors
LDY / MoveNet-based yoga sets	Limited pose inference in real time Pipeline Deployable	Edge-friendly, deployable pipelines	edge friendly Coverage bias (small taxonomy)	overconfident predictions
FHIBE	Fairness evaluation benchmark	Consent + global diversity; fairness auditing for pose estimation	Not yoga-specific; needs task adaptation	Bias auditing of pose-estimation backbones
LDPose	Inclusive pose estimation	Explicit disability inclusion; new task definition	Not yoga-specific; specialized keypoints	Accessibility lens + inclusive keypoint redesign

This table explained Four datasets are compared and how they are utilized in the chapter. Yoga-82 is primarily applied to identify numerous varieties of yoga postures and where models cannot apply or become biased. This is demonstrated using LDY / MoveNet yoga sets which demonstrate how the real-world yoga practice can be left out using a system with few labels of pose. The FHIBE is also present to test the fairness of pose-estimation models across individuals based on region and background, although it is not concerned with yoga. The LDPose is called upon to import an accessibility view, since the tool is meant to be used with individuals with limb differences and specify new keypoints to their bodies. Yoga-82 and LDY / MoveNet are used to aid the discussion of accuracy and cover of yoga poses, whereas FHIBE and LDPose are used to aid the discussion of fairness and inclusion.

Figure 3. Algorithm 1 Yoga Data Family Detection Comprehensive Bias Detection (Dataset D, Metadata M, ModelFamily F).

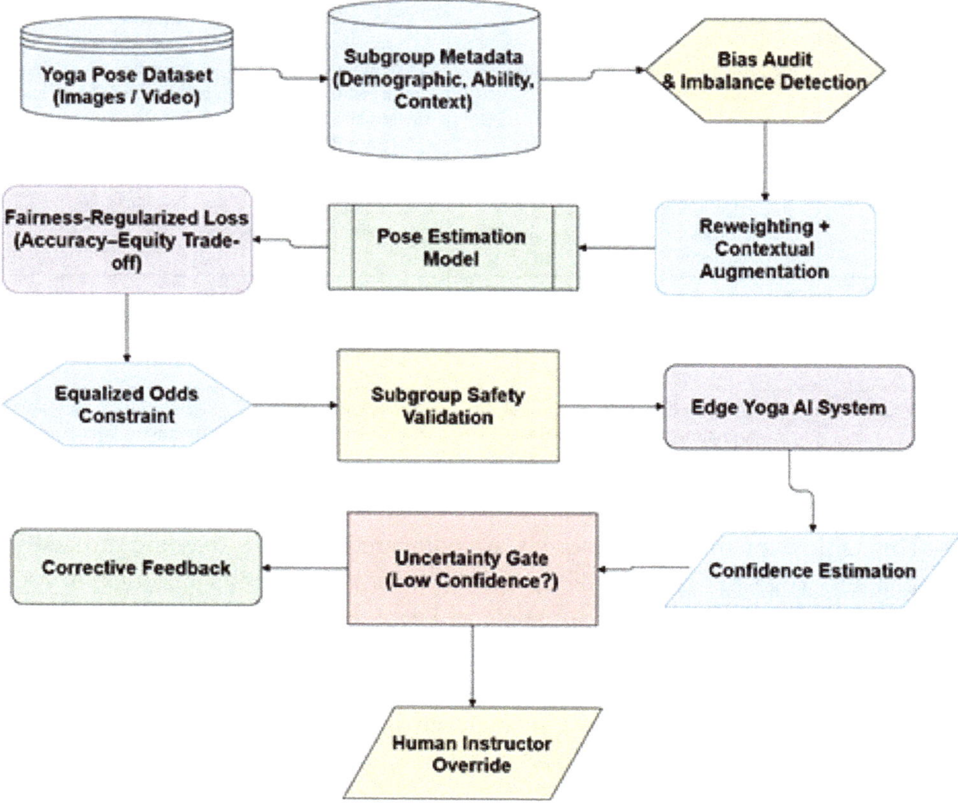

Algorithm 1 measures equity and bias on a pose estimation model. First, it purges the data and cohorts samples into singleton and intersectional subgroups (such as gender x skin tone). The data is then divided into training, validation and test set. The training of a baseline model is conducted using "F" that is the selected model family. The algorithm, then, calculates global measures of accuracy, true/false positive, and calibration error on the test set. It considers each of these metrics separately for every subgroup and compares them to the worldwide values to compute bias metrics: Demographic Parity (DP), Equalized odds (EO) and Calibration gap (Cal).

4. DISCRIMINATION REDUCTION METHODS OF NON-DISCRIMINATIVE AI-BASED YOGA

4.1 Reasons to Reduce bias in Yoga AI

The identification of bias will not be enough to develop inclusive AI systems. Having identified representation, annotation and algorithmic biases, systematic mitigation strategies should be included in the AI lifecycle. Mitigation is especially crucial in yoga AI since wrong or prejudiced feedback may cause bodily harm, user rejection, and cultural dismissal, which is a direct contradiction to the core value of yoga, which is universal access. Inclusive yoga AI mitigation strategies should thus meet three requirements:

1. Fairness of representation - equitable performance between the demographic and cultural, as well as ability-based subgroups.
2. Practical deplorability - compatibility to real-time, edge-based coaching systems of yoga.

In this regard the techniques of mitigation are classified into data-level, algorithm-level and post-model (decision-level) mitigation techniques.

4.2 Data-Level Mitigation Techniques

The major cause of bias in yoga AI is dataset imbalance. One such mitigation strategy is reweighting, in which samples of underrepresented subgroups of the training are given greater weight.

Let

$$D = \{ (x, y, g) \},$$

Where,

x is the input image or frame added by user

y is the pose label,

g Represents subgroup membership.

The reweighted empirical risk minimization loss is defined as:

$$L\_(weighted) = sum\_(i = 1)\^n\ w\_(g\_i)*l(f(x\_i), y\_i)$$

Where $\ell(\cdot)$is the pose classification or regression loss.

The subgroup weight is defined as:

$$w\_g = \frac{1}{sqrt(|S\_g|)}$$

where |S_g| size of testing dataset (samples) of subgroup g. This model makes minorities more dominant and makes training more stable.

In the case of fairness, generic image augmentation is inadequate. The AI systems in yoga need to be contextually augmented to mimic the diversity of practice in the real world, such as variation in clothing, change in lighting, change in camera angle, and change in pose. The process of augmentation may be stated as follows:

$$x' = T\_theta(x),\ theta \sim P(Theta\_(context))$$

where T_theta is a transformation selected according to a context-dependent distribution Θ context instead of random distortions of images. This enhances the strength of practitioners who practice yoga in the non-studio settings.

Figure 4. Inclusive Yoga AI Systems based on Bias-Aware and Safety-Critical Architecture.

Input:

$D = \{(I_i, Y_i, M_i)\}_{i=1}^{n}$; I_i: image/video frame; Y_i: pose label

$M_i = \{$age, gender, bmi, ethnicity/skin_tone, ability, attire, lighting, device$\}$

Model family F (e.g., PoseEstimator + PoseClassifier)

Thresholds $\tau_{DP}, \tau_{EO}, \tau_{Cal}$ (e.g., 0.10), min_size (e.g., 50)

Output:

$B = \{$SubgroupStats, DP_violations, EO_violations, Calib_violations, WorstGroups$\}$

Preprocess & validate metadata

$D_{clean} \leftarrow$ REMOVEMISSINGCRITICALFIELDS(D)

$G \leftarrow$ DEFINEGROUPS(M)

$G_{single} \leftarrow \{$age bins, gender, bmi bins, ethnicity/skin_tone, ability$\}$

$G_{intersection} \leftarrow \{$(gender × skin_tone), (age × ability), (attire × lighting), …$\}$

Split dataset

$(D_{train}, D_{val}, D_{test}) \leftarrow$ STRATIFIEDSPLIT$(D_{clean}$, by $= Y$, key metadata$)$

Train baseline system

model $\leftarrow$ TRAIN(F, D_{train}, D_{val})

Compute global metrics

global_acc $\leftarrow$ ACCURACY(model, D_{test})

$(\text{tpr}_{global}, \text{fpr}_{global}) \leftarrow$ TPR_FPR(model, D_{test})

$\text{ece}_{global} \leftarrow$ EXPECTEDCALIBRATIONERROR(model, D_{test})

Initialize report containers

SubgroupStats $\leftarrow \emptyset$, Violations $\leftarrow \emptyset$

For each subgroup slice g

for all $g \in (G_{single} \cup G_{intersection})$ **do**

  $S_g \leftarrow \{x \in D_{test} \mid x.\text{metadata} \in g\}$

  if $|S_g| <$ min_size **then**

    continue

  end if

  $\text{acc}_g \leftarrow$ ACCURACY(model, S_g)

  $(\text{tpr}_g, \text{fpr}_g) \leftarrow$ TPR_FPR(model, S_g)

  $\text{ece}_g \leftarrow$ EXPECTEDCALIBRATIONERROR(model, S_g)

  Compute gaps

  $\text{DP}_g \leftarrow \dfrac{|\text{acc}_g - \text{global\_acc}|}{\max(\text{global\_acc}, \varepsilon)}$

  $\text{EO}_g \leftarrow \max(|\text{tpr}_g - \text{tpr}_{global}|, |\text{fpr}_g - \text{fpr}_{global}|)$

  $\text{Cal}_g \leftarrow |\text{ece}_g - \text{ece}_{global}|$

  SubgroupStats$[g] \leftarrow \{\text{acc}_g, \text{tpr}_g, \text{fpr}_g, \text{ece}_g, \text{DP}_g, \text{EO}_g, \text{Cal}_g, n_g = |S_g|\}$

  if $(\text{DP}_g > \tau_{DP}) \vee (\text{EO}_g > \tau_{EO}) \vee (\text{Cal}_g > \tau_{Cal})$ **then**

    Violations $\leftarrow$ Violations $\cup \{g\}$

  end if

end **for**

Summarize worst-case bias

$\text{DP}_{max} \leftarrow \max_g \text{DP}_g$

$\text{EO}_{max} \leftarrow \max_g \text{EO}_g$

$\text{Cal}_{max} \leftarrow \max_g \text{Cal}_g$

WorstGroups $\leftarrow$ TOPK(SubgroupStats, key = weighted$(\text{DP}_g, \text{EO}_g, \text{Cal}_g)$)

$B \leftarrow \{$SubgroupStats, Violations, DP_{max}, EO_{max}, Cal_{max}, WorstGroups$\}$

return B (TRAIN(F) + —G—EVAL)

The figure shows a complete end-to-end, bias-aware system of yoga-based artificial intelligence systems that can be deployed safely in real-time and in safety-critical systems. The framework will combine data-level, algorithm-level, and decision-level mitigations strategies to provide fair performance of demographic, ability-based, and contextual subgroups of yoga students. Discovered differences are addressed by reweighting and context-aware data augmentation that will allow better representation of the underrepresented practitioners and non-studio practice settings. The learning aspect has learning performance goals, using fairness-sensitive objectives with task performance and subgroup-sensitive objectives. The loss functions that are fairness-regularized and equalized odds-based error alignment are used to minimize the difference in the performance of subgroups and still assure a high level of overall pose estimation accuracy. Uniqueness of subgroups safety validation as a gateway to avoid the deployment of models that will have disproportionately harmful impacts on minority users. During inference time, trained model is used on edge-based yoga coaching systems to facilitate the provision of real-time feedback. Uncertainty-based decision gating and confidence estimation provide a way to guarantee that only when the predictions of the system are accurate are corrective feedbacks given.

4.3 Mitigation Techniques at an Algorithm Level.

In order to avoid performance differences between subgroups, the fairness constraints are directly introduced into the training goal. The fairness-regularized loss objective is given as:

$$L_{total} = L_{task} + \lambda * sum\_\{g\ in\ G\}\ (Acc\_g - Acc\_\{global\})^2$$

where:

- Acc_g is subgroup of g and specific accuracy,
- $Acc\_\{global\}$ is global accuracy,
- λ (lambda) accuracy and fairness with learning rate.

Equalized odds regularization is a way to ensure the similarity of safety behavior in subgroups by punishing differences in true and false positive rates.

The equalized odds penalty is becomes as:

$$R\_(EO) = sum\_(g\ in\ G)(|TPR\_g - TPR| + |FPR\_g - FPR|)$$

The final objective of training defines:

$$L\_(EO) = L\_(task) + beta * R\_(EO)$$

This fact is critical particularly in yoga AI, where wrong feedback may cause harm or pain.

The inclusive yoga AI system also includes the option of reject to avoid the undesirable overconfidence on new or modified poses. The rejection criterion is set to be:

$$max\_y\ p(y|x) < tau$$

When the confidence that is predicted falls lower than the threshold τ, the system does not give any corrective feedback but rather asks to be modified or guided by a human.

4.4 Post-Model (Decision-Level) Mitigation Techniques

The subgroups must have a similar accuracy of prediction. Subgroup-conscious calibration is used to do this. The ECE (Expected Calibration Error) of subgroup g is computed as;

$$ECE\_g = sum\_(k = 1)\wedge K\ (|B\_k|/n\_g)*|acc(B\_k) - conf(B\_k)|$$

To subgroup-specific correct temperature scaling is applied as:

$$p\_g\wedge(cal)(y|x) = softmax(z(x)/T\_g)$$

where T g is optimized separately within each of the subgroups.

Figure 5. Algorithm 2 End-to-End Fairness-Aware Fairness-Conscious Yoga AI Training and Calibration Process

Input: Dataset $D = \{(x_i, y_i, g_i)\}_{i=1}^{n}$, model family F, confidence threshold τ
Output: Mitigated model F^* and calibrated feedback module
Step 1: Rationale-Aware Initialization
Identify biases in representation, annotation, and model behavior.
Ensure mitigation aligns with inclusivity principles:
(a) Representation fairness, (b) Safety awareness, (c) Deployability.
Step 2: Data-Level Mitigation
(a) Rebalancing and Reweighting:
Assign subgroup weight $w_g = \frac{1}{|S_g|}$ and minimize

$$\mathcal{L}_{\text{data}} = \sum_i w_{g_i}\, \ell(F(x_i), y_i)$$

(b) Context-Aware Data Augmentation:
Generate augmented samples $x_i' = T_\theta(x_i)$ where $\theta \sim \Theta_{\text{context}}$
simulates clothing, lighting, angle, and adaptive pose variation.
Step 3: Algorithm-Level Mitigation
(a) Fairness-Regularized Objective:

$$\mathcal{L}_{\text{fair}} = \mathcal{L}_{\text{data}} + \lambda \sum_g |\text{Acc}_g - \text{Acc}_{\text{global}}|$$

(b) Equalized Odds Alignment:

$$\mathcal{L}_{\text{EO}} = \sum_g (|\text{TPR}_g - \text{TPR}_{\text{global}}| + |\text{FPR}_g - \text{FPR}_{\text{global}}|)$$

Combine as $\mathcal{L}_{\text{train}} = \mathcal{L}_{\text{fair}} + \beta \mathcal{L}_{\text{EO}}$
(c) Uncertainty-Aware Rejection:
If $\text{Conf}(x_i) < \tau$, reject prediction and request human guidance.
Step 4: Post-Model (Decision-Level) Mitigation
(a) Subgroup-Specific Calibration:

$$\text{ECE}_g = \sum_{b=1}^{B} |\, \text{acc}(b, g) - \text{conf}(b, g) \,|$$

Optimize T_g per subgroup using temperature scaling:

$$p'(y|x, g) = \text{softmax}(z/T_g)$$

(b) Variant-Tolerant Feedback:
Classify output using:

$$f(x) = \begin{cases} \text{Correct}, & d(x, r) \le \delta_1 \\ \text{Safe Adaptation}, & \delta_1 < d(x, r) \le \delta_2 \\ \text{Potential Risk}, & d(x, r) > \delta_2 \end{cases}$$

Return: Fairness-regularized model F^* with calibrated and safe feedback policy.

Algorithm 2: Integrated Bias Mitigation Framework of Inclusive Yoga AI Systems is created to in any case be fair, safe, and accessible in the AI lifecycle of yoga coaching models. It starts with the creation of inclusivity principles founded on the fairness of representation, safety awareness, and deployability. On the data level, it uses reweighting to provide increased importance to underrepresented subgroups and context-aware augmentation to approximate the practice conditions in the real world including varying lighting, dress, and body differences. An uncertainty-sensitive rejection mechanism at the algorithmic level limits inaccuracies and demographic equity at the same time, using fairness-regularized loss functions and equalized odds constraints, and discourages unsafe and overconfident reactions. Post-model methods also help to optimize behavior by subgroup-specific calibration that equalizes the confidence levels of demographic groups, and variant-tolerant feedback rules that group poses as either correct, safe adaptations or potentially risky.

4.5 Summary of Mitigation Techniques

Table 2. Inclusive Yoga AI Reducing Measures

Mitigation Level	Technique	Bias Addressed
Data-level	Sample reweighting	Representation bias
Data-level	Context-aware augmentation	Environment & visibility bias
Algorithm-level	Fairness-regularized loss	Accuracy disparity
Algorithm-level	Equalized odds regularization	Safety-critical bias
Algorithm-level	Uncertainty-based rejection	OOD & adaptation bias
Post-model	Subgroup calibration	Confidence bias
Post-model	Variant-tolerant feedback	Cultural & ability bias

Table 3 lists the most significant mitigation measures that a progressive AI-based yoga system should take to be built, grouping them by the level of data, algorithm, and post-model intervention. Sample reweighting and context-aware augmentation at the data level deal with the challenges of representation and environmental bias by making sure that underrepresented groups of practitioners and situations that are relevant to real-world practice are properly represented in training. Resulting in the reduction of performance and safety differences between subgroups by limiting the learning process and avoiding overconfident predictions in the presence of unfamiliar or adapted poses, algorithm-level methods such as fairness-regularized loss functions, equalized odds regularization, and uncertainty-based rejection mechanisms can be used to achieve performance and safety disparities in subgroups. The post model strategies including subgroup-specific calibration, variant-tolerant feedback policies corrects the misalignment of confidence as well as encourages culturally sensitive and ability cognizant interactions since it differentiates between correct poses, safe adaptation and risks it might involve. Altogether, the table brings out that a multi-layered mitigation strategy that combines data balancing, fairness-conscious modeling, and human-centered feedback design can result in fairness and accessibility in AI in yoga.

5. YOGA AI FAIRNESS MEASURES AND ANALYSIS

5.1 Subgroup Accuracy and Deviation of Demographic Parity

Suppose that $D = \{(x_i, y_i, g_i)\}_{i=1}^{n}$ is a labeled yoga dataset, with x_i being an input image or frame,, y_i is being the ground-truth pose label, and $g_i \in G$ meaning one of the subgroups (e.g. skin tone band, attire type, age group or ability level). The classification accuracy calculate by a pose classifier f on a test set created D_{test} global level is

$$\text{Acc}_{\text{global}} = \frac{1}{|D_{\text{test}}|} \sum_{(x,y) \in D_{\text{test}}} 1\{f(x) = y\}$$

The subgroup accuracy of certain subgroup g is

$$\text{Acc}_{g} = \frac{1}{|S_g|} \sum_{(x,y) \in S_g} 1\{f(x) = y\}, S_g = \{(x,y) \in D_{\text{test}} \mid \text{meta}(x) \in g\}$$

Demographic Parity: Performance deviations in the style of Demographic Equilibrium The deviation of subgroup accuracy compared to that of the entire population:

$$\text{DP}_{g} = \frac{|\text{Acc}_{g} - \text{Acc}_{\text{global}}|}{\max(\text{Acc}_{\text{global}}, \varepsilon)}$$

where $\varepsilon > 0$ avoids division by zero. The subgroups whose τ_{DP} (e.g., 0.10) is used to flag subgroups for which $\text{DP}_g > \tau_{\text{DP}}$, are flagged to signify inequitable performance which could be transferred into systematically lower feedback to those practitioners.

5.2 Odds and Safety-Relevant Gaps of Equalization

In the context of yoga coaching False negatives, i.e., when the potentially unsafe pose is not detected and false positives, i.e., when the safe pose is wrongly identified have varied safety implications based on the subgroup of practitioners. Not all users are equally susceptible to these types of errors since physical ability, age, and adaptations to practice may increase or reduce the risks related to misclassification given by:

$$\mathrm{TPR}_g = \Pr\left(\hat{Y}^{\mathrm{safe}} = 1 Y^{\mathrm{safe}} = 1, g\right),$$

$$\mathrm{FPR}_g = \Pr\left(\hat{Y}^{\mathrm{safe}} = 1 \mid Y^{\mathrm{safe}} = 0, g\right)$$

The equalized odds gap applied in the detection of biases is

$$\mathrm{EO}_g = \max\left(\left\{\mathrm{TPR}_g - \mathrm{TPR}_{\mathrm{global}}\right\}, \left\{\mathrm{FPR}_g - \mathrm{FPR}_{\mathrm{global}}\right\}\right)$$

The fairness version of safety-critical is that a subgroup if $\mathrm{EO}_g > \tau_{\mathrm{EO}}$, because it represents the idea that the error profile of a given group is different to the overall population, and therefore may over-warn or under-warn some practitioners.

5.3 Subgroup Accuracy Chart

This schematic figure depicts the differences in accuracy of the four groups of practitioners, which brings into view the performance gaps that have the potential to sabotage inclusivity despite the global accuracy being acceptable.

Figure 6. Disparities in Subgroup Accuracy and Fairness in the Classification of Yoga Pose.

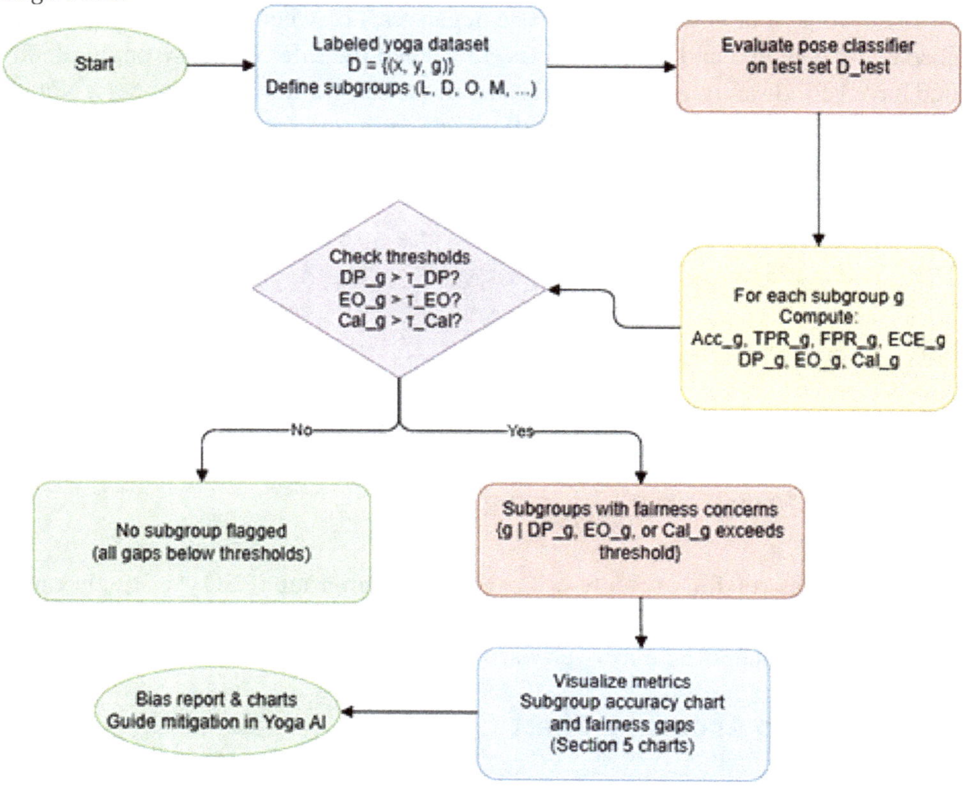

The figure indicates a bar of each of the practitioner subgroups, i.e., L (light-skin, studio attire), D (darker-skin, modest attire), O (older adults), and M (mobility-limited), and their score of individual pose classification accuracy, as well as a horizontal reference line of global accuracy. The visual interpretation of each bar and the global line shows that one group (particularly ones D and M) are significantly below the overall performance, showing that there are differences in demographic parity that are not immediately apparent through a single aggregate metric. These gaps suggest that some practitioners are more susceptible to receiving a wrong feedback, which in the context of yoga may translate to the higher quality of guidance, the higher possibility of having discomfort or injury, and the feeling of being excluded on the part of the user whose body, clothing, or contexts do not conform to the norms in the studio.

6. CONCLUSION

The chapter has given an overall plan of thinking, identifying and diminishing bias in AI systems used to study and teach yoga and it can be seen that the democratizing aspect of yoga AI can only be actualized when the concepts of representation, fairness, and cultural sensitivity are considered as the design principles rather than as the upgrades. Based on this discussion, the chapter proposed a three-pillar concept of inclusive yoga AI representation and governance: yoga datasets typically focus on studio settings, westernized clothing, able-bodied yoga practitioners, and canonical alignment that favors those who practice yoga in other places, practice yoga differently, wear other clothes, and have other adaptations; fairness-conscious algorithm design: yoga data sets that not only mitigate against uncertainty but also incorporate fairness-conditioned objectives, equalized odds penalties, and uncertainty-conditional rejection; and user-centered yoga evaluation and deployment integrate technical fairness metrics The chapter is framed by larger ethical standards and principles such as global health AI principles and risk-management guidelines and the philosophical values of accessibility and non-judgment of yoga, which imply that inclusive yoga AI is both a technical and ethical necessity, and the strategy to develop systems that can deliver high-quality, culturally-respectful support to yoga practitioners, in terms of body, identity, abilities, and contexts.

Future studies on this chapter should be based on development of worldly diversified data sets of consent respecting yoga and fairness standards that contain extensive metadata on body type, mobility, cultural context, and practice setting to make subgroup analysis and bias reduction more solid. This will be critical in developing lightweight edge compatible fairness schemes and uncertainty estimation algorithms such that inclusiveness will not be attained at the cost of real time performance in low resource and mobile deployments. The collaboration between the people working in diverse disciplines must be enhanced, and the AI researchers, yoga teachers who discuss different traditions, therapists, activists, and cultural scholars must collaborate in designing pose taxonomies, feedback solutions, and measurement plans that would be reflective of the lived experiences of diverse practitioners. Additional aspects to be considered are regulatory and governance paths, which would include certain standards of equitable auditing, reporting and responsibility in wellness and movement-coaching use and methods to qualify inclusive yoga AI systems. Finally, longitudinal studies must evaluate the effects of yoga AI in their physical safety and confidence, practices and belonging to local and global yoga communities on the long-term so that the gains of technical fairness could be incorporated into the outcomes of health equity and holistic wellbeing.

REFERENCES

Ashok, B. (2025). *Surendiran, and S. Babu, "Yoga pose estimation using MoveNet deep learning models* (Vol. 50). Sādhanā.

Chamola, V., Gummana, E. P., Madan, A., Rout, B. K., & Coelho Rodrigues, J. J. P. (2024). Advancements in yoga pose estimation using artificial intelligence: A survey. *Current Bioinformatics*, *19*(3), 264–280. DOI: 10.2174/1574893618666230508105440

Chen, I. Y., Joshi, S., Ghassemi, M., & Ranganath, R. (2023). "Probabilistic machine learning for healthcare," *npj Digital Medicine*, vol. 6.

Choudhury, K., ... (2025). "Steganography in the digital age: An in-depth review of techniques," in *ASCIS 2024*, CCIS, vol. 2424, Springer, Cham, DOI: 10.1007/978-3-031-86290-8_24

Doshi, M. (2023). "A comparison of data mining approaches for forecasting sales of FMCG food products," in *Proc. ICCCNT*, Delhi, India, pp. 1–7, DOI: 10.1109/ICCCNT56998.2023.10307432

Doshi, M., Hirapara, J., Ranpara, R., Khachariya, H., Patel, A. K., Jhanwar, K., & Choudhury, K. (2025). Enhancing FMCG sales prediction using recurrent neural networks and economic indicators. *IET Conference Proceedings,* 2025(7), 1223–1230. https://doi.org/DOI: 10.1049/icp.2025.1574

Haridasan, J. T., & Raj, E. D. (2023). Deep learning system for paddy plant disease detection and classification. *Environmental Monitoring and Assessment*, *195*(1), 120. DOI: 10.1007/s10661-022-10656-x PMID: 36399232

Hasanzadeh, F., Josephson, C. B., Waters, G., Adedinsewo, D., Azizi, Z., & White, J. A. (2025). "Bias recognition and mitigation strategies in artificial intelligence healthcare applications," *npj. Digital Medicine*, *8*(1), 154. Advance online publication. DOI: 10.1038/s41746-025-01503-7 PMID: 40069303

Hirpara, J., Doshi, M., Patel, A., & Choudhury, K. (2025). A Study on Machine Learning Algorithms: Forecasting Crop Prices. In Rajagopal, S., Popat, K., Meva, D., Bajeja, S., & Mudholkar, P. (Eds.), *Artificial Intelligence Based Smart and Secured Applications. ASCIS 2024. Communications in Computer and Information Science* (Vol. 2427). Springer., DOI: 10.1007/978-3-031-86299-1_4

Kim, K. K., & Backonja, U. (2025). Digital health equity frameworks and key concepts: A scoping review. *Journal of the American Medical Informatics Association : JAMIA*, *32*(5), 932–944. DOI: 10.1093/jamia/ocaf017 PMID: 39936843

Leslie, D. (2023). *Understanding Artificial Intelligence Ethics and Safety*. The Alan Turing Institute.

Liu, M., Ning, Y., Teixayavong, S., Liu, X., Mertens, M., Shang, Y., Li, X., Miao, D., Liao, J., Xu, J., Ting, D. S. W., Cheng, L. T.-E., Ong, J. C. L., Teo, Z. L., Tan, T. F., RaviChandran, N., Wang, F., Celi, L. A., Ong, M. E. H., & Liu, N. (2025). "A scoping review and evidence gap analysis of clinical AI fairness," *npj. Digital Medicine*, *8*(1), 360. Advance online publication. DOI: 10.1038/s41746-025-01667-2 PMID: 40517148

Miao, Z., Wang, J., & Yu, C. (2024). FairPose: Toward fairness-aware human pose estimation. *IEEE Transactions on Pattern Analysis and Machine Intelligence*.

Mitchell, M.. "Model cards for model reporting," in *Proc. ACM Conf. on Fairness, Accountability, and Transparency (FAccT)*, 2023, pp. 220–229.

Norori, N., Hu, Q., Aellen, F. M., Faraci, F. D., & Tzovara, A. (2023). Addressing bias in big data and AI for health care: A call for open science. *Patterns (New York, N.Y.)*, *2*(10), 100347. DOI: 10.1016/j.patter.2021.100347 PMID: 34693373

Patel, A. K., Doshi, M. V., Hirapara, J. D., & Khachariya, H. D. (2025). Scrutinize Search Engine Optimization Strategies with Artificial Intelligence to Rank a Website. In Rajagopal, S., Popat, K., Meva, D., Bajeja, S., & Mudholkar, P. (Eds.), *Artificial Intelligence Based Smart and Secured Applications. ASCIS 2024. Communications in Computer and Information Science* (Vol. 2427). Springer., DOI: 10.1007/978-3-031-86299-1_3

Ranpara, R., Hirpara, J., Doshi, M., & Shah, D. (2025). A novel Bayesian-inspired framework for proactive detection and mitigation of zero-day attacks in distributed network architectures. *IET Conference Proceedings,* 2025(7), 1168–1175. https://doi.org/DOI: 10.1049/icp.2025.1567

Sadaria, D., Khachariya, H., & Hirpara, J. (2023). Priti, Dr. Haresh Khachariya, and Dr. Jignesh Hirpara. "Exploring the Diverse Applications of Deep Learning Across Multiple Domains.". *Recent Research Reviews Journal*, *2*(1), 183–200. DOI: 10.36548/rrrj.2023.1.16

Shih, C.-L., Liu, J.-Y., Anggraini, I. T., Xiao, Y., Funabiki, N., & Fan, C.-P. (2024). A yoga pose difficulty level estimation method using OpenPose for self-practice systems. *Information (Basel)*, *15*(12), 789. Advance online publication. DOI: 10.3390/info15120789

World Health Organization. Ethics and Governance of Artificial Intelligence for Health: Guidance on Large Multi-Modal Models, Geneva, Switzerland, 2025.

Xiang, , Andrews, J. T. A., Bourke, R. L., Thong, W., LaChance, J. M., Georgievski, T., Modas, A., Rahmattalabbi, A., Ba, Y., Nagpal, S., Papakyriakopoulos, O., Zhao, D., Xue, J., Matthews, V., Gong, L., Hoag, A. T., Cimpoi, M., Sankaranarayanan, S., Hutiri, W., & Spranger, M. (2025). Fair human-centric image dataset for ethical AI benchmarking. *Nature*, *648*(8092), 97–108. DOI: 10.1038/s41586-025-09716-2 PMID: 41193813

Xu, Y., Zhang, Z., & Wang, Y. (2024). *Cross-cultural generalization in vision-based human activity recognition* (Vol. 149). Pattern Recognition.

Xu, Z.. (2024). "Addressing fairness issues in deep learning-based medical image analysis: A systematic review," *npj. Digital Medicine*, *7*, 286. PMID: 39420149

Ying, J.. "LDPose: Towards inclusive human pose estimation for limb-deficient individuals in the wild," in *Proc. IEEE/CVF Int. Conf. on Computer Vision (ICCV)*, 2025. DOI: 10.1109/ICCV51701.2025.00920

Zhou, H., Li, Y., & Huang, K. (2024). AI-assisted physical activity monitoring for personalized wellness. *Sensors (Basel)*, *24*(2).

Chapter 5
Addressing Privacy, Data Security, and Consent in Yoga AI Applications

Yagnik Dave
http://orcid.org/0000-0003-0506-9536
Marwadi University, Rajkot, India

Ankur Khant
http://orcid.org/0009-0004-8492-2615
Marwadi University, Rajkot, India

Hemangkumar Sudhakarbhai Jani
http://orcid.org/0000-0002-8475-7558
Ganpat University, Gujarat, India

Ashish Ashish Kakkad
http://orcid.org/0009-0006-9291-4839
Marwadi University, Rajkot, India

Brijesh Verma
Marwadi University, Rajkot, India

Mrunal Harle
http://orcid.org/0009-0004-6842-3664
District Civil Hospital, Amravati, India

ABSTRACT

The chapter of the book is the critical analysis of the ethical principles of the Artificial Intelligence-based yoga practices with the specific emphasis on the privacy, trust, cultural integrity, and sustainable adoption. It states that AI systems in yoga practice exist in a unique moral and embodied sphere, and data governance and data consent as well as system design can not be reduced to technical or regulatory issues. The chapter is based on the concept of privacy-preserving design as an ethical value system rather than a functional constraint due to yogic principles, including ahimsa, satya, viveka, and collective responsibility. It discusses technical approaches, including federated learning and culturally sensitive and ethical user experience design to illustrate how innovation and ethical integrity could go together. Moreover, the chapter puts trust in a socio-technical and ethical framework, which is built through transparency, accountability, and involvement of community over time.

DOI: 10.4018/979-8-2600-2463-8.ch005

INTRODUCTION

The introduction of artificial intelligence in yoga practice can be said to be among the most significant experiences of the ancient embodied principles with modern digital structures. Historically based on close teacher-student interactions, self-disciplined practice and experience-based knowledge transmission, yoga is being placed on AI-mediated platforms, which are offering personalized learning, real-time feedback, and global access in a way never before seen. These developments are often presented by creators of the fast-growing digital wellness economy as neutral, progressive, or even emancipatory innovations that will democratize the practice of yoga. However, this account of technological good-will hides some more fundamental change in the way yoga is practiced, experienced, and governed.

1.1 Appearance of AI-based Yoga Apps.

The emergence of AI-based yoga apps should be interpreted in the context of the further growth of digital health and wellness technologies. The development of the computer vision, mobile computers, wearable biosensors, and machine learning has facilitated the systems that can monitor the alignment of posture, estimate the joint angle, detect the variation in heart rate, and even learn breathing patterns. Numerous modern applications depend on the cameras of smartphones to decode asana performances and provide the user with correctional feedback in the form of visual overlay, haptic feedback, or synthesized voice guidance. Others combine physiological information of smartwatches and fitness gadgets to produce adaptive sequence using stress signals, fatigue signs or other recovery measures. Generative AI systems increasingly are simulating conversation, providing motivational hints, reflective inquisition, and pedagogical accounts, which reflectively believe human instruction(Jain et al., 2025).

Nevertheless, such a model is strikingly different as compared to classical yoga pedagogy. Classical yoga as expressed in the philosophical text and maintained over the generations of embodied teachers favors experiential knowledge developed over the course of interpersonal relationships. This model of guru-sisya is not only instructional but ethical, which is based on trust, discernment and situational sensitivity. In modern secularized yoga, where the practice is considerably more balanced, teaching performance is still largely reliant on the teacher to sense subtle body-related responses, emotional conditions and situational elements that cannot be formalized. The process of learning occurs by being present, refining, and becoming conscious of the self instead of measuring and judging yourself against others.

Conversely, AI-powered platforms have to work based on abstraction, standardization and quantification. Christ and complicated body and mental conditions are simplified to datasets that may be processed, ordered, and forecasted. Although this allows feedback on a large scale to be automated, it also renegotiates yoga as performance to be assessed and not a practice that can be explored internally. The metric often has the form of scores, streaks, optimization metrics, and, thereby, external validation and comparison are subtly promoted. Such reframing brings up fundamental questions regarding what gets changed, displaced or lost once yoga is subjected to algorithmic mediation. The more critical question is then not merely whether AI can be successfully used to teach yoga, but how in that case the ethical, experiential, and philosophical currents of the practice as such is reconfigured(Sinha & Sinha, 2024).

The problem of Privacy, Data Security, and Consent in Yoga AI Applications.

Introduction Yoga, Artificial Intelligence and Ethical Datafication.

The introduction of artificial intelligence in yoga practice can be said to be among the most significant experiences of the ancient embodied principles with modern digital structures. Historically based on close teacher-student interactions, self-disciplined practice and experience-based knowledge transmission, yoga is being placed on AI-mediated platforms, which are offering personalized learning, real-time feedback, and global access in a way never before seen. These developments are often presented by creators of the fast-growing digital wellness economy as neutral, progressive, or even emancipatory innovations that will democratize the practice of yoga. However, this account of technological good-will hides some more fundamental change in the way yoga is practiced, experienced, and governed.

The central process in this change is the datafication, which is the methodical conversion of the movement of the body, its breathing, attention, affect, and the pattern of behavior into machine-readable information. Wearable sensors are used to capture the yoga practice in order to make it legible to algorithmic systems, which classify, assess, and optimize the embodied experience through computer vision, predictive analytics, and computer vision. This change does not simply introduce new tools of instruction, it restructures yoga as an object of calculation and control. Consequently, there are basic ethical issues of autonomy, dignity, trust, and the circumstances under which autonomy is developed.

According to this chapter, the concepts of privacy, data security, and consent cannot be sufficiently comprehended as the fringe technical safeguards or regulatory requirements in the context of AI-mediated yoga. Instead, they need to be placed as ethical issues that are inherent to the philosophy of yoga. Yoga is not a physical regime that is value neutral but an ethical discipline that aims at self-control, awareness acuity and action restraint. Ethical considerations will be inseparable of the integrity of practice when AI systems are used to mediate practices that involve a constant extraction, analysis, and repurposing of intimate data. Based on this, this introduction places AI-based yoga platforms in the larger socio-technical changes and constructs a moral frame through which forthcoming analysis is set in place(Ganesh & Ramudhin, 2024).

1.2 Incompatibility of Yogic Practice with Algorithms in Ethics.

Ethical issues are further enhanced by data security. The information that is connected with yoga is not limited to common fitness indicators but also includes the trends of susceptibility, pressure, and mental instability. Illegal use, access or secondary exploitation of such data may cause actual damages, such as emotional exposure, stigmatization, or loss of trust. A more hidden power, the fact that we can be surveilled or our data abused may discourage openness in practice, so that we might not be willing to experiment or explore by means of bodies. In the spirit of ahimsa, or non-harm, technological systems to aid in yoga should not only reduce physical risk, but also psychological and moral harm. Security failures are consequently ethical breaches as opposed to a technical neutral lapse(Hanwari et al., 2024).

This chapter is based on the assumption that responsible yoga AI needs to adopt an integrated ethical framework that integrates AI ethics, wellness studies, legal regulation, and yogic philosophy. Sensitivity of yoga-related data, privacy and security issues involved in AI systems, weaknesses of current consent models, and the normative advice presented by the yogic moral principles are explored in the sections that follow. The chapter aims at promoting a more critical, prudent, and responsible approach to artificial intelligence in yoga practice by placing technical design and regulatory debate in a wider ethical and philosophical framework(Venkatasubramanian, 2023).

2. SENSITIVITY AND NATURE OF DATA IN YOGA AI SYSTEM

The ethical implications of yoga AI applications are the most acute when the nature, the scope, and epistemic implications of the data produced and processed by such systems are looked at. As opposed to most digital wellness tools, which focus on the externalization of actions or other performance indicators, yoga AI systems can be described as function on the intersection of the body, physiological response, emotional sensitivity, and contemplation. They render machine-readable streams of data out of embodied and introspective dimensions of practice, through gradual sensing and algorithmic interpretation. This datafication makes highly personal things about the experience of the practitioner have a new form of visibility, analysis, and can be controlled through the technical apparatus. As a result, the stringent awareness of the delicacy of the yogic data must form the basis of any substantive discourse of the issue of privacy, security, and consent in the yoga practice mediated by AI.

This paragraph pushes the discussion forward to the point that information produced in yoga AI data sets is a new form of ethic that cannot be effectively resolved through governance systems that are developed in relation to generic fitness, lifestyle, or consumer health apps. The section by methodically analyzing the nature of data at stake and putting their context into the philosophical and cultural framework of yoga, explains why the increased ethical scrutiny is not only justified but also necessary.

Intuition and Sensibility of Data in AI Ranging in Yoga.

The morality of yoga AI systems usage is most significant when this is considered by analyzing the type, extent, and epistemic nature of the data that is produced and processed by the system. Yoga AI systems work at the intersection of the body, physiology, emotions, and consideration, unlike most digital wellness technologies, which largely measure experiences of externalization (behavior) or performance indicators. They are embodiment and introspective dimensions of practice which are converted into machine readable data streams through constant sensing and algorithmic interpretation. This datafication makes highly personal parts of the practitioner experience visible, measurable and even manageable by technology. In turn, the strict interpretation of the sensitivity of yogic information is an essential precondition of any meaningful debate on the privacy, security, and consent in yoga practice mediated by AI.

It is this section that pushes the argument that the data produced by systems in yoga AI is a unique category of ethical concern that cannot be sufficiently dealt with by governance systems that are meant to be used to address generic fitness, lifestyle, or consumer health applications. Through the systematic analysis of the nature of data at work and its placement, in terms of a philosophical and cultural basis of yoga, the section identifies the necessity and importance of increased ethical scrutiny(Gosalia et al., 2024).

2.1 The data in Yoga AI Applications can be classified into two categories namely Classification of Data in Yoga AI Applications.

Ambivalent and a particularly ethically sensitive place of emotional data in yoga AI ecosystems is a particularly problematic situation. Most applications request the self-reported mood or stress measurement prior to and after the sessions, whereas others are trying to estimate the affective state based on the voice, face recognition, or physiological indicators. Such practices put the line between wellness support and psychological profiling. In classical yoga, the emotional state is developed by the means of introspective observation and ethical self-control, not by the external measure and algorithmic categorization. The objectifying of emotional data in the process of capture and measurement is dangerous to inner experiences, which are contextual, fluid and highly personal(Verma et al., 2023).

Yoga AI data is even ethically complex due to its cumulative and longitudinal nature. Yoga is generally a long-term activity (months and years) where data constantly supplies adaptive machine learning models. With increased richness in datasets, algorithms can draw out correlations and predictions that were never intentionally revealed and in fact consciously identified even by the practitioners themselves. This inferential expansion changes the yogic evidence into forecasting and classifying tools out of the accounting evidence. These changes cast a deep uncertainty regarding autonomy, agency, and self-determination, especially when we learn about something using data that is impenetrable to the users and hard to challenge or put into context(Pal et al., 2023).

Figure 1. Ethical implications of yoga AI system

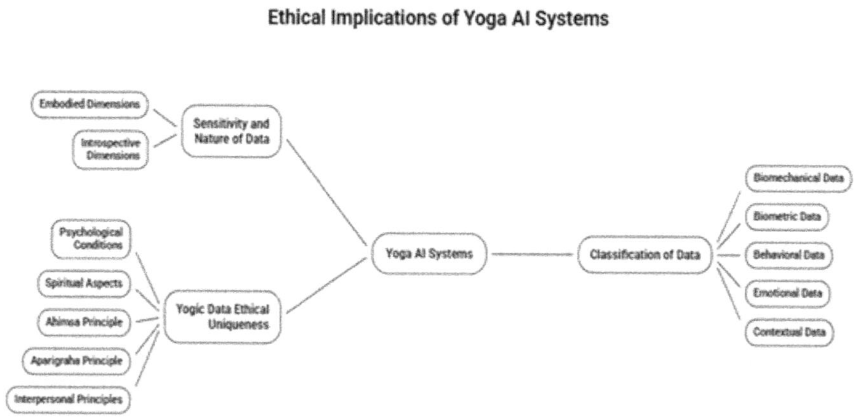

2.2 Yogic Data Ethical Uniqueness.

The ethical environment is also complicated by spiritual aspects. Although modern practitioners do not clearly articulate their practice as a spiritual one, the philosophical tradition of yoga focuses on the change of consciousness and the development of moral virtues. Information, which indicates meditative profundity, regulation of emotions, or consistency of practice, can be perceived as reaching into issues of id, meaning, and moral self-concept. Such data storage and algorithmical processing provokes the issue of dignity and respect that are not sufficiently addressed by the existing data protection paradigms. In contrast to fitness measures, yogic data can be viewed as disclosing aspects of self that can be disclosed only in confidential relational settings that the practitioner would want to preserve or share with his or her trusted associates(Bavli et al., 2025).

Overall, yoga AI systems handle data that is not only sensitive in technical aspects of its nature but also filled with morality and charged in a manner unlike other types of wellness data. The comprehensive categorization of the types of data has shown the scope and level of information involved and the ethical analysis has explained why the yogic data necessitates extra safeguarding and sensitivity to the context. This understanding of what is unique is critical in dealing with the privacy issues, security threats and consent dilemmas discussed in later chapters, and in designing governance and design solutions that are respectful of the ethical, cultural, and philosophical premises in the practice of yoga(Dhinakaran et al., 2025).

3. AI IN YOGA: PRIVACY ISSUES IN ARTIFICIAL INTELLIGENCE

The introduction of the use of artificial intelligence into the yoga practice exacerbates the long-standing privacy issue by offering qualitatively new data-gathering methods, algorithmic meaning, and international distribution. Unlike in the conventional yoga practices, where disclosure of personal information is done selectively, situationally, and in relationships based on a sense of trust, AI-based yoga apps are defined by a consistent stream of data that is not easily discernible. These flows are not merely organized by technological architectures, but also by commercial interests, platform economies and algorithmic logics more or less unreachable to the practitioners. The issue of privacy in yoga AI cannot be perceived as a rare technical failure or a lack of regulation, but it is a component of the structural conditions that redefine the autonomy of practice, self-reliance, and confidence of the practitioners.

Attached to yogic ethics, the developments reveal a deep contradiction between algorithmic governance and the main yogic principles, including intentionality and mindfulness and respect to the integrity of embodied experience. Privacy in AI Ethics of yoga goes beyond the informational control to the configuration of subjectivity itself based on mediation with data. Privacy therefore is a focal point where the Technological power meets ethical self-cultivation(Singh & Vats, 2025).

3.1 Opacity, Algorithmic Inference and the Erosion of Autonomy.

One of the main privacy risks in AI based yoga app is data practices being opaque. The practitioners do not often receive a clear or detailed picture of the information being gathered, its retention, processing, and ultimate disclosure to whom. The platforms might formally disclose data practices by means of a privacy policy or consent interface, however, these measures are usually legalistic, discontinuous and not representative of how yoga practice actually exists in reality. On the ethical level, this lack of transparency negatively affects informed participation and the ability of the practitioner to engage in intentionality. The growth of ethics in yoga cannot be separated by the cultivated awareness, the systems that blur the terms of involvement thus directly conflict with the ethos on which yoga is built.

This is hypocrisy, which algorithmic inference, which is the essence of modern AI systems, adds to. Yoga AI systems are not just data processors taking as input data that has been entered by users literally; they create a new type of personalized information by inducting attributes out of the pattern of postures, motions, breathing, physiological differences, and interaction behavior. The implied qualities can be measures of flexibility, risk of injuries, emotional condition, amount of stress or dedication to exercise regimes. Such processes can be described as personalization or optimization, but in reality, it broadens the scope of surveillance even beyond what can be revealed by the practitioners. The ethical issue in this case does not just pertain to the truth of these inferences but pertains also to their epistemic and moral condition: the practitioners are made knowable to the system in surpasses of their self-understanding and conscious agreement(Chittimalla & Potluri, 2025).

Combined with the conditions that should be in place to make meaningful consent and self-determination, opacity, algorithmic inference, and secondary data undermine the circumstances to do so. The practitioners might also feel empowered whenever the personalized feedback is provided without them knowing the presence of the larger surveillance system within which their practice falls. This inequality of knowledge and power turns voluntary participation into acquiescent participation. Such a transition in yogic terms turns out to be a loss of intentional agency which is essentially contradictory to the discipline of ethical action and mindful restraint(Biswas et al., 2025).

3.2 International Data Transfers and the Weakness of Faith.

The sharing of the data of the third parties also enhances this deterioration of the trust. Yoga software is often based on off-the-shelf analytics solutions, cloud service operators and advertisers, forming complicated data networks that go way past the original application. Even to the extent that single data points seem harmless, their existence in the hands of various organizations increases the chances of profiling and inference and re-identification. To practitioners, the understanding that intimate features of body movement, emotional conditions and the day-to-day routine can flee into obscure business connections can be distressing and betraying. Such violations of trust are especially destructive in actions that require psychological safety and unrestrictedness(Irfan et al., 2025).

Overall, the issues of privacy in AI-powered yoga apps are related to the complex interaction of the principles of transparency, algorithmic inference, general data flow, and commercial amalgamation. These procedures undermine the autonomy of practitioners, mindfulness, and confidence by putting a barrier between people and control over their embodied data. Upon the application of the yogic ethic, the breach of privacy does not manifest itself in the form of abstract breach of compliance but presents itself as direct offence of the values of awareness, non-harm and respect of integrity of the self. This does not mean that such issues can be resolved solely through modifying the policy on an incremental level; it implies a fundamental shift in design, governance and ethical commitment prioritizing practitioner dignity and relational integrity as the core of the technological innovation(Vallabhaneni & Prabhavathy, 2021).

4. DATA SECURITY RISK AND TECHNOLOGICAL VULNERABILITIES

On a technological level, yoga artificial intelligence software is built on the technological systems, which tend to be interconnected and opaque networks involving mobile phones, wearable gadgets, cloud computing, machine learning algorithms, and third-party analytics solutions. The vulnerability of each layer creates very specific vulnerabilities, and the fact that they are interdependent increases systemic risk. The concentration of incredibly sensitive individual, action, and psychological information on distributed infrastructures broadens the attack surface in a manner that cannot be entirely predicted or safeguarded. The risks are made even more acute by the innovation culture projected by the digital health and wellness startups, in which speed and market differentiation often overshadow careful security-by-design. This speed-ethical responsibility tension is especially decisive in the yoga settings, where people can rightfully expect that technologies associated with contemplative practice reflect a degree of care and high-attentiveness that does not necessarily correspond to the technical make up of a given technology(Alonge & Isreal, 2025).

4.1 Cyber Attacks within Yoga AI Systems.

These risks are also increased by cloud-based storage and processing. Yoga AI solutions would often store user data in large amounts on centralized servers to be analyzed longitudinally, personalized, and refined into models. Although cloud infrastructures are efficient and have the benefit of scalability, they also introduce risk that is ethically consequential. Lack of appropriate configuration of storage environment, inadequate access control, or vulnerability of shared cloud architectures, may reveal whole datasets of scale. Additionally, the use of third-party cloud providers creates layers of dependence which are often non transparent to the developers and the users. The practitioners might not know where their data is kept, who has access, or what legal jurisdictions regulate such data. This obscurity compromises a knowledgeable engagement and makes accountability difficult, which is a significant ethical issue of consent and autonomy in the practice of digital yoga(Chelishcheva, 2023).

The other and highly dangerous vulnerability is data poisoning. In this type of attack, adversaries actively inject adversarial data or corrupted data into the training pipeline, and as such this manipulates model behavior in a negative fashion. In the case of yoga AI systems, poisoned data would lead to systemically incorrect posture measures or potentially dangerous recommendations that are disproportionately applied to one type of body, ability, or health status. These dangers are particularly acute in inclusive or therapeutic yoga, where yoga practitioners can rely on the assistance of AI to customize practices to injury, disability, or age-related limitations. Not only does a compromised model significantly inhibit technical reliability, it would also be considered a breach of the ethical imperative to give supportive, equitable, and safe guidance which would lead to diminishing trust in the technology as well as the practice that the technology mediates(Özsezer & Mermer, 2025).

4.2 Embodied, Psychological, and Practice-Level Harms.

Altogether, the technological vulnerability and the issue of data security in the yoga AI systems represent a significant ethical edge. Not only technical issues are hacking, data interception, cloud-based exposures, model inversion, data poisoning; these are moral concerns that have direct physical safety, mental wellbeing, and integrity implications of the yogic practice. The solution to these risks should be based on a complex approach, which integrates both sophisticated approaches to cybersecurity and ethical thinking based on the philosophy of yoga. Stakeholders can shift to yoga AI systems that actually contribute to human flourishing as opposed to unwillingly undermining it by acknowledging data security as a form of care and non-harm(Tripathi, 2025).

5. INFORMED CONSENT IN AI IN YOGA

Here, the section intensively questions dominant systems of consent which yoga AI websites use and proves them to be ethically inadequate. It states that mainstream paradigms, which are mostly pre-platform economy existing, do not embrace the inferential power of AI, sensitivity of data relating to yoga, and normative commitments ingrained in yogic cultural. In reply, the section proceeds to a re-conceptualization of the informed consent as a continuous, ethics-based relationship based on the yogic principles of awareness, intentionality, autonomy and self-governance(Sikarwar et al., 2025).

5.1 Weaknesses of the Modern Consent Mechanisms.

These moral shortcomings are also exacerbated by the inferential nature of AI systems. Machine learning models produce new knowledge types by means of probabilistic inferences unlike conventional data-processing infrastructures which use only explicitly disclosed information as their predominant source of data. It is possible to tell whether a person is in a certain emotional state, whether he is stressed, whether he is adhering to certain cues, whether he is prone to certain amounts of messages, or whether he is vulnerable to specific forms of messages based on ostensibly neutral signals like micro variations in posture, breathing rhythms or consistency of a session. Most importantly, such implied qualities are hardly ever clearly explained in consent processes, even though they can have serious consequences in regard to privacy, autonomy, and psychological comfort. As a result, the consent given at the time of the data collection does not tend to hold any significant breadth to the entire extent of data practices and downstream implications made possible by AI-driven inference(Jebamikyous et al., 2023).

Regarding yogic ethical perspectives, these defects cannot be considered procedural flaws but rather moral lapses. The conscious option, reflection, and deliberate taking of actions that are part of ethical lives are preconditioned within the traditions of Yoga. These values cannot be supported by any uninformed, coerced or clouded by complexity consent. Instead of this, it threatens to re-organize practitioners in the role of passive data subject and reduce embodied self to extractive logics of surveillance. This way, these models of consent risk turning yoga as an experience of conscious self-development into a location of domified actions. The inefficiency of current consent systems, therefore, demands a groundbreaking reconsideration of the conceptual understanding and implementation of consent within the yoga AI systems(Sharma & Sharma, 2024).

Figure 2. Weakness of modern consent mechanism in Yoga AI

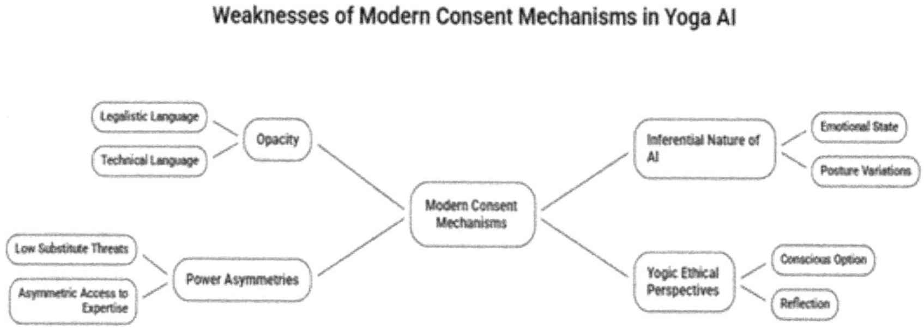

6. THE CONGRUENCE OF THE MORAL WITH THE YOGIC PRINCIPLES

Ethical analysis of AI-based yoga applications cannot be provided satisfactorily with the abstract models of digital ethics. Although such principles like fairness, accountability, and transparency are essential in the context of the modern AI governance, they are deprived of meaning when they are not connected to the moral ontology of yoga itself. Yoga is not some physical postures or therapy but an ethical-philosophical complex that is directed at developing the awareness of the self, restraint and harmony with the self, others and the world of existence. Therefore, in case the artificial intelligence mediates the yoga practice based on data-intensive and algorithmic infrastructures, the artificial intelligence does not simply bring technical mediation, but rather intersects with and, possibly, changes ethical bases of the practice.

The main ethical dilemma is not, however, confined to the statements of whether yoga AI systems meet the rules of the external regulatory norms or abstract standards of digital ethics. Instead, it is the matter as to whether these systems are ethically aligned with the internal values that make yoga a living tradition. In this case, moral congruence is the agreement between technological activities and the ethical goals on which yoga aims to develop. Here, the alignment considerations will be explored through the prism of core yogic beliefs of ahimsa (non-harm), satya (truthfulness), aparigraha (non-possessiveness), and mindfulness and their consistent application to data practices, algorithmic decision making, and commercial logics built into the yoga AI systems. It states that a lack of data practices by misalignment does not only produce technical inefficiencies and legal vulnerability: it also alters the reality and cultural integrity and purposeology of yoga as such, turning a matter of self-development into a terrain of full-fledged harm and moral depletion(Shaumya & Kumar, 2025).

6.1 Ahimsa and Satya in Data and Algorithmic Ethics

The ethical issues are aggravated with the context that the algorithmic feedback systems are insensitive to context. Artificial intelligence systems which are trained in standardized datasets often do not consider the differences in the body, prior injuries, cultural diversification in practice, or varying mental conditions. Where these systems recommend or testure postures without proper precautions or interpretive plasticity, they dangerously promote postures that result in strain, aggravate or belittle previous disorders, or be counterproductive to embodied recognition. Yogic perspective does not help to reduce harm with the help of good intentions and technical expertise. Instead, ahimsa requires proactive moral accountability: those involved in designing and providing yoga AI require to anticipate and avoid the predictable harms of mediation of embodied practice by means of data. In this regard, data safety and model integrity is not just a technical issue but an ethical imperative because the safeguarding of data integrity cannot be the same as the safeguarding of the well-being of practitioners(Murphy et al., 2025).

Intimately connected with ahimsa is the value of satya or truthfulness. Similar to the meaning of satya in yogic ethics, satya does not mean factual accuracy, but alignment between the representation and intention with the lived reality. The issues of satya in the context of yoga AI systems are algorithmic opaqueness, overstated intelligence or personalization, and strategic deception of system capabilities. Numerous applications represent themselves as smart teachers or dynamic tutors without explicitly stating what the boundaries of their model are, what assumptions their training data include and what uncertainties there may be about the procedure of the algorithmic inference. These representations can create an illusion of trust and inspire practitioners to trust systems that might not be prepared to meet their unique body, psychological, and cultural requirements.

Satya also reaches the area of transparency of data. In cases where practitioners do not have detailed information as to what data is being collected, how it gets processed and the eventual purpose of the data end use the ethical basis of the practitioner-system relationship is undermined. The intransparent nature of data pipelines, proprietary algorithm, and hidden secondary data purposes lead to a gap between the practitioner knowledge and the actual functioning of the system. This dissent is a breach of satya where the partial, strategic, or ambiguous disclosure is replaced with a truthful disclosure. Synoptically, this cloudiness interferes with the cultivation of awareness and discernment, substituting thinking activity with the reliance on systems the inner mechanics of which remain obscure.

In addition, satya is presented with a particularly difficult challenge by algorithmic inference. AI systems are more and more providing predictive insights into practitioners that go beyond plainly known data, such as the inferences about emotional state, habits, or vulnerabilities. Although such inferences can be technically advanced, they present ethical issues when they are dealt with as objective and authoritative truths. Satya warns against confusing the outputs of the algorithm and the reality on the ground, pointing out that information between data is situated, partial and interpretive in all times. Provided yoga AI systems offer inferred understandings without the proper contextualization or the epistemic humility, they are likely to reify computational interpretations as the ultimate truth, which will mislead practitioners in their self-understanding and destroy the reflective intentions of yoga practice(Dsouza et al., 2024).

6.2 Aparigraha, Mindfulness, and Opposition to Data Extractivism.

AI systems should not and cannot ethically aligned design support mindful engagement but instead enhance it. This involves the opposition to the intrusive data practices that disaggregate attention or cause enduring evaluative stress. It is also the design of consent, feedback and interaction, which is not based on compliance but reflection. Yogic viewpoint The mindfulness is not solely able to thrive in a setting that conceals power hierarchies, submerges the participants with data streams, or emphasizes unremitting quantification over the experiences. Transparency, restraint and deliberate design are therefore, not only considerations of usability but ethical necessities that are based on the development of awareness(Haryanto et al., 2024).

A combination of ahimsa, satya, aparigraha, and mindfulness makes up a complete and internally-rooted system of ethics to discuss the moral congruence of yoga AI applications. They show that data misconducts in ethics are not the fringes or fringe benefits but hit at the very center of what yoga strives to achieve: non-harm, veracity, restraint, and awareness. The AI systems threaten the integrity of yoga practice by infringing on these values via opaque surveillance, over-collecting data, misinstruction, and misrepresentation, which removes the trust among yoga. Making data governance and system design consistent with yogic ethics, on the other hand, makes the prospect of technologies that actually help to promote well-being without sacrificing moral integrity. This alignment goes hand in hand with a long-term and ongoing ethical personal contemplation and institutional engagement and acknowledges that yoga AI is not only a technological innovation but also a moral discipline that exists through a dense and longstanding tradition of philosophical thought(Jain et al., 2025).

7. YOGA AI REGULATORY AND LEGAL PROVISIONS

The issue of privacy, data safety, and consent in AI-based yoga is not solvable using moral philosophy, nor a technical design, but rather is explicitly influenced by legal and regulatory contexts in which these systems are created and implemented. Since AI-based yoga platforms are becoming available to run in different jurisdictions and to process intimate embodied and affective data, and to blur traditional lines between health, wellness, education, and cultural practice, governance issues are inevitable and complicated. The current regulatory frameworks have been mostly designed to accommodate the established medical technologies or well-established processes of data-processing, and they are ill-suited to accommodate the hybrid nature of yoga AI systems. It is in this section that the suitability and inadequacy of the existing data protection and AI governance frameworks is critically assessed and that the failures of these frameworks have prompted the application of the domain-sensitive regulatory solutions that acknowledge the ethical, embodied, and cultural particularity of yoga as a practice mediated by artificial intelligence(Setiawati et al., 2020).

7.1 Applicability and Limits of Existing Data Protection Laws.

The most powerful and well-rounded regulatory framework that is currently in place is the General Data Protection Regulation (GDPR), which is widely used as a reference point of ethical AI practices regarding the worldwide arena. Its fundamental values, including lawfulness, fairness, transparency, purpose limitation, data minimization, accuracy, storage limitation and integrity, seem, at least in theory, to be appropriate in alleviating most of the privacy risks involved in yoga AI platforms. It is specifically relevant to the provisions that cover special types of personal data, such as biometric and health-related data, as such data is physiological, behavioral, and even psychological and processed by these systems. The focus of GDPR on informed consent, data subject rights and institutional accountability therefore presents an apparently strong platform on which the data exploitative, opaque, or unsafe practices in yoga can be guarded.

However, a more in-depth look shows that there are substantial weaknesses when trying to use GDPR to apply to yoga AI ecosystems. One of the main challenges is the ambiguity of the legal status of yoga-related data. Although some of the data sets, including heart rate variability, posture tracking, or injury-related coordination, may be considered health data in accordance with GDPR, a significant part of what yoga AI produces lies between wellness, lifestyle, and self-optimization in the regulatory gray area. Most platforms specifically place themselves as not part of the medical field in order to escape increased regulatory attention, despite the fact that they are conducting constant tracking of body movement, breathing, and mental conditions. The given strategic placement will allow yoga AI providers to enjoy a relatively reduced weight of regulatory obligations yet still process the data that can significantly influence the physical security and psychological wellbeing of users.

The constraints of GDPR are even more intense when they are regarded with respect to AI-based inference. Despite the fact that GDPR demands the consent be informed and specific, its dominant model of consent is tied to various discrete data collection points. In comparison, yoga AIs constantly create new knowledge using machine learning, and their inferred data either includes the emotional state, the profile of stress, behavioral inclination, or performance prediction. Such inferences can be new personal information, which was not directly given by the practitioner or was not reasonably predictable at the time of consent to them. Although GDPR has a clause that deals with profiling and automated decision-making, its functional mechanisms to control the practice of continuous, on-the-fly inference are under-developed, especially in technologies aimed at consumers that implement wellness where enforcement is not consistent and has been sporadic(Sharma & Sharma, 2024).

These challenges are further worsened by cross-jurisdictional operation. Yoga AI platforms are often traffic-gathered by users in various countries, are based on cloud systems located all over the world, and are composed of third-party analytics or advertising services which can be subject to different legal frameworks. In places where GDPR is claimed to have extraterritorial application, as opposed to non-European organizations, it is hard to enforce. The disjointed national strategies of data protection and AI regulation allow regulatory arbitrage and unequal protection of users. Ethically, this disintegration compromises the yogic quality of satya, or truthfulness, in that it renders unclear the reality of the data processing, sharing and protection(Setiawati et al., 2020).

7.2 Governance Fissures and Regulatory Domain Requirements.

Cultural sensitivity is another aspect that is mostly unavailable in traditional forms of regulation. Yoga AI systems tend to codify specific understandings of yoga as a set of uniform algorithmic frameworks, which may be rather discriminatory of other traditions and pedagogies. This issue could be solved through governance structures that promote participatory control measures, which will entail yoga practitioners, teachers, cultural scholars and ethicists. Even though these participatory models are not widespread in data protection law, they echo with yogic cultures of collective learning, reflexivity and shared responsibility(Alanezi, 2024).

After all, the argument of domain-specific governance of yoga AI is based on the fact that law is not just a risk management tool, but an articulation of values. Regulatory frameworks should be sensitive to the ethical imperatives that define yoga to ensure that the introduction of yoga AI systems will not compromise the real wellbeing but enhance it. This necessitates some form of legal imaginations that will traverse technology, morals and cultural insights. With the recognition of the distinctive moral field of yoga AI, regulators can contribute to the pursuit of innovation in a way that does not contradict human rights as well as yogic principles and, therefore, preconditions the creation of trusting, culturally sensitive, and sustainable usage in the digital era(Silas, 2024).

8. PRESERVING YOGA AI SYSTEM PRIVACY

With the continued multiplication of yoga AI apps into consumer wellness and clinical and mixed pedagogical systems, ethical issues related to privacy, data safety, and consent require more anticipatory, than reactive, answers. Post hoc and regulatory compliance, being the relevant elements of responsible deployment, are still inadequate at dealing with the more profound moral consequences of integrating artificial intelligence into the set of practices that are already embodied, introspective, and transformative in nature. In this respect, privacy-preserving design does not appear as a technical approach but as an ethical value system--a system that places the respect of practitioner autonomy, respect and wellbeing at the heart of system design and interactional rationality(Zaheer, n.d.).

This designing paradigm is a radical break with the previously held concept of privacy as an external limitation to the more recent concept of privacy as a defining feature of ethical practice. In yoga AI systems, where data capture is no longer confined to observable behavior, but also to biometric indicators and affective states, and reconstructed patterns of embodiment, design decisions have an active role in defining the moral conditions with which practice is practiced. Such decisions are not ethically neutral as seen through the eyes of yoga. They are formulations of value, in which values like ahimsa (non-harm), mindfulness, and aparigraha (restraint) are put into computation. In turn, privacy-preserving design should be perceived as a balance between technological innovation and ethical integrity, which conforms the functionality of a system to ethical obligations that characterize yoga as a wholesome practice(Akashi, 2024).

8.1 Privacy and Security by Design Technical Strategies.

Federated learning builds upon the informational concept of decentralization; however, it allows AI models to be trained on distributed devices without having to unify raw data in a central location. Rather, the model updates are exchanged on a local basis and the privacy of individual data points can be maintained whilst facilitating collective learning. This style in yoga AI systems provides an attractive trade-off between customization and confidentiality where systems can be tailored to various bodies, capabilities, and traditions without collecting intimate information about practitioners. In theory, federated learning is consistent with the yogic principles of group development that acknowledges individual wholeness. However, it is not unethically simple. The problems with the spread of bias, the security of communications, and decreased transparency should be maintained through constant monitoring to make sure that decentralization does not stretch accountability and blur responsibility(Liu & Guo, 2024).

All these technical approaches show that privacy and security do not have to be considered as a trade-off to the effectiveness of a system. Instead, they demonstrate that ethical design can be a strong source of innovation, which can create yoga AI systems that are both resilient, reliable, and philosophically consistent with the ethical principles of practice(KB, 2025).

8.2 Culturally Sensitive System Design and Ethical UX.

The feedback mechanisms also require special attention of ethics. Artificial intelligence-based yoga systems often transpose bodily movement into the continuous assessive responses, remedial information, or performance measures. Although this type of feedback can be helpful in learning and injury prevention, it comes with the dangers of creating dependency, anxiety or self-surveillance when it is implemented without reflection. Ethical UX design attempts to reconcile direction and freedom, such that the feedback is used to encourage self-knowledge, as opposed to outside opinion. The harmony is a reflection of the yogic goal of developing inner discernment (viveka), which places AI in the role of assistant and not judge. Privacy-preserving design is linked to this goal because it minimises the use of excess data mining or black box inferential results(Conde & Svantesson, 2024).

The last, but not the least, the privacy-preserving design in yoga AI systems can be perceived not as a limited number of methods but as an ethical approach that incorporates technical architecture, user experience, and cultural sensitivity. Developers can design AI-mediated systems by incorporating the yogic values in the system logic and interactional design, which, at the same time, honor the intimacy of the practice without being reckless in utilizing technological affordances. Such integration creates the basis of trust, sustainability, and ethical legitimacy and proves that the privacy-saving design is something that the future of the digital era yoga cannot do without(Ng et al., 2024).

9. BELONGING, SUSTAINABLE ADOPTION AND TRUST

The usage of artificial intelligence in yoga practice cannot be sufficiently explained in terms of usability, efficiency, or technical accuracy. Instead, it is an inherently moral and social process where trust is used to mediate between the practitioners, digital systems and the communities where yoga is practiced and transmitted. In contrast to the traditional consumer-facing technologies, yoga AI platforms touch on very personal spheres of human experience, including physiological processes, embodied movement, emotional regulation, and, in certain instances, spiritual self-exploration. This increased intimacy makes trust a prerogative of adoption and not an incidental result of technical performance(Yoga Ratnam, 2025).

In this context, trust is beyond operational conceptions of system reliability or functional correctness. It is rather a socio-technical and ethical creation, which is informed by transparency, accountability, cultural legitimacy, and consistency with the moral underpinning of yoga. The sustainability of yoga AI then lies not in technological advancement only, but the ability of the systems to foster a sense of belonging, continuity and wellbeing. Devoid of such ethical and social foundation, even technically sophisticated platforms will be left to be marginal, superficial, or disruptively active to the true practice of yoga(Rachakonda et al., 2020a).

Figure 3. Privacy-preserving design in yoga AI systems

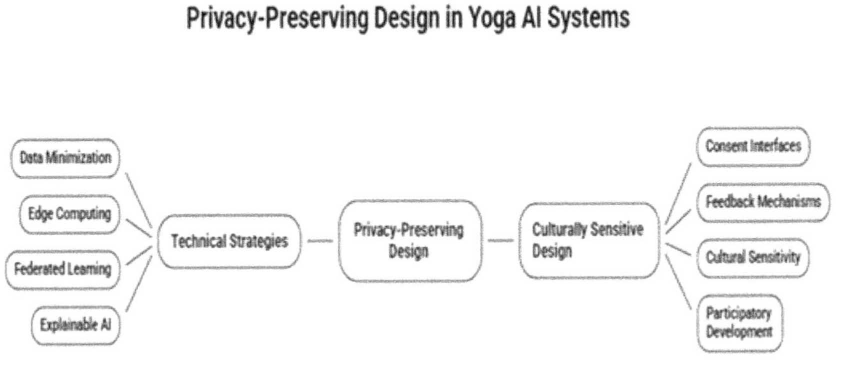

9.1 Trust as a Social-Technical and Ethical Construct

The levels of trust in yoga AI systems exist in interdependent technical, ethical, and social dimensions, which support or deny each other. At the closest level, technical trust assumes the stable and correct system performance. Algorithms need to be able to give accurate posture, breath and physiological practices interpretation to provide contextually suitable feedback that is physically safe. Mistakes in posture detection, incorrectly set breathing instructions, or incorrect biometric information interpretation may not solely decrease user confidence but also cause a physical harm or mental suffering. In embodied practice like yoga, technical failure therefore has ethical impacts, which is where the line between system error and harm to a practitioner is merged.

However, technical reliability as much as it is needed is not adequate to maintain trust in the long run. The ethics of trust depends on the manner in which channels gather, handle and regulate yoga related information, most of which is in a unique form of sensitivity and inference. The practitioners should be assured that their physical, emotional, and behavioral information are used ethically, are not misused, and do not become the subject of unknown and unannounced monetization or third-party usage. In the case of unclear data practices or simply procedural consent mechanisms, trust will be broken, and the ethical integrity of the platform will be questioned. In this regard, ethical trust cannot exist without the meaningful transparency and the clear respect to the practitioner autonomy.

A social-technical approach also adds to the argument that trust is not necessarily enshrined in algorithms alone, but is constructed through constant interaction between users, technologic systems and social environments on a larger scale. Relational authenticity, intentionality and moral coherence are attributes which yoga communities, both of the traditional and digitally mediated nature, attribute a higher value to. To receive trust in such circumstances, the work of AI systems has to be readable and morally appealing. Explainable AI (XAI) strategies are especially important in that respect because they make it possible to make algorithmic processes understandable to users. By having the ability to perceive how posture adjustments are being made, reasons behind the preference of certain feedback, and the types of conclusions being made on their behalf by the technology, users are in a better position to interact with it in a more thoughtful manner than in a passive one(Rajendran & Sethuraman, 2023).

More importantly, the confidence in yoga AI is also measured in the terms of the ethical standards set by the yogaic philosophy itself. Like ahimsa (non-harm) and satya (truthfulness), principles serve as normative points of reference in a manner in which a practitioner evaluates digital systems. These values are more aligned with platforms that provide non-obtrusive guidance, do not engage in manipulative engagement strategies, and have accuracy and honesty in the feedback they provide. On the other hand, systems that promote engagement measures, commerce optimization, or overuse of data mining at the expense of practitioner wellbeing run the risk of flouting fundamental ethical anticipations. This kind of misalignment does not only damage trust in the technology, it also criticizes the perceived authenticity of the practice that it mediates.

Trust is then to be perceived as relational and temporal as opposed to being static. Initial acceptance can be affected by branding, endorsements, or credibility but long term acceptance will be as a result of ethical performance over time. The ongoing ethical relationship is through responsiveness to the concerns of the users, clear communication on updates to the system as well as the provisions of feedback and redress mechanisms. It is important to note as well that this temporal aspect of trust reflects the gradual, repetitive development of awareness that is at the core of the traditional yoga practice. A platform that does not recognize this relationship continuity may experience shallow interaction, premature abandonment or instrumentalization of work, thus contributing to the failure of long-term sustainability(-Fabbrizio et al., 2023).

9.2 Community Development and Long-term sustainability.

One of the ways of enhancing this collective trust is through the involvement of governance mechanisms. Sites which seek practitioner feedback on policies of data governance, algorithmic agendas or content curation imply respect to user agency and collective ownership of practice. These techniques of participation are compatible with the relational spirit of yoga culture that can bring the values of conversation and responsibility into the digital realm. Through the integration of practitioner insights into design and control, platforms are able to increase the social legitimacy and generate ethical loop-backs that can respond to emerging issues(Dittakavi et al., 2022).

Altogether, ethical alignment, relational engagement, and cultural legitimacy should be involved in the trust of yoga AI. It requires technical dependability, but equally long-term consideration of moral and social aspects of embodied practice. Through the development of trust as a socio-technical and ethical category, as well as the establishment of a sense of belonging and collective wellbeing, the AI yoga system can assist the types of adoption that are not only sustainable, but also loyal to the integrity and dignity of yoga itself. Ethical AI in this field is thus a necessity and not an add-on or competitive advantage: a basic requirement of the possibility of significant, long-term interaction with technologies that interfere with the most intimate aspects of human experience(Raval et al., 2022).

10. CONCLUSIONS

The fast development of artificial intelligence in the practice of yoga has put the issue of ethics at the edges of the technological discussion and brought it to its core. Convergence of AI with yoga, as this chapter has illustrated, requires an integrative paradigm through which ethics, technology and economy of yoga are constitutive elements of designing, governing and adopting such literature. Privacy, data security, and consent cannot be pushed to the regulatory checklists or technical appendix, instead, they serve as preconditions of the maintenance of the moral, bodily, and spiritual integrity of yoga as such. The issue of AI-mediated yoga, as opposed to most other aspects of digital innovation, directly involves the body, mental conditions, and self-reflection of the practician, which makes the breach of ethical standards especially meaningful. Ethical stewardship, though, cannot simply stay within the procedural compliance or algorithmic optimization but operate in relation to the relational, experience and philosophical aspects that state yoga as a whole practice.

REFERENCES

. Akashi, A. (2024). Inner landscapes: An autoethnographic journey of meditation and AI-generated digital artworks from an yoga psychology perspective

Alanezi, F. (2024). Assessing the Effectiveness of ChatGPT in Delivering Mental Health Support: A Qualitative Study. *Journal of Multidisciplinary Healthcare*, *17*, 461–471. DOI: 10.2147/JMDH.S447368

. Alonge, M., & Isreal, O. (2025). Fine-Tuning Big Transfer Models for Real-Time Yoga Posture Feedback.

. Bavli, I., Ho, A., Mahal, R., & McKeown, M. J. (2025). Ethical concerns around privacy and data security in AI health monitoring for Parkinson's disease

. Biswas, A. A., Zulfiker, M. S., Rahman, M. M., Jani, M. R., & Anwar, M. M. (2025). Data privacy and security analysis for mental health chatbot applications. 2025 20th ACM/IEEE

. Chelishcheva, E. (2023). Innovation in the Yoga and Ayurveda Industry: Exploring the role of technology and entrepreneurship.

. Chittimalla, S. K., & Potluri, L. K. M. (2025). Enhancing Yoga Pose Recognition Using Large Language Models with Real-World Dataset Integration for Personalized Fitness Assistance.

Conde, J., & Svantesson, D. J. B. (2024). The five generations of facial recognition usage and the Australian privacy law. *International Data Privacy Law*, *14*(3), 247–258. DOI: 10.1093/idpl/ipae007

Dhinakaran, D., Raja, S. E., Jasmine, J. J., Kumar, P. V., & Ramani, R. (2025). The Future of Well-Being: AI-Powered Health Management with Privacy at its Core. In B. Bhushan, A. Khanday, K. Aurangzeb, S. K. Sharma, & P. Nand (Eds.)

Dittakavi, B., Bavikadi, D., Desai, S. V., Chakraborty, S., Reddy, N., Balasubramanian, V. N., Callepalli, B., & Sharma, A. (2022). Pose tutor: An explainable system for pose correction in the wild. *Proceedings of the IEEE/CVF Conference on Computer Vision and Pattern Recognition*, 3540–3549. DOI: 10.1109/CVPRW56347.2022.00398

. Dsouza, S. M., Gadwal, J. M., Darshan, S., Rai, R., & Helena, V. (2024). Manas–Weaving Tech and Science for Mental WellBeing-A Survey Paper. Grenze International Journal of Engineering & Technology (GIJET), 10.

. Fabbrizio, A., Fucarino, A., Cantoia, M., De Giorgio, A., Garrido, N. D., Iuliano, E., Reis, V. M., Sausa, M., Vilaça-Alves, J., & Zimatore, G. (2023). Smart devices for health and wellness applied to tele-exercise

Ganesh, K., & Ramudhin, A. (2024). Leveraging AI to Mitigate Risks in Yoga Practice: A Real-Time Posture Correction Application. *Proceedings of the 12th International Conference on Sport Sciences Research and Technology Support*, 241–250. DOI: 10.5220/0013063300003828

Gosalia, M., Dedhia, R., Doshi, S., Sharma, R., & Mangla, M. (2024). Individualized Guidance in Yoga Practice: A Comparative Analysis of Technology Solutions. *2024 International Conference on Electrical Electronics and Computing Technologies (ICEECT)*, 1, 1–6. DOI: 10.1109/ICEECT61758.2024.10739307

Hanwari, E., Kanani, J., Bhavsar, Y., & Shah, N. (2024). AI Based Personal Yoga Assistant. *2024 IEEE International Conference on Interdisciplinary Approaches in Technology and Management for Social Innovation (IATMSI)*, 2, 1–5.

Haryanto, C. Y., Vu, M. H., Nguyen, T. D., Lomempow, E., Nurliana, Y., & Taheri, S. (2024). SecGenAI: Enhancing Security of Cloud-based Generative AI Applications within Australian Critical Technologies of National Interest (arXiv:2407.01110). arXiv.

Irfan, N., Zafar, S., Shakil, K. A., Wani, M. A., Kumar, S. N., Jaiganesh, A., & Abubeker, K. M. (2025). Integrating AI predictive analytics with naturopathic and yoga-based interventions in a data-driven preventive model to improve maternal mental health and pregnancy outcomes. *Scientific Reports*, *15*(1), 23878. DOI: 10.1038/s41598-025-07885-8

Jain, I., Srivastava, R., Srivastava, V., Sinha, V., & Juneja, A. (2025). Ethical Decision-Making in Yoga Posture Detection through AI: Fostering Responsible Technology Integration. In Juneja, S., Dhanaraj, R. K., Juneja, A., Sathyamoorthy, M., & Shaikh, A. (Eds.), *Ethical Decision-Making Using Artificial Intelligence* (1st ed., pp. 99–123). Wiley. DOI: 10.1002/9781394275311.ch5

Jebamikyous, H., Li, M., Suhas, Y., & Kashef, R. (2023). Leveraging machine learning and blockchain in E-commerce and beyond: Benefits, models, and application. *Discover Artificial Intelligence*, *3*(1), 3. DOI: 10.1007/s44163-022-00046-0

. KB, L. S. (2025). TECH YOGA: THE SMART MAT REVOLUTION. I-Manager's Journal on Embedded Systems, 13(2).

Liu, S., & Guo, L. R. (2024). Data ownership in the AI-powered integrative health care landscape. *JMIR Medical Informatics*, *12*, e57754. DOI: 10.2196/57754

Murphy, A., Bowen, K., Naqa, I. M. E., Yoga, B., & Green, B. L. (2025). Bridging Health Disparities in the Data-Driven World of Artificial Intelligence: A Narrative Review. *Journal of Racial and Ethnic Health Disparities*, *12*(4), 2367–2379. DOI: 10.1007/s40615-024-02057-2

Ng, J. Y., Cramer, H., Lee, M. S., & Moher, D. (2024). Traditional, complementary, and integrative medicine and artificial intelligence: Novel opportunities in healthcare. *Integrative Medicine Research*, *13*(1), 101024. DOI: 10.1016/j.imr.2024.101024

Özsezer, G., & Mermer, G. (2025). Real-Time Prediction of Correct Yoga Asanas in Healthy Individuals With Artificial Intelligence Techniques: A Systematic Review for Nursing. *Nursing Open*, *12*(8), e70278. DOI: 10.1002/nop2.70278

Pal, R., Adhikari, D., Heyat, M. B. B., Ullah, I., & You, Z. (2023). Yoga meets intelligent internet of things: Recent challenges and future directions. *Bioengineering (Basel, Switzerland)*, *10*(4), 459. DOI: 10.3390/bioengineering10040459

Rachakonda, L., Bapatla, A. K., Mohanty, S. P., & Kougianos, E. (2020a). SaYoPillow: A Blockchain-Enabled, Privacy-Assured Framework for Stress Detection, Prediction and Control Considering Sleeping Habits in the IoMT (arXiv:2007.07377). arXiv.

Rajendran, A. K., & Sethuraman, S. C. (2023). A survey on yogic posture recognition. *IEEE Access : Practical Innovations, Open Solutions*, *11*, 11183–11223. DOI: 10.1109/ACCESS.2023.3240769

Raval, H. Y., Parikh, S. M., & Patel, H. R. (2022). Self-maintained health surveillance artificial intelligence assistant. In Handbook of Research on Lifestyle Sustainability and Management Solutions Using AI, Big Data Analytics, and Visualization (pp. 168–184). IGI Global Scientific Publishing. DOI: 10.4018/978-1-7998-8786-7.ch010

Setiawati, D., Hakim, H. A., & Yoga, F. A. H. (2020). Optimizing personal data protection in Indonesia: Lesson learned from China, South Korea, and Singapore. *Indonesian Comparative Law Review*, *2*(2), 95–109. DOI: 10.18196/iclr.2219

Sharma, A. K., & Sharma, R. (2024). Comparative Analysis of Data Protection Laws and ai Privacy Risks in brics Nations: A Comprehensive Examination. *Global Journal of Comparative Law*, *13*(1), 56–85.

. Shaumya, S., & Kumar, R. (2025). Artificial Intelligence in Ayurveda: A Systematic. Journal of Ayurveda and Naturopathy, 2(2), 05–19.

Sikarwar, K., Venu, N., Dubey, A., & Bisen, D. (2025). AI-Based System for Real-Time Yoga Pose Detection and Correction. 2025 IEEE International Students' *Conference on Electrical, Electronics and Computer Science (SCEECS)*, 1–6.

. Silas, N. (2024). AI in Chemistry: The Future of Scientific Discovery. The Scientific Spectrum of AI Enhancing The Future, 192.

Singh, A., & Vats, A. (2025). Safe and Trusted Artificial Intelligence: Privacy as the cornerstone for digital transformation in Traditional Medicine. *International Journal of Ayurveda Research*, *6*(4), 286–292. DOI: 10.4103/ijar.ijar_340_25

Sinha, N., & Sinha, R. K. (2024). Harnessing the Potential of Artificial Intelligence in Yoga Therapy. *International Journal of Yoga*, *17*(3), 242–245. DOI: 10.4103/ijoy.ijoy_124_24

Tripathi, R. L. (2025). AI Meets Mindfulness: Redefining Spirituality and Meditation in the Digital Age. *The Voice of Creative Research*, *7*(1), 17–26. DOI: 10.53032/tvcr/2025.v7n1.03

Vallabhaneni, N., & Prabhavathy, P. (2021). The analysis of the impact of yoga on healthcare and conventional strategies for human pose recognition. *Turkish Journal of Computer and Mathematics Education*, *12*(6), 1772–1783. DOI: 10.17762/turcomat.v12i6.4032

Venkatasubramanian, A. (2023). A digital health trust framework guided by values from the science of yoga. *Oxford Open Digital Health*, *1*, oqad007. DOI: 10.1093/oodh/oqad007

Verma, P., Sharma, R., & Rajput, N. S. (2023). Enhancing yoga practice through real-time posture detection and correction using artificial intelligence: A comprehensive review. *NeuroQuantology : An Interdisciplinary Journal of Neuroscience and Quantum Physics*, *21*(6), 1053.

Yoga Ratnam, K. K. (2025). Generative artificial intelligence in public health research and scientific communication: A narrative review of real applications and future directions. *Digital Health*, *11*, 20552076251362070. DOI: 10.1177/20552076251362070

Zaheer, S. (n.d.). Designing Emotion-Aware UX: Leveraging Sentiment Analysis to Adapt Digital Experiences. Retrieved January 13, 2026

Chapter 6

Exploring the Impact of AI on the Growth of Yogasana as a Global Competitive Sport

Tanya Gandhi
Lovely Professional University, India

Harmanpreet Kaur
Lovely Professional University, India

Amrik Singh
http://orcid.org/0000-0003-3598-8787
Lovely Professional University, India.

ABSTRACT

With its wellness and spiritual origins, Yogasana is fast becoming a competitive sport in the world. Along with this change, there is the necessity of precision, fairness, and training approaches that are scientifically oriented. Artificial Intelligence (AI) is becoming an effective solution to fulfill these needs because it allows moving tracking, real-time posture correction, performance evaluation based on data, and automated judges. AI-driven applications and wearable technologies are used to deliver individualized training plans, avoid injuries, and improve the accuracy of scoring, and online platforms increase the accessibility of the sport around the world by hosting online competitions and communicating in different languages. Even though the studies involving AI usage in yogasana are scarce, the experience

DOI: 10.4018/979-8-2600-2463-8.ch006

of other sports involving precision proves that it can transform the sphere of athlete development, increase the consistency of judges, and assist with international promotion, even with an opportunity to participate in the Olympics.

INTRODUCTION

Yoga has a history of development, starting around 5,000 years ago, in the Indus valley, and being deeply embedded in the religious and cultural traditions of the ancient Indians (Dhankhar & Sharma, 2023). Initial yoga disciplines were around ancient sages who led sedentary lives of performing ritual activities, such as meditation and yajna, with their diet made predominantly of forest vegetarian food (Padhi, 2016). After 200 BCE, Patanjali codified classical yoga and created moral codes of practice, yoga poses (asanas), breathing (pranayama) and meditation (Dhankhar & Sharma, 2023). Over the centuries, yoga was differentiated into different schools such as Hatha, Bhakti, Jnanayoga and Karma yoga (Dhankhar & Sharma, 2023). Its international fame started to emerge at the end of the 19th and the early 20th centuries, with the help of such personalities as Swami Vivekananda or Paramahansa Yogananda (Dhankhar & Sharma, 2023). The contemporary yoga has developed into a popular practice in the global market, but there are various modernized forms of the practice, and it has been scientifically acknowledged to have therapeutic effects within health care systems (Dhankhar & Sharma, 2023; Jugran, 2024). Yogasanas are now used in the treatment of different conditions, and gynecological disorders are amongst them (Jugran, 2024). The introduction of the Yogasana as a competitive sport has its origin in its ancient Indian form besides its adaptation to the athletic environment. In the 20th century, postural yoga was modernized, legitimizing yoga practice, which previously did not focus on postural practice, and was made accessible by Shri Yogendra and Swami Kuvalayananda (Singleton, 2013). The modern studies also emphasize that yoga helps athletes to develop muscle balance, flexibility, and prevent injuries, offers better mental attention and stress reduction due to breathwork and connection with the mind (Rahul, 2023; Basireddy et al., 2023). Yoga has been adopted as an addition, a remedial, and restorative aid in sports training, which helps in warm-up, cool-down, and total performance. These advances have led to the acceptance of Yogasana as competitive sport in terms of physical and psychological benefits to the sporting athletes. The transformation of yogasana as a traditional wellness program to a full-fledged competitive sport has been a well-formulated process with the aim of preserving the culture and an urge to expand to different parts of the world. Whereas traditional Yoga is a holistic combination of spiritual, psychological, and physical practices, the introduction of Yogasana Sport involves a synergy of the physical expression of the asanas (pose) based on its challenge, balancing, mastery, flexibility, and stamina. The official change has received considerable momentum, with the policy acknowledgement in India, specifically, in December 2020, the ministry of Youth Affairs and Sports officially acknowledged yogasana as a competitive sport. The main move that was made with the consultation of the Ministry of AYUSH allows the given discipline to enjoy governmental funding, be featured in the national sporting plans, and have the infrastructure and approaches that are implemented in relation to other officially recognized sport types ().

The key element in the sport institutionalization is the National Yogasana Sports Federation (NYSF) that was formed to preserve and develop yogasana as a competitive sport and is accredited by the ministry of youth affairs and sports. Structuring the competition, including the creation of an exhaustive rulebook, a syllabus and an automated scoring system is a critical task that has been undertaken by the NYSF and its international counterparts, World Yogasana, to bring about objectivity and professionalism to the competition. This framework establishes different categories of events of both the male and female gender, including Traditional Yogasana, Artistic Yogasana (Single and Pair), and Rhythmic Yogasana (Pair and Group), with certain numbers of medals suggested. It is a critical component needed to make this structure acceptable in large-scale events (Sharma et al., 2024). Yogasana Sport is an actively seeking organization in its global expansion using its presence at major national multi-sport events and a long-term international presence objective. Yogasana has also been introduced into the Khelo India Youth Games and the National Games which has been an exposure to the emerging athletes and has helped the sport gain more popularity, especially among the youth. Internationally the setting up of World Yogasana body and hosting events such as the Asian Yogasana Championship, and the proposed World Yogasana Sport Championship are some of the important strategies to expand internationally. The final goal is to make yogasana an Olympic-style sport with the ancient Indian tradition positioned as a competitive sport around the world and an effective tool in spreading health and wellness, as well as a flourishing wellness economy, to the whole world.

REVIEW OF LITERATURE

Artificial Intelligence in the Sporting Performance

The field of sports performance analysis and training is being transformed by artificial intelligence in numerous aspects. The application of AI technologies, such as machine learning algorithms, computer vision systems, and predictive analytics, is changing the way athletes and coaches view the process of performance optimization

(Pisaniello, 2024). Such systems improve the accuracy of performance monitoring of athletes, facilitate real-time coaching decision-making, and optimize the injury prevention process on the basis of biomechanical data (Pisaniello, 2024; Sharma et al., 2024). Artificial Intelligence is also disrupting the sports game as it changes the training, strategy and health of athletes through the latest analysis of data. In its simplest form, AI is based on Machine Learning and Computer Vision to process speedy loads of data (collected by wearable sensors and high-speed cameras) to provide unexpectedly better insights than humans can. Within the scope of performance analysis, AI can follow all the movements of a soccer player and sprint speed or position to a baseball player and the mechanics of its swings to see even the slightest technical errors and the ability to improve. Importantly, currently, AI models play a significant role in injury prevention, examining the workload, fatigue rate, and injury history of an athlete to forecast a greater risk of getting a soft tissue injury so that coaches could make proactive changes to the training and recovery regimen. In addition to the individual athlete, AI optimises game strategy via analysis of extensive historical video footage to determine the presence of complex opponent tendencies and simulating game situations to provide teams with a convincing competitive advantage. Basically, AI is a performance companion, an objective, and end-all-seeing robot that takes the sporting capabilities of human beings to the extremes by making training smarter, safer, and more accurate. AI applications in team sports contribute greatly to the management of training load, analysis of sport performance, injury prevention, recognition of talents, and the monitoring of the well-being of athletes (Mateus et al., 2024). In the case of individual sports, machine learning, deep learning, and computer vision can be used to provide personalized training programs, performance feedback, and assessment of the risk of injuries (Bodemer, 2023). The ecological dynamics model shows how AI can be used to read patterns of sport performances and calculate effective practice situations in different sports such as football, golf, and climbing (Araujo et al., 2021). Although such innovations exist, there are also issues with the interpretability of the AI model, data privacy ethics, and the need to balance between automated systems and human knowledge (Pisaniello, 2024; Mateus et al., 2024).

Technology in Yogasana Practice

The use of technology in the practice of yogasana has become one of the focus of research and has taken advantage of artificial intelligence and computer vision to supplement the traditional yoga teaching. The latest research shows the combination of deep learning models such as PoseNet, OpenPose, and LSTM networks to the systems of real-time pose recognition and correction (Tyagi et al., 2024). The concept of technology is deeply engaging with and enriching the age-old exercise of Yogasana and making it more user-friendly, customized, and more specific to the contemporary student of the practice (Nuong et al., 2024). This incorporation is largely motivated by the Artificial Intelligence (AI) and affiliated Internet of things (IoT) gadgets. AI, particularly, Computer Vision, and Machine Learning algorithms are applied to posture real-time detection and correction. The system can scan joint angles and position, comparing the pose of the user with an ideal model to stop injuries and perfect technique, which is a feature traditionally available through one-on-one instructions, but which the system can perform using a smartphone camera or embedded sensors on a smart yoga mat. In addition, wearable technology, e.g., smartwatches and rings, is a seamless one as it tracks such physiological indicators as heart rate, breathing patterns, and stress levels during a session. Through this information, AI will be able to create hyper-personalized yoga practices that will self-adjust to the user based on the current level of physical effort or fatigue or on the user's particular health targets. In addition to the practice at home, Virtual Reality (VR) and Augmented Reality (AR) are developing immersive environments, which enable users to train with AI teachers in simulated peaceful settings, which increase concentration during meditation and make the practice more interactive (Nuong et al., 2024). In reality, technology serves as a smart and non-invasive mirror and a coach, and the information it offers offers an enhanced level of self-awareness and maximizes the physical and mental advantages of yogasana.

Bibliometric analysis demonstrates the consistent increase in the number of researches devoted to this interdisciplinary sphere with the higher contribution of India and the USA, still, there are gaps in the identification of subtle postures and long-term outcomes (Raj et al., 2025). Examples of practical applications are the IoT-driven physiological parameter monitoring systems with body sensors to measure blood pressure, temperature, and heart rate with demonstrable positive effects on health indicators of practitioners (Mani et al., 2017). Convolutional neural networks and transfer learning-based deep learning methods have shown good performance, and systems can identify a yoga pose out of an image and a video frame with an accuracy of 85 percent (Jose & Shailesh, 2021).

AI Training and Athlete Development

Artificial intelligence has become the revolution in the industry of athletic training and athlete development and is transforming the conventional methods with new technologies. AI applications utilize machine learning, computer vision, and data analytics to improve on a number of areas in sports performance (Zhao et al., 2025). The application of AI is fundamentally altering the training and development of para-athletes by offering unprecedented amounts of personalization and precision that is particularly important in terms of the overall variety of body functions and mobility among para classifications (Nuong et al., 2024). It employs such technologies as Computer Vision (video processing) and wearable sensors to conduct real-time biomechanical analysis of movement recognizing minor inefficiencies in technique, such as force distribution on a prosthetic or a wheelchair push, which a human coach would overlook. This data is used as an input to Machine Learning models to produce adaptive training plans, and dynamically change workouts, rest, and select exercises to eliminate overuse injuries, which is a primary issue among para-athletes, and maximize long-term health. Moreover, AI can be used to identify talent by objectively evaluating performance and potential using a large amount of data and can be used to plan strategies by analyzing the behavior of opponents, which, in the end, is a potent tool and can facilitate elite-level coaching and make it more accessible, data-driven, and person-centered. These technologies make it possible to make training schedules personalized so that they maximize performance and minimize the risk of injuries, wearable devices can give real-time physiological data to make immediate adjustments to training (Biro et al., 2024). AI can be used in talent identification and predicting performances through analyzing large volumes of data to identify unseen trends, evaluate injury risks, and offer a customized training program, especially in track and field (Raveena & Rathod, 2024). AI-based applications also provide holistic services such as biomechanical information, refinement of technique with gait analysis, cognition training to make better decisions, and monitoring of well-being (Biro et al., 2024). The level of AI application in individual sports training is beneficial in the form of a personal training program, analysis of performance, and injury prevention models (Bodemer, 2023). The developments presented here indicate how AI is relevant in assisting coaches and athletes to ensure the best performance results (Nuong et al., 2024).

AI in Judging and Performance Scoring

Studies of AI in judging and performance scoring show the areas of opportunities and challenges in various fields. In employee performance appraisal, AI is more consistent and efficient, but with human supervision over aspects of qualitative nature such as leadership and cultural alignment, this results in hybrid models that integrate AI and human judgment (Novrianto et al., 2025). AI is changing the performance scoring and judging of sports particularly those that are based on subjective human judgment such as gymnastics, figure skating, and diving through Computer Vision and 3D sensing technology to offer objective and data-driven assistance. Such systems as the Judging Support System (JSS) created by the International Gymnastics Federation (FIG) record a performance in multiple angles, then convert provide the complex motions of an athlete into numerical form (including joint angles, rotations, and body position), and compare them with a large database of official scoring rules in close real-time. The purpose of using this AI aid is to drastically decrease the human factor and error, enhance technical scoring accuracy, and provide uniformity and fairness in different competitions. Although AI is more of a support, rather than an uprooting tool, to supplement, but not to replace, human judges who still need to determine artistic and subjective merit it provides a valid, real-time frame of reference to coaches contesting a score or officials in split-second scenarios. The same can be stated about competitive sports where there are contradictory tensions associated with the adoption of AI-based evaluation systems, especially in terms of accuracy, objectivity, and the protection of the art of judging (Mazurova et al., 2021). The evidence-centered design models applied in educational assessment are useful in maximizing automated scoring powered by AI by harmonizing construct definitions with AI capabilities and limitations (Ercikan & McCaffrey, 2022). Interpretable AI systems based on rubric-informed segmentation can be used in sports action quality assessment to successfully mimic Olympic judges with clear explanations that build user acceptance and trust (Matsuyama et al., 2023). All these studies are united by the need to preserve the human touch and make AI-based evaluation systems more transparent.

DISCUSSION AND INTERPRETATION

Yogasana: AI Tools and Technologies:

Pose Estimation and Computer Vision Software

The software of computer vision and pose estimation has come up as strong tool of analyzing human movement and posture in most applications. Human pose estimation is a task of estimating and classifying human body joints with the help of deep learning algorithms and has found applications in medicine, sports, augmented reality, and video games (Vyshnivskyi et al., 2023). Computer Vision (CV) is an area of Artificial Intelligence that lets computers read and comprehend data in digital images or video clips, which is essentially training a computer to visually perceive the world around us and be able to process it. The pose estimation software is a dedicated CV application, based on Deep learning, that will identify and localize the position and orientation (a pose) of an object most commonly the human body by precisely identifying a collection of salient points (elbows, knees, wrists, etc.) in two-dimensional or three-dimensional space. These points of detection are linked in the software to form a virtual skeletal structure, which can then be used to analyse movement, posture and action recognition markerlessly either in real-time or on a pre-recorded video. Applications based on this technology are used in several industries, such as performance optimization in sports analytics, rehabilitation exercise monitoring in physical therapy, motion capture in gaming and augmented reality, and others. The discipline contains numerous methodological tools such as model-based, feature-based, direct, hybrid and deep learning-based techniques, each possessing different strong and weak points based on the needs of the application (Sulong & Randles, 2023). More recent applications apply computer vision systems such as OpenCV and MediaPipe to identify pose landmarks on real-time and videos captured in advance. The study by Shah et al. (2023) demonstrated that the BlazePose GHUM 3D model can estimate multi- persons using the model with high accuracy of 96.9% in detecting landmarks. Its practical applications are fitness guidances that give users real-time feedback on exercise posture to allow them to maintain posture and avoid injuries (Rai et al., 2024; Sharma et al., 2024). All these improvements in precision and strength keep establishing progress in robotics, human-computer interaction, and healthcare sectors ().

Smart Sensors and Wearable

The use of wearable sensors and smart devices are becoming common in the practice of yoga in order to improve monitoring and feedback. Several other researchers have come up with IoT-based systems that use body sensors to track such parameters as pressure, temperature, humidity, blood pressure, and heart rate during yoga training (Mani et al., 2017; Prasanna et al., 2017). Yoga is becoming safer, more convenient, and personal with the help of modern technology, which is being built into regular devices with advanced sensors and artificial intelligence (AI). A good example is smart yoga mats, which have pressure sensors and can detect the weight distribution, balance, and posture of a yoga practitioner in real-time and correct the posture immediately through an app or voice recognition or visual visualization to avoid any injury. Along with the mats goes wearable sensors and smart clothing, including yoga theyalands, special bands with Inertial Measurement Units (IMUs) and flex sensors, which detect angles of the joints, positioning of the limbs and micro-movements, with haptic (vibrating) feedback occasionally used to make minor corrections. Moreover, devices are also being specialized in details on yoga, including respiration sensors to track Pranayama (breathing) methods, EEG-enabled headbands to scan the brain to enhance mindfulness and meditation. In the future, AI-based personalization, real-time Virtual Reality (VR) and Augmented Reality (AR) development with 3D instructors, is likely to provide a fully guided, adaptive, and highly engaging practice according to the unique needs of an individual and real-time physiological health. These systems analyze information using smartphones or smart devices and offer real-time recommendations and feedback to practitioners, and the research shows that blood pressure and heart rate have improved following yoga sessions (Mani et al., 2017; Prasanna et al., 2017). High-end applications have smart yoga mats that have pressure sensors, accelerators, and gyroscopes that track movement in positions, balance, and body pressure distribution, which also provide real-time feedback through application interfaces and cloud-based data storage (Pavithra et al., 2025). Other wearable products have been made with specific techniques to track the yogic techniques of breathing such as pranayama, heart rate, posture and breathing patterns to ensure that the techniques are performed correctly (Puranik & K. M, 2019).

VR/ AR Applications

The applications of Virtual Reality (VR) and Augmented Reality (AR) technologies are getting more and more widely used in the healthcare and wellness field. VR involves developing computer-generated simulations that enable dealing with artificial environments in 3D and interprets with specialized equipment, whereas AR superimposes the digital content on real objects in the real world. VR-based systems have been designed in yoga practice, which detects, classifies, and corrects poses, and uses AI in conjunction with immersive experiences, allowing users to receive real-time feedback of poses such as Bridge, Mountain, Downward Dog, and Warrior II . Both Virtual Reality (VR) and Augmented Reality (AR) are transforming yoga in terms of being able to make it more immersive, more accessible, and guide-based, but in different ways. VR provides a headset to take the practitioner to the world of a calming beach or a mountain top, completely simulated and devoid of distraction, making it ideal to enhance the attention in the process of meditation (mindfulness) and relaxation exercises such as Yoga Nidra by eliminating every external stimulus. VR devices are commonly characterized by 3D teacher and avatars allowing one to see their own movement in the virtual reality, even though the total visual block offers safety issues with the risks of dynamic balancing. In comparison, Augmented Reality superimposes the digital environment onto the physical surrounding of a user, normally through a smartphone or smart glasses, which can be considered a powerful benefit regarding safety since it does not blur the real-life awareness. The AR technology is the best to provide an accurate and real time feedback with features such as displaying a 3D holographic instructor or visual attractions on the floor to be followed by foot and hand positioning and proper alignment in asanas (poses). Finally, although VR can give the full immersion to the mind-body connection, AR can offer more practical and visually guided instructions at the home environment, as the two technologies will help bring the future of yoga practice to a more personalized and engaging experience (Ansari & Singh, 2024). In cardiac rehabilitation, VR/AR has a wider medical purpose, using it as a complement to the conventional methods of patients with rehabilitation programs and intensive care. Healthcare uses touch anatomy education, surgery education, pre-procedural planning, intra-surgery guidance, rehabilitation, pain management, and psychology and FDA has started approving clinical applications.

AI for Athlete Development:

Identification of Talents using AI Analytics

Recent studies show that AI use in analyzing the yoga postures and identifying talents has a lot of potential. Yoga machines with AI capabilities are capable of detecting and correcting their pose in real-time, and researchers found that they are highly accurate in recognizing different yogasanas. Convolutional neural network and transfer learning-based deep learning methods were able to predict the yoga postures with 85 percent accuracy on image recognition on 10 different yoga poses. The possibility of AI use in posture analysis in yoga is revolutionary, with computer vision and deep learning as its main opportunities. The pose estimation models (such as OpenPose or MediaPipe) are AI-powered systems that can be used to track key body parts in real-time video streams. Algorithms are then used to process this information to assess joint angles and the relative alignment of the practitioner to the correct and correct orientation of a certain yoga pose (asana). Real-time corrective feedback is the most important application, as the system can become a virtual instructor, whereby immediate feedback is displayed (visual or audio) to correct the faulty alignment and thereby make the practice safe and effective and minimize the risk of getting injured. In addition to correction, AI can allow personalized yoga experience by tracking it, pointing out frequent mistakes, and offering customized practices or adjustments due to physical abilities and limitations of an individual (Nuong et al., 2024). Essentially, AI democratizes the access to expert-level advice which means that quality and personalized yoga instructions can be offered to every user equipped with a camera, thus increasing the safety and ease of home practice. Machine learning can be very effective, as Random Forest Classifiers were able to identify the pose of a yoga person with a 99.04% accuracy using a feature of joint angles obtained as a result of applying the tf-pose estimation algorithms on datasets of more than 5,500 images (Yash Agrawal et al., 2020). Although there seems to be very few studies on the subject of talent identification in yoga using AI analytics, similar studies in the field of track and field have shown the potential of AI in talent detection and predicting performance based on physical endowment, bio-mechanism, and response (Raveena & Rathod, 2024).

Individualized Fitness and Nutrition:

Fitness and Nutrition Plans

The personalized nutrition and fitness applications powered by AI are becoming the revolutionary approach to managing health individually. The systems will use the whole user information such as their age, weight, height, activity, diet type, and health status to come up with the personalized recommendations (Vijayalakshmi & Dharshni, 2025). Machine learning algorithms are used to manipulate complicated datasets that include genetic, phenotypic, and behavioral data to generate highly personalized diets and exercise routines (Ngugi, 2024; Sharma & Gaur, 2024). The field of personalized nutrition and personalized fitness is changing fundamentally due to Artificial Intelligence which is using advanced machine learning (ML) and data analytics to generate more dynamic and highly personalized health plans. These AI-based applications go way beyond sterile, generalized advice and incorporate extensive amounts of personal information, such as goals of the user, preferences in the foods consumed, and instant biometric reading obtained through wearables (heart rate, sleep, activity). With this detailed profile, the AI then applies two fundamental services: hyper-personalized meal planning and adaptive fitness coaching. In nutrition, AI employs such methods as computer vision to simplify food logging based on photo recognition, approximates nutritional values, and continuously changes meal recommendations after learning about the user and their metabolic activity (). To achieve fitness, the system will generate routines that become more challenging (progressive overload) over time and can even estimate poses through the camera of a device to give a real-time and corrective feedback on exercise form, which will dramatically reduce the risk of injury. Simply put, these AI systems provide 24/7, scalable virtual coaching, which provides the sort of ongoing, data-driven assistance that previously could only be achieved through the human one-on-one coaching, or at great expense, and consequently make effective, personal wellness coaching available to a significantly larger population.

The innovative features are the ability to track posture in real-time using such technologies as Mediapipe, progress tracking, and adjustable recommendations, which change according to the feedback of its users. The assessment studies indicate positive outcomes, where systems show 90 percent congruence with professional health plans and 85 percent user satisfaction. Nonetheless, there are still such issues as the privacy of data, model interpretability, variations in tracking accuracy, and the necessity of a strong regulatory framework (Ngugi, 2024; Sharma & Gaur, 2024). The evolution in future can also incorporate genomics and microbiomics, as well as wearable to be even more accurate (Sharma & Gaur, 2024).

Mental Conditioning and Stress Management

Recent studies indicate that AI-based mental health technologies have been made to achieve remarkable progress in terms of stress management and conditioning. Mental Health AI is a full-scale solution as it makes use of deep-learning to determine stress levels by combining various data types such as physiological measurements, sentiment-analysis of social media posts, and demographic data (Bharathi et al., 2024). Anxiety and depression management using AI have the potential to be effective due to chatbots, mobile apps, wearables, virtual reality, and large language models, which provide affordable and customized solutions to complement standard treatment (Pavlopoulos et al., 2024). The use of AI-driven technology is essentially reinventing the mental health landscape by providing the ability to scale and customize mental health stress management and emotional conditioning as never before. These services are mostly relying on Natural Language Processing (NLP), which then analyzes the user input in their chat history, their mood journal, or even voice recorded data to determine sentiment and identify early signs of distress, as well as individual emotional stimuli. At the very heart of their operation is the idea that they will serve as 24/7 virtual coaches/therapists (such as Woebot or Wysa) that provide evidence-based interventions, such as Cognitive Behavioral Therapy (CBT) and mindfulness practices, which are dynamically adjusted in response to the real-time emotional state and progress of the user. Moreover, the wearable device can be integrated with the AI to monitor biometric data, including heart rate variability and sleep quality, which is an objective measure of stress that can be used to supplement self-reported information. This is an iterative data-driven process of feedback that allows the system to condition emotional resilience by offering individualized coping mechanisms and relaxation methods at the time when they are most required, ensuring that effective mental health support is made accessible to everyone and stigma-free everywhere (Al-Romeedy & Singh, 2025). Physiological and behavioral monitoring can be used to identify stress in real-time by integrating IoT devices with AI, although issues have been raised on accuracy, scalability, and privacy of data. Artificial intelligence (AI) stress-sensing applications that track health indicators via sensors and bracelets are effective in an organizational setting as they are beneficial in workplace well-being by the presence of chatbots, virtual therapists, and biofeedback devices. These technologies prove to have the potential of changing mental health support and only human monitoring is needed.

CASE-STUDIES AND REAL-LIFE APPLICATIONS

AI-Based Yoga Apps

Recent studies indicate that there are great improvements in AI-based yoga programs to detect, correct, and individually instruct on postures. In their systematic review of AI-based yoga posture recognition devices, Verma et al. (n.d.) discovered that real-time posture recognition and posture-correcting technologies such as OpenPose and Convolutional Neural Networks are significantly accurate. The COVID-19 pandemic advanced the use of AI-supported yoga applications, and apps offered personalized experiences and feedback to home users in real-time (Agarwal et al., 2022). The use of AI-based yoga apps is transforming the home practice by providing real-time, personalized coaching that greatly improves safety and efficacy, which effectively provides a balance between the pre-recorded video learning and a real teacher. These complex applications use Computer Vision and frequently include applications such as PoseNet or Mediapipe, to scan a live video stream of a user in real-time, accurately tracking key body features and joint angles. The AI will immediately detect any deviation of the posture of the user against the ideal asana (pose) position and provide corrective feedback in real-time, usually via voice-based messages or visual overlays, as in the case of straighten your back or lift your hips higher. In addition to correction, AI algorithms assess user data, such as physical abilities, intentions, and even wearables data such as heart rate to dynamically create personalized yoga routines and plans, making them challenging but safe and changing with the progress of a practitioner. Such a combination of intelligent feedback and hyper-personalization, also applied to such features as progress tracking, customizable duration of classes, and AI-led meditation instructions, transforms expert-level yoga instruction into a highly accessible and affordable service to yoga practitioners of all levels and eventually leads to a more consistent and mindful home practice through self-evaluation and biofeedback processes. In addition to the posture detection, Parab et al. (2023) proposed a new strategy where a personalized yoga recommendation is developed with the help of Game Theory, so that the proposed recommendation is based on the needs of an individual (medical conditions, level of experience, and lifestyle objectives) and is not a one-size-fits-all solution. All these emerging trends make yoga more accessible, safe, and efficient by means of smart technological implementation.

Virtual Yogasana Championships

The virtual yoga presented during the COVID-19 pandemic became one of the most important sources of physical, mental, and spiritual health in the conditions of lockdown. Virtual yoga was done through the use of different digital platforms such as YouTube, Facebook, Instagram, Zoom and any other online media to unite the practitioners during social distancing. The onset of the COVID-19 pandemic and the consequent global lockdowns instigated a vital shift in the competitive Yogasana and the traditional physical championships had to be relocated to the virtual arena to guarantee the survival of the sports. Federation of sporting clubs such as the International Yogasana Sports Federation had to adapt by organizing major events such as the World Virtual Yoga Sports championship where participants around the world participated in the sport despite travel bans. This transition demanded that the sportsmen would do complicated asanas (postures) at their homes or personal training areas and be evaluated remotely using video recordings or live streams. Although the virtual environment enabled competitions to continue and offered the much-needed release to athletes, such as the example of Indian athletes capturing medals in the 2021 virtual competitions, it also presented judges with new challenges of determining members of perfect alignment, stability, and difficulty without being able to see them in three-dimensional view. Finally, the online platform in times of COVID-19 proved the strength and flexibility of the Yogasana community. Keeping the competitive spirit up alive, and opening the way to the further recognition of the sport and its international scope, though physical events later returned to their usual course (Nuong et al., 2024;). These online interventions were actually needed since the pandemic caused a lot of stress and anxiety among people, especially among the workers and those at risk, and it had the potential to undermine immune systems due to disrupted sleep (Sharma et al., 2020). The practice of yoga is highly beneficial during the pandemic because it enhances immunity, minimizes stress and anxiety, or improves lung health - especially when the upper respiratory tract is the gateway to SARS-CoV-2 (Srivastava et al., 2020). Online meetings equipped with breathing exercises, asanas, pranayamas, and meditation offered convenient channels of attaining physical and mental health in the conditions of social distancing (Sharma et al., 2020; Srivastava et al., 2020).

Pilot Projects in AI Judging

The latest studies have been oriented to the development of yoga pose recognition and correction systems based on the use of computer vision and deep learning technologies equipped with AI. Lavanya et al. (2024) built a yoga pose detector based on CNNs and TensorFlow Movenet that allows giving instant feedback in the form of visual and audio feedback when poses are done right. Implementation of Artificial Intelligence (AI) to adjudicate in competitive sports has left the discussion phase and entered live national and international pilot programs, especially in sports with a high level of subjective scoring. The most significant of them is Judging Support

System (JSS) which was co-developed by the International Gymnastics Federation (FIG) and Fujitsu. Employing 3D sensing technology to record and analyze the movement, angles of the joints and pose of a gymnast in real-time without markers, this system has been officially in a supportive role at Artistic Gymnastics World Championships since 2019, including all events of the championships as of 2023. Although it does not entirely exclude human judges, it offers objective, data-driven support system which human judges can review and confirm technical aspects of the case by trying to eliminate human error and bias.

Outside of gymnastics, other judged sports are also coming up with similar pilot projects. Indicatively, AI scorecards have been tested, unofficial in judging snowboarding halfpipe runs at the X Games to determine future possibilities, and an artificial intelligence-based training system by Baidu has been used by the Chinese diving team to score diving moves in real-time to offer accurate and objective feedback to coaches. The Olympic Games 2024 in Paris, shots were also integrated by the international Olympic Committee (IOC) into its strategy which saw AI serve in collaboration with other companies such as OMEGA and Alibaba to produce advanced data graphics in diving events and to run multi-camera replay systems in various sporting activities, further showing it was not used as a replacement of human judgement but as a decision-support tool. In Yogasana, although full competition judging is developing, research and development on AI models based on deep learning and pose estimation (such as PoseNet) to correctly detect and correct postures in real-time is underway, a step towards eventually having AI-assisted scoring of competitive Yogasana.

Likewise, Waghmode et al. (2023) developed YogaAI that provides visual and audio feedback on the poses in real-time, tutorials on how to perform each pose step by step, and track progress. A systematic review by Verma et al. (n.d.) investigated the literature of 2019-2023 and identified considerable accuracy in AI-based posture detection models and concluded that different methods such as OpenPose, CNNs, and Long Short-Term Memory networks have been developed to successfully estimate and correct yoga poses.

Yogasana Tech in Yogasana:

In recent years, the intersection of technology and yoga practice has evolved from simple video tutorials to sophisticated systems that assist practitioners in performing Yogasanas (yoga postures) more accurately and safely. Central to this evolution are two major technological trends: pose estimation using computer vision and wearable sensor-based systems. Together, these technologies form what might broadly be called "Yogasana Tech," focused on consolidating data from cameras and wearable parts to assess, classify, and ultimately improve yoga posture performance.

Pose Estimation in Yogasana

Pose estimation refers to the computational process of detecting and tracking human body joints and limb orientations from images or video streams. In the context of yoga, this means recognizing complex postures such as Vrikshasana (Tree Pose) or Adho Mukha Svanasana (Downward Dog) by extracting skeletal keypoints of a person's pose. Modern pose estimation models such as MediaPipe, OpenPose, and PoseNet are commonly used to detect major body joints in 2D or 3D coordinates, which can then be analyzed to determine if the practitioner is aligning correctly with the target posture. A typical pipeline might first extract keypoints representing elbows, shoulders, hips, knees, etc., and then feed these features into machine learning classifiers (like Support Vector Machines or Random Forests) to accurately identify the yoga posture being performed. Expansion of this basic approach into real-time systems like those developed in recent research allows the system not just to recognize a pose but also to provide immediate visual or audio feedback to the user.

Wearable Parts and Sensor Integration

While camera-based systems are powerful, wearable technology adds another dimension by capturing motion directly from the body. Wearables usually include Inertial Measurement Units (IMUs) sensors that track angular velocity and acceleration often placed on limbs or joints. These devices can precisely measure joint angles and orientation in 3D space without being affected by lighting or camera angle issues. One notable study used 11 IMUs attached to various body parts (e.g., forearms, thighs, waist) to recognize and evaluate yoga postures quantitatively. In this wearable setup, data from the sensors feeds into a classifier and a Bayesian network to not only identify the pose but assess how standard that pose is relative to an expert model. This approach can pinpoint deviations in specific limbs and give easy-to-understand feedback like "straighten your right forearm" or "lift your left leg higher," enhancing self-guided learning.

Case Studies: Combining Vision and Wearables

Vision-Only Systems: Projects like DeepYoga leverage deep learning and computer vision to classify yoga postures in real time, offering visual feedback on alignment and reducing injury risk in at-home practice.

Wearable-Only Systems: Wearable packages with IMUs detect posture and quantify correctness beyond what the camera sees. These systems are especially useful in occluded situations (e.g., when the camera can't fully view a posture).

Integrated Approaches: Cutting-edge applications merge both strategies using camera-based pose estimation for overall posture detection and wearable sensors for precise joint angle feedback. Early work in this hybrid direction shows promise for fine-grained alignment correction and personalized recommendations, making yoga instruction more accessible and effective for a wider range of users.

Yogasana Tech that consolidates pose estimation and wearable parts is reshaping how yoga is practiced and taught. By combining AI-driven vision systems with wearable sensor feedback, these solutions can provide accurate posture recognition and actionable guidance bringing expert insights into everyday fitness routines while reducing risk and enhancing performance. Investigation and refinement of these integrated systems continue as research and commercial applications expand.

CHALLENGES

Combining artificial intelligence into the practice of yoga poses some important opportunities and challenges. The technical and philosophical concerns surrounding the realization of the journey to introduce Artificial Intelligence (AI) into the evaluation of Yogasana as an international competitive sport are challenging, and the prominent one is the question of the need to balance objective measurement with subjective art. The technical challenge is to come up with an Automated Scoring System which is effective and solid enough in measuring a performance. This would necessitate real-time 3D pose estimation with computer vision which is a complicated activity considering the fact that asanas are subtle and complex due to necessitating accurate joint angle, spinal curve, and segment perpendicularity. The AI models would need to be trained with various data sets so that there is fairness and generalization of the models with different body types, clothing, and lighting conditions, which is a significant challenge because there is no single standardized large-scale Yogasana dataset yet. More so, the problem of the AI being robust to misalignments of the camera, or an actual obstruction, in a dynamic competition scenario remains an object of continuing engineering efforts (Sharma et al., 2024). The challenge is even more philosophical and ethical. Yogasana competitions embrace aspects such as Artistic Yogasana and Free Flow/Group Yogasana that are not only judged based on technical accuracy but also flow, grace, emotional outpouring and presentation aspects which an Artificial Intelligence can hardly read. Scoring needs to devise a method of objectively quantifying subjective standards, or it will be operating as nothing more than a mechanical exercise and thus losing the authenticity and traditional aspect of the sport, an all-encompassing practice aimed at inner awareness and mastery of breathing. This poses a paradoxical paradox that a correct AI can be seen as being too precise or even being prejudiced due to the fact that it disregards the human factor.

Lastly, the adoption of AI brings about important ethical and governance concerns to a wellness-based practice (Nuong et al., 2024). The use of cameras and sensors to capture biometric and visual data to be judged poses risks of data privacy and security which should be regulated by clear policies and a high level of protection and especially internationally. Human control is also essential since the black box aspect of AI may result in the absence of transparency and the inability to establish the reasons behind a score, which may jeopardize the judgement of the integrity of the competition and, consequently, the position of human judges and coaches.

These technical, artistic and ethical dilemmas must be overcome in order to succeed in expanding Yogasana all over the world by establishing a system that promotes fairness without subjecting the soul of the practice to any compromise. Computer vision methods demonstrate the possibility of human pose recognition in yoga, but they have not been extensively used in the health and exercise sphere where very little literature is specifically focused on yoga solutions.

FUTURE DIRECTIONS

The introduction of the Artificial Intelligence to the competitive yogasana is in its infancy and has immense capabilities of innovations and advances. The scoring systems may be standardized and be fair in the international competitions in the next several years through the creation of widely accepted AI-based judging programs. The development of the motion tracking and biomechanical analysis with the help of 3D scanning and deep-learning models will allow detecting micro-movements, muscle involvement, and balance precise and help athletes improve their techniques and reduce the risks of injuries. It is possible that AI-based talent development tools could be created to bring in perspectives of prospective athletes early on by observing them in video recordings of their performances and evaluation of their competition statistics, and that individual coaching interfaces can showcase the current advancement and suggest specific areas of focus. Integrating AI and immersive technologies, including Virtual Reality (VR) and Augmented Reality (AR), will generate the environment of hybrid training, which will enable athletes to train with holographic trainers or virtual trainers despite geographic restrictions. Simultaneously, the multilingual interface using AI and low-cost mobile apps will help make yoga more globally accessible, introducing competitive yoga to the rural communities and underserved populations. As technology however advances though, the spiritual and philosophical aspect of yoga will be necessary. The future innovations should be based on ethical issues connected to data privacy, AI transparency, and responsible use of performance data. Through these developments, AI may be instrumental in making yogasana recognized in the Olympics through the consistency and credibility that it gets through the development of AI.

CONCLUSION

The artificial intelligence is already turning out to be a game changer in the way the yogasana is changing to be more of a healthy activity of the past to a competition-based sport today. Allowing to analyze the posture accurately, conduct unbiased judging, design individual training plans, and reach the whole world digitally, AI helps to bridge the divide between tradition and innovation. Precision-based sports can prove that AI can enhance fairness, accuracy, and the safety of athletes, and the first applications in the yoga field prove that AI can be actively used in real-time correction and monitoring of performances. However, in the world of ever evolving technology that is defining competitive yogasana, there is a need to retain the holistic principles of yoga, focusing on mindfulness, discipline, and inner equilibrium. The future of the yogasana will be in the ability to achieve a delicate balance between tradition and technology to coexist in harmony. When applied wisely, AI can, in addition to increasing the level of competition in the yogasana sector, bring it to a greater recognition on the global arena, motivate future generations of sportspersons, and assure its global presence, perhaps as an Olympic sport.

REFERENCES

Agrawal, Y., Shah, Y., & Sharma, A. (2020, April 1). Implementation of Machine Learning Technique for Identification of Yoga Poses. DOI: 10.1109/CSNT48778.2020.9115758

Al-Romeedy, B. S., & Singh, A. (2025). Reimagining Customer Relations Through AI Innovation. In Darwish, D., & Kumar, S. (Eds.), *Utilizing AI and Machine Learning in Financial Analysis* (pp. 351–368). IGI Global Scientific Publishing., DOI: 10.4018/979-8-3693-8507-4.ch019

Ansari, A. I., & Singh, A. (2024). Growth and Opportunity of Medical Tourism in the Indian Healthcare Sector: A Critical Review. In Hassan, V., Albattat, A., & Basheer, S. (Eds.), *Impact of AI and Robotics on the Medical Tourism Industry* (pp. 290–301). IGI Global Scientific Publishing., DOI: 10.4018/979-8-3693-2248-2.ch013

Araujo, D., Couceiro, M., Seifert, L., Sarmento, H., & Davids, K. (2021). Artificial Intelligence in Sport Performance Analysis. New York: Routledge, 2020.: Routledge. DOI: 10.4324/9781003163589

Basireddy, R., Reddy, K. R. S., & Pakkiraiah, Y. (2023). Complimentary and Supplementary Yoga in Sports. *International Journal for Multidisciplinary Research*, *5*(4), 5928. Advance online publication. DOI: 10.36948/ijfmr.2023.v05i04.5928

Bharathi, S. T., Raj, F., Krishnan, R. S., Rajalakshmi, V., Kumar, V. V., & Anchitaalagammai, J. V. (2024). MentalHealthAI: Utilizing Deep Learning for Accurate Stress Level Prediction. 1705–1712. DOI: 10.1109/ICACRS62842.2024.10841747

Attila Biró, Antonio Ignacio Cuesta-Vargas, & László Szilágyi. (2024). AI-controlled training method for performance hardening or injury recovery in sports. DOI: 10.1109/SAMI60510.2024.10432911

Dhankhar, A., & Sharma, R. (2023). Evolution of Yoga. *International Journal of Physiology Nutrition and Physical Education*, *8*(2), 510–513. DOI: 10.22271/journalofsport.2023.v8.i2g.2846

Ercikan, K., & McCaffrey, D. F. (2022). Optimizing Implementation of Artificial-Intelligence-Based Automated Scoring: An Evidence Centered Design Approach for Designing Assessments for AI-based Scoring. *Journal of Educational Measurement*, *59*(3), 272–287. Advance online publication. DOI: 10.1111/jedm.12332

Jose, J., & Shailesh, S. (2021). Yoga Asana Identification: A Deep Learning Approach. *IOP Conference Series. Materials Science and Engineering*, *1110*(1), 012002. DOI: 10.1088/1757-899X/1110/1/012002

Jugran, S. (2024). Yogasanas and Their Importance in Stree Rog. *International Journal of Advanced Research, 12*(04), 877–890. DOI: 10.21474/IJAR01/18627

Lavanya, V., Premkumar K, & Rohith R. (2024). AI Enhanced Yoga Pose Detection And Alignment Using Deep Learning. DOI: 10.1109/INOCON60754.2024.10512108

Mani, P., Thangavelu, A., Sharma, A., & Chaudhari, N. (2017). A Real Time Monitoring System for Yoga Practitioners. *International Journal of Intelligent Engineering and Systems, 10*(3), 85–93. DOI: 10.22266/ijies2017.0630.10

Mateus, N., Abade, E., Coutinho, D., Ángel Gómez, M., Peñas, C. L., & Sampaio, J. (2024). Empowering the Sports Scientist with Artificial Intelligence in Training, Performance, and Health Management. *Sensors (Basel), 25*(1), 139–139. DOI: 10.3390/s25010139 PMID: 39796930

Matsuyama, H., Kawaguchi, N., & Lim, B. Y. (2023). *IRIS: Interpretable Rubric-Informed Segmentation for Action Quality Assessment. ArXiv*. Cornell University., DOI: 10.1145/3581641.3584048

Mazurova, E., Standaert, W., Penttinen, E., & Tan, F. T. C. (2021). Paradoxical Tensions Related to AI-Powered Evaluation Systems in Competitive Sports. *Information Systems Frontiers, 24*(3), 897–922. Advance online publication. DOI: 10.1007/s10796-021-10215-8 PMID: 34867076

Novrianto, A., Gustion, D., & Rahmawati, E. (2025). AI-Powered Performance Appraisal: Balancing Automation with Human Judgment in Performance Management Systems. Journal of Economics and Management Scienties, 389–396. DOI: 10.37034/jems.v7i3.163

Nuong Deri, M. ., Singh, A., Zaazie, P. ., & Anandene, D. . (2024). Leveraging Artificial Intelligence in Higher Educational Institutions: A Comprehensive Overview. Revista De Educación Y Derecho, (30). DOI: 10.1344/REYD2024.30.45777

Padhi, M. M. (2016). Evolution of Yoga and Physiotherapy. *Journal of Yoga and Physiotherapy, 1*(2). Advance online publication. DOI: 10.19080/JYP.2016.01.555556

Pavithra, S., Dhanya, R., Dharshana, M., Fathima, I. N., & Soundariya, S. (2025). Tech yoga: The smart mat revolution. *I-Manager's Journal on Embedded Systems, 13*(2), 46. DOI: 10.26634/jes.13.2.21490

Pavlopoulos, A., Rachiotis, T., & Maglogiannis, I. (2024). An Overview of Tools and Technologies for Anxiety and Depression Management Using AI. *Applied Sciences (Basel, Switzerland), 14*(19), 9068–9068. DOI: 10.3390/app14199068

Pisaniello, A. (2024). The Game Changer: How Artificial Intelligence is Transforming Sports Performance and Strategy. Geopolitical. *Social Security and Freedom Journal*, *7*(1), 75–84. DOI: 10.2478/gssfj-2024-0006

Prasanna, M., Arunkumar, T., & Arunkumar, S. (2017). A Mobile Application Based Smart System for Supporting Yoga Activities and Health Monitoring. *Research Journal of Pharmacy and Technology*, *10*(11), 3863. DOI: 10.5958/0974-360X.2017.00701.6

Rahul, M. (2023). Fitness and Yoga in Sports. *International Journal for Multidisciplinary Research*, *5*(6). Advance online publication. DOI: 10.36948/ijfmr.2023.v05i06.9428

Rai, D., Kumar, A., & Baghel, A. (2024). Pose Detection Using OpenCV and Media Pipe. 1–6. DOI: 10.1109/ICIC3S61846.2024.10603040

Raveena, N. M., & Rathod, L. L. (2024). ROLE OF AI IN TALENT IDENTIFICATION AND PERFORMANCE PREDICTION IN TRACK AND FIELD. *ShodhKosh Journal of Visual and Performing Arts*, *5*(7SE). Advance online publication. DOI: 10.29121/shodhkosh.v5.i7SE.2024.5878

Shah, M., Gandhi, K., Pandhi, B. M., Padhiyar, P., & Degadwala, S. (2023). Computer Vision & Deep Learning based Realtime and Pre-Recorded Human Pose Estimation. DOI: 10.1109/ICAAIC56838.2023.10141279

Sharma, K., Anand, A., & Kumar, R. (2020). The role of Yoga in working from home during the COVID-19 global lockdown. *Work : A Journal of Prevention, Assessment, and Rehabilitation*, *66*(4), 731–737. DOI: 10.3233/WOR-203219 PMID: 32925134

Sharma, S. K., & Gaur, S. (2024). Optimizing Nutritional Outcomes: The Role of AI in Personalized Diet Planning. *International Journal for Research Publication and Seminar*, *15*(2), 107–116. DOI: 10.36676/jrps.v15.i2.15

Singleton, M. (2013). Transnational Exchange and the Genesis of Modern Postural Yoga. Transcultural Research - Heidelberg Studies on Asia and Europe in a Global Context, 37–56. DOI: 10.1007/978-3-319-00315-3_2

Srivastava, R., Khanna, P., & Anand, A. (2020). Digital Yoga Interventions in Social Distancing Era. *Annals of Neurosciences*, *097275312094516*. Advance online publication. DOI: 10.1177/0972753120945165 PMID: 34733049

Sulong, G. B., & Randles, N. M. (2023). Computer Vision Using Pose Estimation. *Wasit Journal of Computer and Mathematics Science (Print)*, *2*(1), 54–58. DOI: 10.31185/wjcm.111

Vijayalakshmi, P. S., & A, D. D. (2025). The Personalized Fitness and Nutrition Coach. *International Journal of Research Publication and Reviews*, *6*(4), 6822–6826. DOI: 10.55248/gengpi.6.0425.14155

Vyshnivskyi, D., Liashenko, O., & Yeromina, N. (2023). HUMAN POSE ESTIMATION SYSTEM USING DEEP LEARNING ALGORITHMS. *Navigation and Communication Control Systems Collection of Scientific Papers*, *2*(72), 75–79. DOI: 10.26906/SUNZ.2023.2.075

Waghmode, P., Shitole, A., Telrandhe, M., & Bide, P. J. (2023, May 1). Real-time Yoga Pose Classification and Correction: YogaAI. DOI: 10.1109/INCET57972.2023.10170599

Yenishettil, S., Karajkhede, G., & Panat, L. (2024). Virtual Yoga Teacher With AI Model For Yoga Posture Correction For Good Health. 1–8. DOI: 10.23919/ITUK62727.2024.10772930

Zhao, X., Zheng, H., & Zhang, Q. (2025). Modern Advances in Artificial Intelligence Across the Athletic Domain. *Concurrency and Computation*, *37*(9-11), e70068. Advance online publication. DOI: 10.1002/cpe.70068

Chapter 7

Artificial Intelligence Applications in Subtle Energetic Systems of Nadis and Chakras

Ashutosh Bhardwaj
http://orcid.org/0009-0008-3311-8335
Poornima University, Jaipur, India

Nikhil Kumar Goyal
http://orcid.org/0009-0007-4532-8033
Noida International University, Greater Noida, India

Sumit Kumar Dave
http://orcid.org/0009-0005-9618-0206
Poornima University, Jaipur, India

Anmol Chaturvedi
Poornima University, Jaipur, India

ABSTRACT

This chapter talks about the possibility of artificial intelligence to facilitate the study and knowledge of subtle energetic systems, namely the Nadis and Chakras explained in the traditional science of yogic practices. Lighting up the models of the ancient energy with the aid of modern computational, the AI helps to identify patterns, conduct predictive analyses, and objectively estimate physiological, emotional, and energy states. Artificial intelligence algorithms, bio-signaling, and multi-modal data-hypothesis receive aid in the detection of relationships amid breath rate, neurophysiological response and electromagnetic difference, as well as chakra or

DOI: 10.4018/979-8-2600-2463-8.ch007

nadi-activation model. The chapter underscores how AI-based simulations, biometric sensing, and digital twin solutions could provide a new understanding of the nature of energy flows and assist in understanding individualized wellness measurements and populace science and knowledge.

1: INTRODUCTION

1.1 Understanding the Traditional Subtle Energy Framework

The original classical theories of subtle energy systems are found in yogic, tantric and Ayurvedic traditions in which the human person is considered to be a multi-dimensional being comprised of the physical layers, emotional layers, mental layers and spiritual layers. Nadis are said to be invisible systems that transmit prana, the life giving energy that provides stability and energy. It is estimated that ninety two thousand nadis are discussed in ancient literature, and special reference is paid to Ida, Pingala and Sushumna, which were first channels which predetermined a human consciousness and physiological harmony. Chakras are connected with the spinal axis and are, in the conceptual approach, the energy centers which manage numerous life experiences of human beings such as survival instincts and higher senses. This traditional interpretation of the systems has been grounded on meditative inquiry in the sense of intuitive insight and experience but not scientific validation (Iyengar, 2010).

Spiritual practitioners too have developed elaborate systems of meditation, pranayama and visualization to either stimulate or balance chakras or smooth-line the engine of energy down the nadis over centuries. These traditions demand an inner clarity, breathing and fine perception to adjust the body-mind complex to the high levels of clarity and vastness. Although these thoughts have been transmitted by the generations of teacher and pupil, they are rather linguistic, symbolic, and subjugated to the subjective experience.

The models of these ancient models in the frames of physiology, neuroscience and bioenergetics are becoming more popular among researchers and specialists today. One way the traditional and the scientific point of view may enter a point of contact may be that the correspondence of the chakras and the endocrine glands and nerve plexus like that of the heart and nerve plexus. Similarly, the breathing modes linked to the Ida and Pingala activation are related to the results that can be measured in the autonomic nervous system. These relations do not put themselves forward as complete validations of the traditional models but are suggestive of possible points of contact at which the ancient wisdom and the science of the present day may ease each other into a clearer comprehension. The introduction of advanced technologies in the research of subtle energy is preconditioned by the knowledge of these basics (Mallinson & Singleton, 2017).

1.2 Scientific Discovery of Energetic Pathways

During the past several decades, subtle energy studies have transformed their gossip level into a scientific discipline encompassing the fields of physiology, psychology, biophysics and the study of consciousness. Areas that scientists have investigated as potential correlates of energetic activity as described in yogic literature include bioelectric fields, thermal differences, galvanic skin responses, and heart brain coherence. The comparison of the electroencephalograms (EEG) reveals particular trends, which are attributed to the meditative condition, which is conventionally connected to the chakra activation, and the outcomes of the research related to the difference in the heart rate variability (HRV) indicate the strong connection between the regulation of breathing and auto-regulation. The advances offer promising opportunities of mapping delicate energetic processes on measurable biological signals.

Subtle energy systems have also found other applications in psychophysiological research, where body-wide energetic coherence effects were investigated using the emotions, attention and mental state. Studies into the effects of deep meditation, breathwork and counseling of mindfulness have reported the possibility to reach cardiac, respiratory and neurological systems pattern synchrony which in theory coincides with more expensive flow and chakras balancing. These results do not affirm directly traditional descriptions, however, there are signs that they are dynamics which can be measured which can impersonate the physiological expressions of subtle states of energy (Sharma, 1997).

The thermal image, photoplethysmography, photoplethysmography, new sensors of electromagnetic fields, a wearable biosignal sensors that can provide a more detailed and continuous reading of the small discrepancies all over the body are all new technologies. Along with these changes, comes an opportunity to objectively exploit virtually the phenomena whose exploration had previously been confined to subjective discovery. Along with the recognition of such scientific breakthroughs, researchers could begin suspicious work on combined methods which are capable of combining old models of energy with newer physiology knowledge and create a strong foundation around which AI analysis may be implemented (Woodroffe, 1974).

1.3 Applications of AI in Interpreting Subtle Energy System

The artificial intelligent will be a groundbreaking approach to studying subtle systems of energy since it will be possible to identify complex and non-linear trends in any type of physiological data. In the occurrence of energetic phenomena, where a number of biological systems interact simultaneously, a phenomenon that would be considered hard to capture in usual scientific practices is the dynamism of this phenomenon, not to mention its complexity. It is possible to however train machine learning algorithms on input of multimodal data including EEG, HRV, electrodermal activity, respiration and movement patterns, and thermal data to establish associations and support the observation of correlation between the two concerning different energizing states as reported in classical literature. The computing capacity provides AI with the capacity to resolve the subjective and the quantifiable physiological pointers.

Figure 1. AI-Driven Workflow for Subtle Energy Interpretation

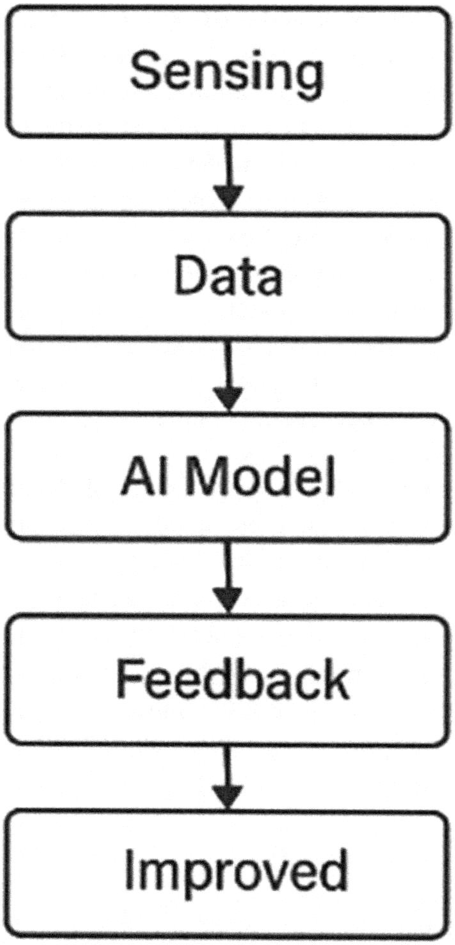

The successfulness of the AI-based models has been achieved in the vastness of the recent literature in categorizing the meditative states, predicting autonomic responses and alongside investigating fine changes in emotional and energy balance. These skills make it possible to map shapes connected to the opening of the nadis, the positioning of the chakras or the flow of the pranic energy in a detail that was not possible previously. Training models using synchronized practitioners with experience on the use of yogic methods can also start to induce the physiological expressions of subtle energetic methods, and compare it with the description of those experiences presented in traditional literature (Gray's Anatomy, 1997).

The introduction of AI into subtle energy studies also allows assessing energy and improving ways of wellness individually and optimally. As an example, the algorithms can propose a specific distribution of the breathing practices, meditation, or posture due to analyzing data in real-time and, thus, helping people acquire balanced energetic states. As the systems develop over time, they are able to make informed guesses about individual patterns and a person can get more precise information about their energy preferences. It is a great transition as compared to generalized spiritual teaching to information-driven, personalized advice.

2: AI-DRIVEN PHYSIOLOGICAL MAPPING AND THE QUANTIFICATION OF SUBTLE ENERGY

2.1 Integrating Biosignals to Explore Energetic Phenomena

The science of subtle energy systems has been short of direct measuring equipment able to detect the subtle physiological changes that are coupled with such a practice as pranayama, chakra meditation and practice of energy healing. The artificial intelligence allows a novel methodological approach to be used through the combination of various biosignals into integrated analysis systems. Continuous monitoring in heart rate variability, respiration depth, brainwave activity, skin conductance, gradients in micro-temperature and muscle tension is now possible using wearable and ambient sensors. Each of these metrics provides a partial view of bodily activity, but as a subset composed of all the metrics, one gets a multifaceted high-dimensional depiction of the inner body state. Such multimodal sets of data are best handled with AI models, which can find subtle correlations, which could relate to the energetic processes discussed in standard literature.

Figure 2. Energy Mapping State

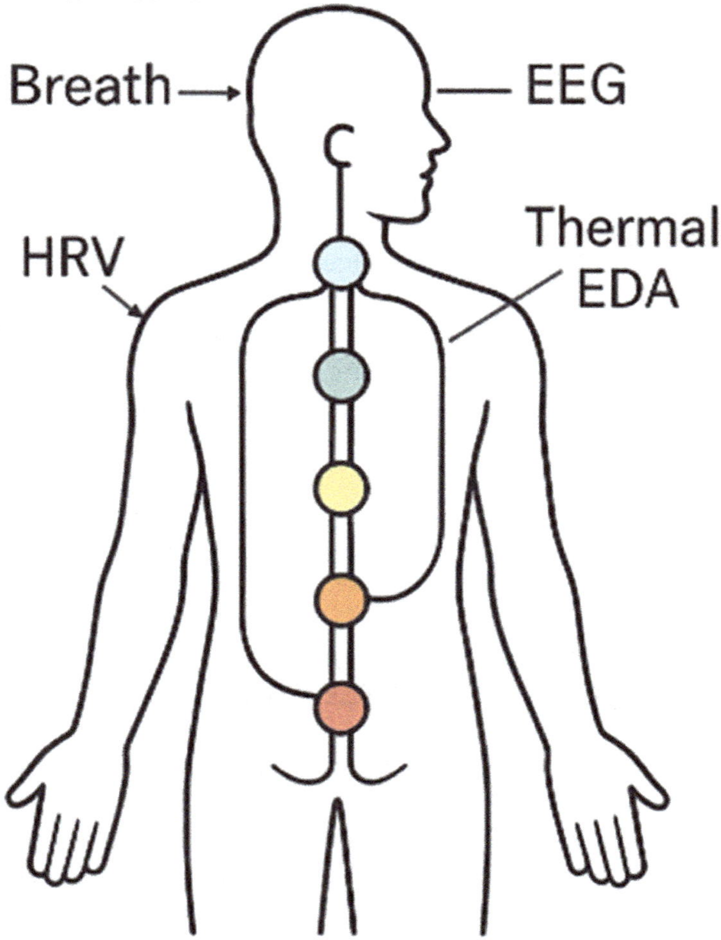

Nadi proxies Given the information about the breath symmetry, nasal airflow dominance, and autonomic balance, one can have measurable proxies of Ida and Pingala activity. As an example, the change in parasympathetic dominance can be usually correlated with Ida nadi-related activation, and the patterns of sympathetic arousal can be correlated with Pingala-related stimulation. Equally, the notion of Sushumna orientation - a concept traditionally associated with state of cognitive clarity and meditative absorption - can be associated with the states, in which physiological measures approach coherence and stability (Thatte, 2016).

2.2 Models of machine learning used to detect trends of Chakra Activation

Machine learning enables an extra potent technique to examine patterns which vary all the time throughout meditation, breathwork or energy-centered work. The classical accounts of chakras dwell on their unique psychological, emotional and energetic peculiarities. AI is able to investigate the possibility of these traits being expressed in distinct physiological forms. As an illustration, events connected with the root chakra, which can be linked to grounding and physical stability, could be linked with decreased fluctuations of variability of heart rate and an advancement of muscular immobility. Practices, on the other hand, with functioning on the heart chakra could be more coherent in conjunction of heart beats and breathing, which is the regulation of emotions and the composition of the parasympathetic (Grimes, 1996).

Kingdom new method What is These supervised learning methods, like a neural network or gradient boosting model, can be trained on labeled data composed of experienced meditators practicing guided chakra practices. The model is trained to determine the physiological habits that are associated with every meditative focus. With time, the algorithm has the ability to assign new sessions on the basis of the learned energetic signatures giving the prediction of the probabilities of chakra being activated. Unsupervised learning techniques, like clustering algorithms or dimensionality-reduction methods, can additionally help to gain greater understanding, by providing an insight into unmarked groups of the data (Lochtefeld, 2002).

2.3 Computational Mapping of Energetic Flow and Psychophysiological Coherence

The ability to research dynamic processes in real time can be viewed as one of the most radical contributions of the AIs to the research of subtle energy. Where heavily design stimulative descriptions in vivo tend towards discrete states e.g. an opened chakra or balanced nadi, AI has the ability to trace the dynamic formation of physiological signals in practice continuum. Methods such as time- series modelling, hidden Markov, and recurrent neural networks enable the system to follow the progression of energy related states, stabilize, vary, or decay throughout a session. These time-changing models give an idea of the possible correspondence of the pranic flow to the changing patterns of neural, cardiac and respiratory synchrony.

As an illustration, when in the state of deep meditation, AI systems tend to recognize coherence increasing along physiological pathways, such as synchronized breathing, regular heart rates and less variability in brainwave synergies. Such states can be related to the levels of description of pranic alignment or opening up of central energy channels. On the other hand, in another practice, where the intention is to activate specific chakras, AI can record localized body physiological modifications, including change of temperature in hands, chest, and forehead, which in the perception of practitioners can be termed as energetic sensations. These calculation mappings do not warrant the being of the metaphysical assertions and this is because of the reason that they affirm the fact that the demands of the energetic experiences are equivalent on environmental indications that are recognizable on the physiological plane (White, 2012).

Personalized energy profiles myself could be created through the assistance of constant training based on AI, and I would demonstrate the person how his or her body reacts to various practices. It is easy to use in meditative education, psychotherapeutic intervention and health monitoring. The system can suggest breathing patterns or focus points depending on the reaction of each user that will put oneself into a state of coherence and reduce stress or bring more stability. Such kind of individual guidance may be regarded as the strong step to include the old wisdom of power with the new evidences (Pradhan, 2014).

3: AI INTERPRETATIONS OF ENERGETIC PHENOMENA

3.1 Modeling Subtle Energy Through Computational Metaphors

As a concept, artificial intelligence provides the only conceptual framework in the re-definition of classical systems of energy such as nadis and chakras under the metaphor of computations. Even though subtle energy cannot be directly observed with the assistance of sensors or other scientific apparatus, artificial intelligence structures allow the researcher to estimate complex human conditions in light of patterns and signals and hypothetical reasoning. As a case in point, fluctuations in the variability of heart-rate, emotional coloring in the speech or coherence of the brainwaves can be researched and analyzed using algorithms to present dynamic patterns that loosely depict the flow and harmony of traditional energetic ideas. Such computational representations will not claim to be in place of well led notions but will instead offer an alike language which will mediate between intuitively generated and scientifically understood notions.

Accordingly, subtle energy can be referred to as a phenomenon of emergence, which occurs on the condition of multiple interacting variables of physiological and psychological nature. Probably, machine learning models will be capable of recalling correlations that are not of interest to humans which will enable one to come to a more nuanced answer regarding what kind of nature have dynamics of change in energy lead to changes in behavior, emotion, and thinking. To the degree that AI processes these multidimensional signals, its outputs give an insight that is similar to those already done of intellectual currents of energy such as filling up of stress, emotion free stable or impaired mind coherence. Hence, AI is incapable of recognizing prana, nadis, but it shows patterns that would be functionally comparable to the ones presented in ancient literature (Brennan, 1988).

Moreover, computational metaphors provide the reason why mind-body practices do carry measurable effects on health (Brennan, 1993).

3.2 Machine Learning in Biofield Research

Biofield science tries to discover the patterns of non-invasive energy or information around the human body that are subtle, and machine learning provides powerful technologies to research these multifaceted processes. Even though the biofield is not universally accepted in the mainstream science, the studies of electromagnetic radiation, thermal changes, and the frequencies of neural waves provide the abundance of data, which can be analyzed with the help of AI. Machine learning models have the ability to detect minute variations, latent correlations, and interactions among multiple signals which may not be noticeable when using traditional statistical techniques. Consequently, scholars can have a better understanding of how painful feelings, mental activity, and physical responses are unified to create the foundation of what is referred to as dynamic fields in ancient traditions.

The models are especially effective in explaining the data of such practices as Reiki, qigong or the yogic meditation. In the instances that the practitioners practice these techniques, sensors tend to measure the alteration in the heart coherence, skin conductance, and neural coherence. The analysis of the signals by AI can forecast the changes in relaxation, stress, or cognitive clarity, and offer the current perspective through which practices guided by energy can be viewed in modernity. Although this is not tantamount to quantification of prana per se, it shows how subtle balance and imbalance effects can be observed physically by becoming measurable (Eden, 1998).

3.3 Neural Correlates of Chakras and Energy Centers

The chakra system is one of the organized approaches which help conceive a psycho-energetic functioning, and the research done by AI-based neuroscience new direction which can be represented in relation to neural work and feelings processing. Even though chakras are not part of the anatomy, most of their functions are similar to parts of the nervous system, endocrine glands, and network centers in the brain. Brain imaging data decoded using AI models has been used to identify groups of neural activity that are linked to an emotional, intuitive or motivational condition, which is historically linked to this or that chakra. This does not support that chakras are physical structures, but indicates that there are functional analogies that would increase interdisciplinary awareness.

As an example, AI-based analysis of meditative sessions, in which one is guided to look at particular chakras, will likely show specific patterns of neural activity. Focus on the heart center could be linked to greater coherence of the parasympathetic nervous system whereas the exercises involving the third-eye center could stimulate the regions related to introspection and eye-sensory fusion. Such correlations serve to understand why chakra based practices tend to lead to quantifiable psychological outcomes, such as lower anxiety, increased emotion, and cognitive ability (Govinda, 2002).

The correlation of different energetic states and psychological well-being is also the area where AI would be applicable. Analysing the activity of thousands of shrunk neural samples, machine learning can determine the relationship between emotional blocks, motivational loss or mental exhaustion and the neural connection pathology. These distortions mean the nature of energetic imbalances experienced in the traditional systems which denotes that the traditional systems are talking about the same underlying human processes though with different perspectives. With centuries-old philosophy of the chakra system, AI-managed neural research can therefore offer a more detailed, balanced observation of the functioning of the human body without being disrespectful of scientific and conventional data.

4: AI-ENHANCED VISUALIZATION OF ENERGETIC PATHWAYS

4.1 Digital Mapping of Energetic Flows

Artificial intelligence is changing the way the human energetic systems can be represented so that small physiological data can be turned into meaningful tendencies. Although such idea as nadis and chakras cannot be quantified in actual physical terms, AI software may respond to secondary data (breath, heart rate, stress biomarkers, neural rhythms, and others). These indicators are observed to oscillate irregularly in patterns, which have been conventionally referred to as flow of energy, obstruction and strength or imbalance. Being complex of multimodal signals generated by devices, AI can create dynamic models that contain a visual representation of the way the inner condition of a person evolves during a day or even during a specific practice such as meditation, breathing exercises or yoga. These representations serve as an interpreter of subjective energetics experience and the empirics (Chhabra et al., 2013).

The smarter the AI models are the better they will be able to process raw data to provide meaningful storytelling visually. Heat map, waveforms and resonance diagrams would be examples as a way of illustrating how different parts of the body react to emotional or cognitive changes. This kind of visualization may help users to be more conscious of their inner states and provide the practitioners with valuable messages of how energy-based intervention, like mindful breathing or imagery, changes physiological fluctuations of the body.

Such representations are not aimed at demonstrating and refuting traditional notions of energy. On the contrary, they offer each other a supplementary layer of comprehension. It is aimed at emphasizing patterns that can match patterns described in old sources, but still it will be accepted that the mechanisms involved may be physiological or psychological or a combination of both. In the instances of AI-generated visualizations producing harmonious rhythms or synchronized patterns, people tend to refer to it as a sense of being open, grounded, or clear, which are often referred to as balanced flows of energy. This overlap between the subjective experience and tube montage increases the discourse between technology and tradition (Hammerschlag et al., 2015).

4.2 AI Chakra Pattern Recognition Saudies

The development of machine learning has provided fresh perspective in investigating the connection between the emotional, cognitive, and physiological state and the functions that have always been linked to chakras. Even though chakras are philosophical notions and not anatomical organs, the moods and psychological characteristics associated with any of them tend to be reflected in physical indicators that can be conveniently measured. The AI can process extensive amounts of emotional outperformance, voice change, and heart rates variability and brainwave indications and identify those patterns that fall under these categories. Such insights enable investigators to suggest how some mental or emotional conditions are inclined in the symbolic meanings of particular chakras.

When trained on multimodal data reflecting stress, compassion, confidence, intuition, or groundedness, the machine learning classifiers can be used to differentiate the patterns that are related to stress, compassion, confidence, intuition, or any of the above-mentioned chakra centers. As an example, the states related to the heart chakra can be labeled by the height of the vagal tone, regular rhythm of the breathing, or empathetic speech patterns. On the same note, alpha-wave predominance or a low degree of sensory reactivity could be the outcome of introspective or intuitive states that are linked to the third eye chakra. Correlations are not assertions that prove that chakras are literally physical objects, but prove that there exists a functional parallel which permits these ancient concepts to be scientifically understood (Becker, 1990).

Pattern recognition is also a good tool of personal development owing to the role of AI in pattern recognition. When people can meditate or think about certain chakras, with the help of AI, they can be able to receive feedback on whether their physiological signals are becoming balanced with that of being calm, open, or clear (Beirne et al., 2017).

4.3 Visualization interfaces based on the users

The manner in which the insights, generated by AI are presented into the interface will also be a critical parameter, which will determine how well the information can be interpreted and utilized by the user. The translation of complex physiological data into the ability to make sense in intuitive form that is easy to digest is of concern to the visualization platforms that are targeted at users. Those interfaces usually utilize gradients of colors, moving effects, and concentrated geometrical shapes which respond to the aesthetic of chakras and nadis. The more the fluctuation is presented in this manner in a way that users find meaningful visually, the more they are able to perceive it on an experience-based level and less of an abstract level, thereby increasing the level of engagement and emotional reaction (Bennett, 2019).

The interface is thoroughly designed and while the process of meditating as well as breathing or mindful movements, a user can find out what happens to his or her inner state in real-time. The interface transforms the antique texts of displaying transformation in forms, colors or beat of rhythm. This convincing compatibility creates атроv across the instinctual tradition and the exactness of the digital and the user can feel an instantaneously appeal of some greater energetic narration and as soon as the user can feel the instant connection with the scientifically supported information. Such a two fold influence is supported by the fact that technology does not demand substitution of spiritual structures, on the contrary, it can be employed in enhancing their functions by providing accuracy and feedback.

Moreover, user-friendly interfaces are valuable in the long-term self-regulation and self-development. After the time during which people pay attention to the dynamics of their energy, they start seeing the role the thoughts, habits and emotions play in contributing to the internal harmony. The AI-based visualizations are not trying to give direction but are providing a gentle guidance, reduce the prescriptive authority to the user, letting the system make the user aware and not rather feel evaluated. By constantly learning and reflecting, a person may come up to a more compatible relationship with their bodies and mental states. Consequently, the interfaces become potent in respect of incorporating ancient energetic techniques in contemporary well-being systems (de Goede et al., 2018).

5: INTEGRATING AI WITH TRADITIONAL HEALING PRACTICES

5.1 AI-Assisted Meditation for Chakra Alignment

AI is transforming meditation because it provides some degree of personalization that it previously could achieve with the help of more experienced trainers. Conventional balancing of chakras is relying on subtle sensations, inside images and intuitive awareness and most people are not able to make sense of them. To overcome this discrepancy, the AI-assisted meditation systems can be used to analyze physiological indicators in real-time, including breathing patterns, heart rate fluctuations, and neural activity so that the practitioners could be guided more efficiently. Such systems may adjust speed, intensity and concentration of meditation instructions to the peculiarities of energetic and emotional state of a user and make the exercises more approachable and comfortable.

By referring to patterns and analyzing emotions, AI can identify the point, when a user gets distracted, stressed, or imbalanced. When a person is working with a meditation in the chakra of the solar plexus e.g. trying to balance this chakra by healing a patient, the changes in the breathing or muscle tension can be the sign of resistance to the issues or unpleasant feelings. One of the responses that can be made by AI-guided meditation is to provide grounding cues, modulate the frequencies of the audio, or redirect the meditation into stabilization. This two-way interaction is similar to the responsiveness of the traditional teacher who then tailors the direction based on the status of the student and added advantages of monitoring the student and prompt feedback (Hamblin, 2018).

The AI-aided meditation will also facilitate the process of learning because the user can learn the relationship between internal states and physiological reactions. After some time, the user is able to see their progress with the help of a graph or resonance patterns or color-coded energy flows that can be explained using traditional chakra depictions of the chakras.

5.2 Artificial Intelligence-based Assistance Systems to Energy Healers

Energy healers normally rely on intuition, sensitivity and experience which takes years to diagnose disorders in the system of body energy of a patient. Though they are highly personal and are deeply grounded in intuition, AI-upgraded support system presents an extra experience into the researched subtle-physiological tendency that accompanies different states of energy. The patterns of skin temperatures, heart bursts, micro-expressions, and stress patterns are the options that can be calculated with the help of AI models to form more objective perception of the inner conditions of the client. This data is not the replacement, but the supplement of the intuitive judgment of a healer.

The AI systems can also be used in the long run to help the healers track the success of their intervention. Through the physiological information obtained of a client before a session, and after a session, the healer can have a greater comprehension of the impact of the treatment on the incorporation of the body and its internal operations. The emotional release, deep relaxation or improved coherence cases are detected by AI-based systems and projected on meaningful visualisations. These lessons may help the helpers to better their strategies, develop personalized care plans, and identify trends that might have not been readily identified using the intuition only (Dirlich et al., 1997).

The second important effect of AI on the healing practice is that it is empowering the people who would otherwise not be able to reach an exceptionally experienced practitioner conveniently. Self-healing platforms guided by AI are organized and offered by breathwork, visualization, sound therapy, and led to a relaxation state and comply with the typical chakra themes. These systems do not target the replacement of skills of the trained healers but allow the benefits of the energy-balancing practices to make an even further reach to the audience. AI offers a promising healing journey through the accurate tracking and flexible learning without any limitations in geographical and economic features.

5.3 Making the Traditional and Technological Workflow Intersect

The meeting of AI and antique energetic practice is the collaboration of two worlds which may appear to be contradictory to one another intuition with the spirit and scientific research. This new synthesis exhibits that the new wisdom can build on the previous wisdom rather than regard technology as a threat to the customary knowledge. Conventional systems of chakras and nadis are common systems of tradition, wherein human experience can be analyzed, and AI contributes the power of algorithms and real-time feedback to them. They form a complete concept of the mind-body relationship together.

This process of bridging fosters the respect of the various types of knowledge. Researchers of ancient traditions obtain the instruments that allow justifying and optimizing their practice and researchers of technology learn new avenues of investigation based on the knowledge of millennia on the human mind. The patterns shown with the help of AI allow visualizing the traditional ways of describing the state of energy, and thus, it becomes possible to explore the opportunities of science without diminishing the traditions to simplistic physiological explanations. Rather, the discussion is more complete, with both sides of the argument getting along and enlightening each other (González et al., 2018).

The amalgamation style also ensures individuals gain a more understanding about themselves. The assistance of AI will allow a user to understanding the effect of their traditional methods of meditation such as mantra repetitions or chakra-based meditation better, whether the user wants to supplement those approaches with AI or not. The interaction via this communication enhances a more conscious and disempowering rapport with personal wellness.

6: CYBERSECURITY TOOLS, PLATFORMS, AND THE TECHNOLOGY LANDSCAPE

6.1 Network and Endpoint Security Technologies

The front line protection of the modern organizations is network and endpoint security technologies which strive to interrupt, deter and provide control of the unauthorized access and evil act on the IT environments. There are real-time policy enforcing create a controlled perimeter that sieves bad communication at the network layer and real time inspecting systems on the traffic. Deep packet inspection, traffic correlation and continuous monitoring can assist the defenders in learning the normal behavior of the network in a healthy condition and also to observe the abnormalities capable of reflecting intrusion, lateral movement or loss of data. These features of a network are combined with such architectural choices as microsegmentation and zero-trust designs that reduce the scope of attack and limit the extent of damage that any sort of compromise may lead to.

The endpoint protection is useful to network defenses since they secure the devices, on which users are exposed to corporate resources. Nowadays, its endpoint security is far beyond signature based antivirus, and includes behavioral analytics, process review and automatic reaction. Host-based endpoint detection and response tools are making an attempt to accumulate pull telemetry bearing a lot of knowledge concerning every host as well as allowing security staff to reconstruct attacker activities, confine infected machines and execute remedial measures. The movement to remote working and Brat-you-bring-your- own-iPads has exacerbated the requirement to have hardened endpoint controls that can operate in various operating systems and network environments at the same time maintaining user efficiency (González et al., 2019).

Machine learning is also being added both to network technologies and endpoint technologies to improve the detection of more advanced threats. The behavioural models are able to identify malicious activity patterns which are impossible to detect using simple rule-based systems, reducing the quantity of false positive and shortening the incident triage time. The intelligent augmentation helps companies to manage masses of alerts and guide human experience where it will be needed most. But there are operational problems, such as model drift, adversarial evasion, and model validation and contextual tuning, which also tend to get larger with a dependency on automated models, and in the changing circumstances, the continuous model validation and contextual optimization are likely to become significant.

6.2 Threat Intelligence, Threat Monitoring and Automated Response Platforms

Threat intelligence and central-monitors can provide high visibility in terms of emerging threats hence rendering the achievement of the successful cybersecurity. Gathering logs and telemetry of network devices, endpoints, cloud services and applications will generate a whole systems dialogue to be interrogated by security analysts. Multi-stage attacks would be identified through the matching of streams of different events and would assist in the retrospective investigation. Security information and event management platforms do such correlation in which they offer long term storage, search factors as well as ability to operationalize intelligence in generating actionable detection as well as response signals.

Besides passive monitoring, orchestration and automation tools also allow organizations to code play books of response that will lead to containment and remediation actions being adopted. This will reduce the time to respond and uniformity in responding to normal incidents. The use of orchestration platforms in conjunction with other security controls is to integrate and automate operations such as host isolation, malicious network connections blocking or to enhance alerts with third party intelligence. Automated workflows not only reduce the repetitive work of the analysts, but also enable scaling of the security workflows to the demands of the modern business environment, provided that the governance and sites of manual work are controlled appropriately to prevent the occurrence of an erroneous automated work.

The threat intelligence enhances the surveillance by providing finer details in relation to adversarial tactics, tactics, and procedures and indications of vulnerability. Gathered intelligence could help in giving priority to the examination, screening the investigation, and educating proactive hardening. The operation of effectively implementing intelligence should be put under specific consideration, audit and congruing the performance to the risk profile of the company. Intelligence and detection platforms as well as automation of responses create a feedback loop because in the long run, operational data helps to improve intelligence and intelligence leads to better operational performance due to the creation of security posture (González et al., 2019).

6.3 Vulnerability Assessment and Cloud Security Ecosystems Forensics

Forensic capabilities and vulnerability assessment are the necessary components of a defensible security program and allow the organization to find out the vulnerabilities before them, and redefine the incidents in the case of breaches. Digital forensics tools enable investigators to distill objects in the storage, memory, and network captures to establish the chronology of attacker movement as well as to gather practice materials to be used in the legal or control endeavors. Vulnerability testing and scanning offers proactive testing of systems and applications that deliver prioritized advice on remediation to reduce the exposure to exploitable conditions and informs about patching strategies.

The fast move towards cloud computing presents fresh demands and chances to security tools. The security solutions provided by cloud-native solutions cover the configuration hygiene, identity and access management, workload isolation, and runtime protection, in highly automated ephemeral environments. This is because cloud security posture management assists in the process of keeping configurations safe, whereas cloud access brokers and workload protection platforms are used to protect data flows between IaaS and the SaaS. The main idea in implementing cloud telemetry and incorporating it with other monitoring and forensic systems is to have the visibility and consequently the capability to perform the investigations and respondences to be extended to the hybrid and multi-cloud environments.

In forensics, vulnerability assessment, and cloud security, there is a growing trend in the use of automation and analytics to boost speed and scale only to require a strong governance approach. The tools should be validated, the chain of custody and the results of the tools put into perspectives of the priorities in the business so that efforts should not take the wrong direction. Human knowledge is still necessary in the process of deciphering multi-level signals, risk tolerance judgment, and establishing technical advice in coordination with corporate strategy. With automation, expert practitioners working together as a technical tooling, security programs are in a better position to spot threats and restrain or recover with resilience after cyber-breaches [26].

7: FUTURE DIRECTIONS IN AI-ENHANCED SUBTLE ENERGY RESEARCH

7.1 Emerging Trends in AI-Driven Subtle Energy Mapping

The subtle energy mapping AI is at a transformative stage, whereby more sophisticated computational procedures become capable of handling physiological and energetic indications of the most subtle kind. As various types of multimodal data become increasingly available, AI programs are being trained to mediate between concepts of subtle-energy (blockages or problems in chakra circulation) and physical responses in the form of a biological field, biological temperature or neural activity. The increasing prowess of such has granted researchers a chance to reevaluate the systems of knowledge concerning subtle energy within a scientific system with reverence of their metaphysical foundations. These models in the long-term can culminate into co-creation of hybrid models that utilize the traditional models which are based on energy with scientific empirical models.

In future mapping, the real-time bio-sensing technologies will likely be used to monitor and acquire analyses of the energies to be tracked. Such systems would be an integration of state-of-the-art imaging, wearable sensors, and machine learning algorithms to accomplish achieving getting dynamical images on the movement of energy within the human body. These images would be developed to such a degree that would detect the changes of the dynamic state in the moment to moment level and give the practitioners additional information on healing, meditation or therapeutic intervention. With the increase in computational power, the process of subtle energy mapping can experience a transition towards the predictive modeling which involves AI predicting energy imbalance before it is completely established.

Also, these trends indicate a change of paradigm in the study of subtle energy phenomena. Rather than considering energetic systems as solitary and mystical, future advances in AIs might integrate a system into the interconnected biopsychosocial frameworks acknowledging the impact of emotional, cognitive, environmental and cultural factors. By making these dimensions blend, the concept of subtle energy can be further understood because it will be grounded in holistic and integrative science. Subtle energy mapping will possibly emerge as a research field as interdisciplinary teams become more common with standard datasets and validated models that will bridge existing knowledge systems and new AI (Cervellin & Lippi, 2011).

7.2 The Hypothesis of integrating the Eastern Philosophy and AI Research

The Eastern philosophy and AI research point to the possibilities of the redefinition of scientific knowledge on consciousness and human energetics. Conventional philosophies like Yoga, Ayurveda, Taoism and Tibetan systems of healing do not define energy only as a physical entity but as a combination of mental, emotional and spiritual energy. The integration of these views on contemporary AI systems enables researchers to expand the conceptual scope of any computational modeling and promote the creation of systems that can take into account the qualitative features of human experience. This change can enhance the explanatory capacity of AI by incorporating in the system contextual and experiential knowledge which is generally not well taken into consideration by traditional scientific paradigms.

Through the growing number of interventions between technologists and experts of traditional knowledge, AI systems can soon start interpreting very subtly the patterns of energy as manifestations of deeper consciousness states. As an example, the trains of thoughts may be trained to identify the meditative walks and the indicators of vibrational energy, or emotional reactions and chakras reactions. Graven such incorporations may result in the application of AI in the larger framework of the welfare, psychological and spiritual growth where the technology can awaken discipline of self-awareness devoid of tainting the philosophical integrity of the primesval beliefs. The possible benefits are the individual measure of energy, smart meditation sanhetis and the philosophy-based learning promoted with AI (de Sousa et al., 2012).

However, when assigning these philosophies to AI, it is important to consider in particular, the matters of cultural sensitivity, the ethical considerations, and the risks posed to a simplification of the issue. The ancient notions such as prana, qi or kundalini are extremely metaphysical and cannot be reduced to pure computational interpretations, without taking away some crucial meaning. Responsible integration implementation involves the interdisciplinary discussion, the respect extended to the owners of the indigenous knowledge and the methodologies that fail to harm the excellence of the culture wisdom systems. Having the correct attitude, the AI can be employed as an addition rather than a replacement to the philosophical knowledge where it will positively influence the scientific activity and the religious attitudes.

7.3 Future Epistemic and Scientific Difficulties

The subtle energy systems involving AI represent a very tricky ethical and epistemic problem since the area itself is subject to very personal, spiritual, and culturally-based practices. The problems of privacy, consent, and the fact that AI may be used to obtain considerably personal information that has no permission can appear since AI begins reading the active lifestyles of individuals or the way of their feelings. To make sure that ethical boundaries are observed, it is necessary to make data-handling structures more transparent and provide informed consent; and lay down very strong restrictions on the ways in which energy-based data can be employed in healthcare, wellness, or business. In the absence of those measures, AI-based energy evaluation systems might pose a threat of being insistent or demanding in disrespect to the autonomy of individuals (Einstein, 1955).

The second issue is the problem of epistemic uncertainty because subtle energy systems cannot always be found in the mainstream discourse of science. The reliability of AI models can only comprehend the reliability of the datasets used to train it, and in case subtle energy, the datasets can be limited, unbalanced, or prone to cultural biases. This results to a problem of model validity, biasness and probability of making fallacious statements which appear scientific but do not have due empirical support. This is what researchers must approach with methodological humility and interdisciplinary rigor in this type of research to ensure that the meaning obtained with the help of AI will not create an illusion of certainty and eliminate traditional wisdom as unscientific.

Scientific legitimacy will never be possible in the future without the development of standard forms of data collection, terms and validation. The cross-disciplinary research that includes neuroscientists, AI experts, clinicians, and conventional energy specialists could assist them in integrating culturally sensitive and innately valid in place models. The guidelines can then be implemented to make sure such innovation remains responsible and so that concepts of subtle energy may not be misinterpreted and commercialized as they refine. And finally, the future of AI-assisted subtle energy-based studies requires the creation of the middle-ground of open mind coupled with the pre-destined scientific accountability in that the identical technological inventions will increase worth and not pollute the wisdom of the foresights of the books of subtle energy [30].

CONCLUSION

It is the success of artificial intelligence and subtelene systems (chakras and nadis) they are one of the few applications, where the ancient metaphysics of antiquity are faced with the science of the computers. It is this novel interdisciplinary advantage that comes to bear focus the opportunity of re-defining the human conscious, energy and well-being. Even though the conceptual models always thought of subtle energy as flowing, experience-based and spiritually charged, AI may achieve a chance to examine the regularities, identify correlations and generate dynamic models in such a manner that the dimensions hidden by science could be studied more effectively with the assistance of science. Machine learning, biosignals and multimodal sensing can enable subtle energy state to be graphically perceived in an alternative way which does not just provide the insight of the technology, but it also provides more self-awareness. Such synergy implies that the customary practices are available to avenue where the technology is not replacing the technology but instead, it is making its availability to be more available, decipherable and integration into the extant or current health and wellness constructs.

Over time, as advances in research are made, AI controlled subtle energy systems can help to direct personal measurements of energy, an adaptable meditation app, integrative health treatment, and a scientific study of consciousness. The fusion of Eastern philosophical concept and AI analytical potentiality: It can attain more detailed and multidimensional models, ones that are based on physical, emotional, cognitive, and spiritual experience of a human being. However, with these inventions, morality begins to be put at the center. The vital energy information is strongly personalized, with it having a bearing on identity, emotion and faith, and willingness. The solution to this issue is assuring privacy, respectful use of the data, cultural appropriateness, and methodological integrity to be sure that sacred traditions are not exploited or turned into a reductionist manner. It also has to be a value less extreme so as to pay attention to the richness of subtle energy systems that exist in metaphysical form and use AI as a subsidiary discovery and revelation.

As in the future, one can highlight the fact that the successful evolution of the sphere is based on the interdisciplinary interaction of the long period, enough scientific assumptions, and the desire to make the epistemology of different forms unite. Neither subtle energy traditions nor AI can offer a comprehensive picture of human energetics, but the two provide an opportunity to discover the holistic view of what was impossible to observe previously. As scientists, practitioners, technologists and philosophers converge in this debate, it is hoped that the future of AI-augmented subtle energy research would come in handy to improve both scientific knowledge and the human well being.

REFERENCES

Becker, R. O. (1990). *Cross Currents*. Penguin Books.

Beirne, K., Rozanowska, M., & Votruba, M. (2017). Photostimulation of Mitochondria as a Treatment for Retinal Neurodegeneration. *Mitochondrion*, *36*, 85–95. DOI: 10.1016/j.mito.2017.05.002 PMID: 28499983

Bennett, J. P. (2019). Medical Hypothesis: Neurodegenerative Diseases Arise from Oxidative Damage to Electron Tunneling Proteins in Mitochondria. *Medical Hypotheses*, *127*, 1–4. DOI: 10.1016/j.mehy.2019.03.034 PMID: 31088629

Brennan, B. A. (1988). *Hands of Light: A Guide to Healing Through the Human Energy Field*. Bantam.

Brennan, B. A. (1993). *Light Emerging: The Journey of Personal Healing*. Bantam.

Cervellin, G., & Lippi, G. (2011). From Music-Beat to Heart-Beat: A Journey in the Complex Interactions Between Music, Brain and Heart. *European Journal of Internal Medicine*, *22*(4), 371–374. DOI: 10.1016/j.ejim.2011.02.019 PMID: 21767754

Chhabra, G., Narayanan, A., Samantha, S., & Samanta, S. (2013). "Human Aura: A New Vedic Approach." *International Conference on Mechanical and Industrial Engineering*, 26 May 2013, New Delhi. ISBN 978-93-82208-95-2.

de Goede, P., Wefers, J., Brombacher, E. C., Schrauwen, P., & Kalsbeek, A. (2018). Circadian Rhythms in Mitochondrial Respiration. *Journal of Molecular Endocrinology*, *60*(3), R115–R130. DOI: 10.1530/JME-17-0196 PMID: 29378772

de Sousa, M. C., Caldas, I. L., Rizzato, F. B., Pakter, R., & Steffens, F. M. (2012). Controlling Chaos in Wave-Particle Interactions. *Physical Review E: Statistical, Nonlinear, and Soft Matter Physics*, *86*(1 Pt 2), 016217. DOI: 10.1103/PhysRevE.86.016217 PMID: 23005517

Dirlich, G., Vogl, L., Plaschke, M., & Strian, F. (1997). Cardiac Field Effects on the EEG. *Electroencephalography and Clinical Neurophysiology*, *102*(4), 307–315. DOI: 10.1016/S0013-4694(96)96506-2 PMID: 9146492

Eden, D. (1998). *Energy Medicine*. Penguin Putnam.

Einstein, A. (1955). *The Meaning of Relativity* (5th ed.). Princeton University Press.

González, M. J., Olalde, J., Ward, T. D., & Miranda-Massari, J. R. (2019). Physiological Modulation: The Orthomolecular Explanation of Phytotherapy Based on the Systemic Medicine Approach. *Journal of Orthomolecular Medicine*, *34*(1).

González, M. J., Seyfried, T., Nicolson, G. L., Barclay, B. J., Matta, J., Vasquez, A., D'Agostino, D., Olalde, J., Duconge, J., Hunninghake, R., Berdiel, M. J., & Cintrón, A. (2018). Mitochondrial Correction: A New Therapeutic Paradigm for Cancer and Degenerative Diseases. *Journal of Orthomolecular Medicine*, *33*(4).

González, M. J., Sutherland, E., & Olalde, J. (2019). Quantum Functional Energy Medicine: The Next Frontier of Restorative Medicine. *Journal of Restorative Medicine*, *8*(1), 1–7. DOI: 10.14200/jrm.2019.0114

Govinda, K. (2002). *A Handbook of Chakra Healing: Spiritual Practice for Health, Harmony and Inner Peace*. Konecky & Konecky.

Grimes, J. A. (1996). *A Concise Dictionary of Indian Philosophy: Sanskrit Terms Defined in English*. State University of New York Press.

Hamblin, M. R. (2018). Photobiomodulation for Traumatic Brain Injury and Stroke. *Journal of Neuroscience Research*, *96*(4), 731–743. DOI: 10.1002/jnr.24190 PMID: 29131369

Hammerschlag, R., Levin, M., McCraty, R., Bat, N., Ives, J. A., Lutgendorf, S. K., & Oschman, J. L. (2015). Biofield Physiology: A Framework for an Emerging Discipline. *Global Advances in Health and Medicine : Improving Healthcare Outcomes Worldwide*, *4*(1_suppl, Suppl), 35–41. DOI: 10.7453/gahmj.2015.015.suppl PMID: 26665040

Iyengar, B. K. S. (2010). *Light on Pranayama*. The Crossroad Publishing Company. Chapter 5: Nadis and Chakras.

Lochtefeld, J. G. (2002). *The Illustrated Encyclopedia of Hinduism: A–M*. The Rosen Publishing Group.

Mallinson, J., & Singleton, M. (2017). *Roots of Yoga*. Penguin Books.

Pradhan, B. (2014). *Yoga and Mindfulness-Based Cognitive Therapy: A Clinical Guide*. Springer.

Sharma, R.K. (1997). Fifth Edition. Chaukhambha Sanskrit Series Office, Varanasi. Chapter 30, Shloka 3–4.

Thatte, D. G. (2016). *Elements of Shaarira Rachana* (1st ed.). Chaukhambha Orientalia.

White, D. G. (2012). *Yoga in Practice*. Princeton University Press. DOI: 10.1515/9781400839933

Woodroffe, J. (1974). *The Serpent Power*. Dover Publications.

Chapter 8
Prana-Centered AI Integrating Subtle Yogic Energetics Into Intelligent Wellness Systems

Prabir Mondal
http://orcid.org/0009-0000-3550-0986
Lakshmibai National Institute of Physical Education, Gwalior, India

Sohom Saha
http://orcid.org/0009-0006-9438-1554
Lakshmibai National Institute of Physical Education, Gwalior, India

Bharat Prasad
http://orcid.org/0009-0004-7275-4810
Central University of South Bihar, Gaya, India

Shravan Shaurya Dubey
http://orcid.org/0009-0000-8255-0708
Central University of Punjab, India

Ganesh Shanker Pandey
http://orcid.org/0009-0007-4541-7351
Central University of Punjab, India

Sukanta Das
http://orcid.org/0009-0002-8500-1207
Central University of South Bihar, Gaya, India

ABSTRACT

This chapter introduces Prana-Centered AI, a pioneering framework that blends ancient yogic energetics with modern intelligent wellness technologies. While contemporary AI-powered wearables excel at tracking physiological data, they overlook the subtle dimensions of human vitality described in classical yoga, Prana, Nadis, Chakras, and the subtle body. Prana-Centered AI bridges this gap through multimodal sensing, machine learning, and culturally sensitive interpretive models that translate physiological signals into insights aligned with yogic principles. By integrating HRV, EEG, respiration, thermal imaging, and emotional analytics, the

DOI: 10.4018/979-8-2600-2463-8.ch008

framework enables personalized guidance for breathwork, meditation, and energetic balance. This chapter outlines its architecture, scientific foundations, ethical safeguards, and emerging applications, proposing a transformative, holistic pathway for future intelligent wellness systems.

1. INTRODUCTION

The modern trend of the digital health and wellness systems has seen the greatest expansion in history as artificial intelligence (AI) became a groundbreaking software in the individualized care provision. Over the last few years, wearable health technology, which relies on the use of flexible electronics, has received immense attention due to its appealing characteristics of reduced healthcare costs, continuous physiological monitoring, and large-scale accessibility (Yuan et al., 2022). The capabilities of these AI-based systems to analyze cardiac activity, glucose levels, and other physiological indicators have proved impressive and change the paradigm of healthcare practices to more proactive ones rather than reactive ones. The AIs-controlled wearable devices are changing the remote health monitoring field as they create the potential of diagnostic real-time, customized response, and proactive disease management in a wide range of conditions, such as diabetes, cardiovascular disease, neurodegenerative diseases, mental illnesses, and maternal and infant care (Soumma et al., 2025).

Nevertheless, even with these technological innovations, there is still a vast gap in terms of dealing with aspects of human well-being that are holistic as the ancient traditions of healing explain. The Indian subcontinent yogic sciences provide an advanced system of conceptualizing health beyond the physical body, to include energetic, mental and spiritual domains of health. These approaches revolve around the notion of Prana, or the vital life force energy present in writings as early as prior to 1000 BCE, such as the Chandogya Upanishad (Muktibodhananda, 2012). This subtle energy, also known as qi in Chinese traditions, ki in Japanese tradition, and animal magnetism in Western esoteric traditions, is believed to be the fundamental constituent of all biological systems as well as the fundamental constituent of the subtle body and the whole chakra system.

Combining such ancient wisdom with the modern AI technologies is a challenge with deep prospects and challenges. Biofield science is a relatively new discipline which seeks to offer a scientific basis of complex homeodynamic regulation of living systems (Rubik et al., 2015). The biofield (complicated organizing energy field) concept, which is involved in biological homeodynamics creation, maintenance and regulation, offers the possible solution between the existing energetic schemes and the scientific knowledge. Modalities of energy medicine, such as biofield therapies, like Reiki, therapeutic touch, and external Qigong have been shown to have effects at cellular, tissue, and systemic levels; however, mechanisms are still under research (Moga & Bengston, 2010).

2. PHILOSOPHICAL FOUNDATIONS: THE SUBTLE BODY IN CLASSICAL YOGA LITERATURE

2.1 The Concept of Prana in Vedic and Tantric Traditions

Prana is a Sanskrit word that is composed of 'pra' (forth) and 'ana' (to breathe), which means the source of life force that gives life to living organisms. In yogic philosophy, prana represents the fundamental life force underlying physiological, psychological, and spiritual processes (Frawley, 1999). The Taittiriya Upanishad states that everything is born out of Prana, lives on Prana and goes back to Prana when it dies making it the ultimate rule in life itself. The Hatha Yoga Pradipika, one of the three traditional books on hatha yoga along with the Gheranda Samhita and the Shiva Samhita, says that Prana is the key to all practices related to yoga and mastering it is the fundamental principle of hatha yoga (Muktibodhananda, 1998).

Hatha yoga Hatha yoga includes the Hatha yoga Pradipika, a compilation of earlier texts of hatha yoga composed by Svatmarama in the 15th century (Svatmarama and Svatmarama, 2002). It is explicitly mentioned in the text that hatha yoga, which means the union of ha (denoting the vital force) and tha (denoting the mind, the mental energy), aims at bringing pranic and mental forces together in order to reach the higher levels of consciousness. Such an awareness places the breath control as not only a breathing exercise, but as an advanced technology to control subtle energies.

The subtle energy of pranic nature is scientifically identified and described as a biofield in the present-day research literature. The historical background of biofield therapies (millennium-old and still relevant in modern practice) has been applied to treat a variety of health disorders and prevent ill health, although scientific research and integration of these therapies has suffered due to cultural issues and institutional barriers (Sprengel et al., 2025). The current scoping review identified 353 studies in 352 published reports that investigate biofield interventions such as Reiki, Therapeutic Touch, Healing Touch, intercessory prayer, External Qigong, and Spiritual Healing, indicating the scientific interest in the practices.

2.2 The Subtle Body (Sukshma Sharira) Model

According to classical yoga literature, the human being is made up of many interpenetrating bodies or sheaths (Koshas). Sukshma Sharira (the subtle body) has nineteen components such as the five senses, the five organs of action, the four inner faculties (Antahkarana) and the five pranas (Muktibodhananda, 1998). Developed in the Hatha Yoga Pradipika, Gheranda Samhita, and Shiva Samhita, this model becomes a complex map of human energetic anatomy that has been the basis of the practice of yogic centuries. Kosha model proposes five levels of existence which descend to a dimension of the gross to subtle. Annamaya Kosha is the physical body that the food sustains and it is the most materialistic aspect of human life. Pranamaya Kosha refers to energy body that is associated with flow of pranic energy and energy. Manomaya Kosha is the mental body which harbors thoughts and emotions. Vijnanamaya Kosha is the body of wisdom that is related to intuition and higher knowledge. Lastly, the body of bliss, the Anandamaya Kosha, is the most inner part of the body, pure joy and spiritual consciousness. This complex interpretation is an indication that the interventions of wellness need to focus on several dimensions at the same time, a concept that Prana-Centered AI aims to operationalize using multimodal sensing and unified interpretive systems.

The Hatha Yoga books refer to the body by various other names like Ghatha and Pinda and contain minor concepts like Prana, Nadi, Chakra, Kundalini, Surya (sun), Chandra (moon), and Granthis (psychic knots) amongst others (Pramanik & Singh, 2023). There are two syllables of Ha and Tha correlated with Surya and Chandra which are considered to be the forces that should be balanced to achieve maximum health and spiritual growth. Hatha Yoga does not regard the body as bare matter, or as an obstacle on the way of yoga, but as the visible expression of Supreme consciousness that can become open and receptive to higher consciousness when it is employed as an ideal tool of yoga.

2.3 Nadis: The Subtle Energy Channels

Nadi (channels of subtle energy) is the circulatory system of subtle body. The Hatha Yoga Pradipika and Goraksha Samhita state that there are 72,000 nadis, and Classical yogic texts describe thousands of nadis forming a subtle energetic network throughout the body. The Hatha Yoga Pradipika clearly says that nadi does not refer to nerve but flow, similar to the flow of electricity in a cable and one of the wires carries the negative and other wire carries the positive force (Muktibodhananda, 1998).

These are the three main nadis, Ida (left), Pingala (right), and Sushumna (central) that run down the spine to the head and constitute the main routes of the pranic flow. The Ida nadi, which is lunar, is the movement of consciousness and is functionally parallel to the activity of a parasympathetic nervous system. The solar qualities are linked to the Pingala nadi which is vital energy and is equivalent to sympathetic activation. The Sushumna nadi, which is located along the spine column, the seven chakras of the body, is the neutral path through which spiritual power (Kundalini) may ascend during advanced yoga practice.

According to the text, once Sushumna is united with Ida and Pingala at Ajna chakra, it is known as hatha yoga and once this initial union is done, the energy proceeds to Sahasrara chakra and here the ultimate union is termed as yoga. Cleaning of nadis is a very crucial practice prior to hatha yoga. This is because the Hatha Yoga Pradipika states that upon the purification of the nadis, external signs of success are evident: the body becomes thin and glows which means there is best flow of prana (Svatmarama & Svatmarama, 2002). This focus on nadi purification with exercises like pranayama and shatkarma (six cleansing methods), is an indication that quantifiable physiological effects are present in conjunction with the purification of the body with energy, which are potentially measurable with modern sensing technologies.

2.4 Chakras: Centers of Consciousness

The chakra system is an expression of centers in which the numerous nadis meet each other producing centers of increased power and awareness. Within the varied tantric texts there are various numbers of chakras detailed in the Netra Tantra (six), the Kaulajnanaitnaya (eight) and the Kubjikamata Tantra (seven), although Kubjikamata Tantra (seven) has since become the most popular system of chakras in modern practice (White, 2003). The awakening of Kundalini is the topic of the Hatha yoga with Kundalini moving upwards through the chakras to the realms of higher mental states and ultimately settling in Sahasrara chakra at the crown of the head (Muktibodhananda, 1998). The chakras have a particular psychological state, physiological functions and spiritual states, making it a full map of human experience. The Muladhara chakra at the base of the spine is associated with survival instincts and grounding, Svadhisthana with being creative and fluid emotional, Manipura with personal power and digestion, Anahata with love and compassion, Vishuddha with communication and expression, Ajna with intuition and insight, and Sahasrara with spiritual connection and transcendence. This correspondence indicates possible mappings between chakra states and quantifiable physiological values, which Prana-Centered AI aims to investigate with the aid of state-of-the-art sensing technologies and machine learning, keeping in proper epistemic humility regarding the characteristics of these correlations.

2.5 The Five Vayus: Functional Aspects of Prana

The prana exists in the form of five main functional forms (Vayus), which are the ones that control particular processes, which are physiological and psychological. Prana Vayu is the ruler of inhalation and taking in of energy, making holes in the head and the brain to allow the reception of vital force. The Apana Vayu controls the elimination and downward moving energy and forms openings in the lower-body and regulation of elimination processes. The upward and downward forces are in equilibrium and are controlled by Samana Vayu which controls the digestion and absorption at the center of the navel. Udana Vayu also controls expression, speech and upward moving energy, and it helps in communication and spiritual aspiration. Vyana Vayu is in charge of flow and distribution within the body so that pranic energy flows to every tissue and organ.

The Hatha Yoga Pradipika also lays stress on the connection between Prana and Apana Vayu whereby in Mula Bandha (root lock) Prana and Apana join Nada (inner sound) and Bindu (life energy) to bring perfection in yoga (Svatmarama & Svatmarama, 2002). The text goes further to elaborate that when the Apana goes up and enters the fire sphere, the flame is extended, and Kundalini, which senses the intense warmth, wakes up and straightens himself. This pranic energy functional differentiation offers a subtle framework of comprehending the imbalance of energies and their manifestations, which can be used to guide AI-oriented evaluations and interventions solutions without disregarding the metaphysical aspects of pranic energy that cannot be exhaustively quantified by technological methods.

Although the classical literature of yogurthara explains that prana, nadis, and chakras are subtle energetic principles, recently, science studies them more as their potential physiological counterparts. The control of the breath has an effect on the work of the autonomic nervous system, meditation can change brain waves, and the mood is associated with physical indicators of the state. These physiological indicators do not capture the metaphysical aspects of yogic energetics, but they offer quantifiable proxies through which the current technologies can investigate the possibility of the connection between classical wellness models and biological homeostasis. This new intersection grounds the conceptual framework of Prana-Centered AI offered in this chapter.

3. SCIENTIFIC CORRELATES: BRIDGING TRADITIONAL KNOWLEDGE AND MODERN RESEARCH

3.1 Pranayama and Autonomic Nervous System Modulation

Modern studies have developed strong scientific principles of the physiological impact of the yogic techniques of breathing. Meditative states, stress reduction, and lung capacity are also known to be induced through the millenarian breathing exercises of Yoga, known as Pranayamas, although more physiological evidence is still yet to be explained how these practices adjust the human nervous system

(Campanelli et al., 2020). A systematic review of evidence based on PRISMA guidelines included all the articles published within the period of 2008-2018, and fourteen studies that met the inclusion criteria were found to show consistent changes in the measurements of autonomic nervous system towards parasympathy dominance, and increases in paroxysmal gamma waves and changes in the power and wave expression in the EEG readings.

It has been shown that slow pranayama breathing produces inhibitory signals and hyperpolarizing current by mechanical stretching of tissues that activate the synchronization of the neural components in the central nervous system that leads to changes in autonomic balance in favor of the parasympathetic (Kavitha et al., 2024). In a randomized controlled trial study on the effects of pranayama in the treatment of patients with anxiety disorders, the pranayama group was significantly higher in mean RR intervals ($P < 0.01$), SDNN ($P < 0.001$), RMSSD ($P < 0.001$), NN50 ($P < 0.05$), and pNN50 ($P < 0.001$) in time domain indices; frequency domain indices were significantly higher in HF ($P < 0.001$) and total power These results show that slow pranayama practice will reduce cardiac autonomic functioning and achieve a positive shift in sympathetic-parasympathetic dominance.

A systematic review of psycho-physiological correlates of slow breathing analyzed the publications that studied the alterations in the parameters of physiological activities of the central and autonomic nervous system, as well as the correlation with the outcomes of behavior (Zaccaro et al., 2018). Following PRISMA-guidelines, the review analyzed only studies that have used healthy human subjects with objective measures, and confirmed that slow breathing (less than 10 breaths per minute) techniques are to have a positive influence on the work of the autonomic nervous system and the central nervous system. These results offer an empirical confirmation of the traditional yoga concept that the control of breath makes a difference in the whole psychophysiological system.

A recent systematic review and meta-analysis of the effectiveness of pranayama against mental disorders used randomized controlled trials reported in PubMed, PsycINFO and Central databases until April 2024 (Mutze et al., 2025). The review estimated the standardized mean difference with the 95 percent confidence interval of the symptom severity, health related quality of life and depression outcomes. The results have shown that slow breathing has been linked to elevated alpha power in the electroencephalogram, which is a sign of relaxation and attention, and that pranayama protocols based on the use of slow and controlled breathing methods may enhance the effects of the treatment and reduce adverse events (Mutze et al., 2025).

3.2 Neurological Correlates of Meditation and Contemplative Practices

The studies conducted on electroencephalography (EEG) have already reported unique neural activation patterns that are related to different meditation practices. A comparison of the practitioners of three meditation traditions Vipassana, Himalayan Yoga, and Isha Shoonya with a control group showed that all meditators demonstrated a high parieto-occipital 60-110 Hz gamma amplitude compared to the control subjects as a trait effect during meditation (Braboszcz et al., 2017). This gamma power had a positive correlation with the experience of meditation of the participants and independent component analysis ensured that gamma activity did not arise within eye and muscle artifacts. These results indicate that the common characteristics of more gamma activity might be found in meditation traditions that might be shown as improved attention and brain involvement. Review of literature on mindfulness meditation shows that meditation training has both state and trait behavior on neural activity. Among long-term meditators the parietal-occipital EEG gamma power in non-REM sleep is higher and the effect is more concentrated in the 25-40 Hz gamma range, and is positively correlated with the practice of daily meditation throughout their lifetime (Ferrarelli et al., 2013). Interestingly, the gamma activity of the parieto-occipital regions in sleep was predictable on a daily basis, but not on retreat time, which is the original evidence of a particular effect of everyday meditation on the neuroplasticity of the brain unlike intensive retreat meditation.

Meditation may be theorized as a sequence of control and self-inquiry mental training programs developed towards different purposes, such as the training of well-being and psychological wellness, and growing evidence indicates that meditation training leads to functional and anatomical neuronal adaptations associated with perception, cognition, and emotional processing developments (Ferrarelli et al., 2013). Recent systematic review studies have shown theta waves to be the most prominent in the frontal and middle brain areas during meditation, and probably arise out of reduced attention that observes inner processes, and alpha-waves during meditation arise out of wakeful relaxation, and beta-waves reduce during meditation and rest and so meditators leave the problems to themselves (Lagopoulos et al., 2009).

EEG research conducted has supported the hypothesis that mindful awareness is a spontaneous state of being which brings with it joy, peace, and happiness, and is also linked with spontaneous brain alpha activity of 8-13 Hz (Duda et al., 2024). It is also linked with global changes in oscillatory activity in those who engage in focal attention and open monitoring mediation practices than to meditation-naive adults, and the magnitude of these changes grows with an increment of the duration of meditation training. Although there are correlations between focal attention and open monitoring with enhancement of anterior theta state, there are only focal attention correlations with the alteration of posterior theta oscillations, which indicate practice-specific neural activities.

3.3 Alternate Nostril Breathing and Hemispheric Balance

Studies on Nadi Shodhana (alternate nostril breathing) have led to the provision of evidence about the association between the yogic activities and the hemispheric activity within the brain. The systematic review of forty-four randomized controlled trials revealed that alternate nostril breathing has positive effects on autonomic nervous and cardiopulmonary system, cardiovascular parameters, cognitive functioning, problem-solving, and motor memory retention (Ghiya, 2017). These results are in line with conventional theories of yoga that focus on balancing of Ida and Pingala nadis via alternate nostril breathing techniques. It was already shown that manipulations with the nostril's airflow using hands can selectively influence the brain network oscillations (Zickerick et al., 2020).

The suggested physiological interactions of pranayama are a cascade of activities which start with mechanoreceptors and chemoreceptors of the respiratory system, then mechanoreceptors and chemoreceptors of the circulatory system, then the respiro-circulatory control center of the brain, then the cerebellum, then the limbic system, and then the cerebral cortex (Mondal, 2024). This is a multifaceted model corroborated by seventy-three papers reviewed in accordance with the PRISMA guidelines that can offer a scientific framework of how practices regarding breath control can impact various physiological systems at the same time.

3.4 Yoga Nidra and Deep Relaxation States

Yoga Nidra, or a structured approach to attaining profound physical, mental, and emotional rest and staying awake, has aroused considerable neuroscientific interest. The authors of the first fMRI experiment on Yoga Nidra, the researchers of IIT Delhi, AIIMS Delhi, and Mahajan Imaging Delhi, studied how the functional connections of meditators (n=30) and novice controls (n=31) alter when practicing (Fialoke et al., 2024). The researchers discovered that the experts, in a state of Yoga Nidra, showed decoupling in the default mode network (DMN) connectivity, and beginners showed more DMN connectivity. This deviation could be an indication of the higher skills of the skilled practitioners to control their mind and brain states in the deeper relaxation levels.

Importantly, the length of the meditation practice was also associated with the decrease in functional connectivity of DMN seeds to DMN areas in the course of Yoga Nidra, indicating that the long-term yoga practice results in the long-term alteration of brain patterns of connectivity (Fialoke et al., 2024). The research enhances the comprehension of the neural mechanisms of Yoga Nidra whereby it is demonstrated that there is a decoupling of the DMN connectivity in case of meditators and that this decoupling is associated with meditation and yoga experience. The findings may be potentially indicative of the fact that the experienced meditators have lower mind-wandering than novices since the DMN is linked to self-referential processing and mind-wandering. It has been researched that Yoga Nidra is linked to favorable physiological shifts, such as hematological variables, red blood cell counts, blood glucose levels, and hormonal status (Pandi-Perumal et al., 2022). Previous PET-EEGs found a 65 percent rise in dopamine release during the practice of Yoga Nidra, which is linked to the decrease in striatum activity and executive control, which might trigger positive affect and motivation. Yoga Nidra is practiced in the guided directions and supine position making it open to neuroimaging and clinical studies, allowing repetition of experiments within the context of the practice.

3.5 Heart-Brain Coherence and Neurocardiological Integration

The studies of the cardiac and cerebral activity relationship can give some knowledge about pranic concepts of energetic coherence. Research conducted to investigate the impact of mindfulness meditation on neurocardiological interaction revealed that the practice of meditation modulates the brain waves and heart coherence as well as a significant relationship exists between the alpha peak frequency and the cardiac measures (Gao et al., 2023). Heart coherence of the HRV spectrum, expressed as the peak power/total power of the HRV, measures the extent of similarity between the waveform of the HRV tachogram and a sinusoidal wave, which is the extent of synchronization in autonomic regulation.

Visceral activity is controlled via the autonomic nervous system by the central nervous system, and the majority of visceral organs have distinct circadian rhythms independently (Gao et al., 2023). Wellbeing requires the coherent mind-body activity and circadian rhythms, and disturbances of them may cause dysfunction of the visceral organs. Frontal midline theta rhythm has also been established to be linked with cardiac autonomic processes occurring in attention-challenging meditation processes, indicating that certain brain waves may be used as an indicator of psychophysiological integration. The results can be compared with the yogic ideas of pranic coherence and the unity of various components of the subtle body.

Table 1. Conceptual Mapping Between Yogic Energetics, Physiological Markers, and AI Sensing Technologies

Yogic Concept	Physiological Indicator	Sensing Technology	AI Interpretation
Prana flow	Heart rate variability (HRV), respiration rhythm	ECG, PPG, respiratory sensors	Detection of autonomic balance and energetic vitality patterns
Nadi balance (Ida–Pingala)	Hemispheric EEG asymmetry, nasal airflow	EEG headsets, airflow sensors	AI models identify left–right neural balance patterns
Chakra activity	Emotional state, brain oscillations	EEG, EDA, HRV	Pattern recognition linking emotional regulation with meditation states
Vayu regulation	Breath rhythm, digestive signals, circulation	Respiratory belts, wearable biosensors	AI models detect breathing irregularities and energy imbalance
Meditation depth	Alpha, theta, gamma EEG activity	Portable EEG	Machine learning classification of meditative states

4. TECHNOLOGICAL FOUNDATIONS: MULTIMODAL SENSING FOR SUBTLE ENERGETICS

4.1 AI-Powered Wearable Sensors and Health Monitoring

With the advent of AI-driven wearable sensors, the opportunities of constant health monitoring have never been as robust before. The human health monitoring wearable sensors may be categorized with physical sensors that measure physical and physiological signals, chemical sensors, and biosensors that measure the chemical signals, and such devices can assist clinical and healthcare services to move away of centralized clinical diagnostics to more personalized and individualized home care (Shajari et al., 2023). Federated learning, transfer learning, and edge-AI are machine learning techniques that can improve the processing of these physiological signals, i.e., glucose levels, gait patterns and heart rate variability.

An exhaustive analysis of wearable sensors and machine learning to assess health has discovered that transformer model can handle multi-source sensor signals, exhausting the full capability of self-attention mechanisms and timing expression features to highly decrease the rates of false negative of abnormal states (Chen et al., 2024). Combining knowledge bases with wearable systems is what allows the discrimination schemes that merge the multi-source sensor signals with the expert experience using two-step anomaly recognition plan. This practice is similar to the classical yoga focus on integrating physical observation and wisdom experience. The field of wearable devices is actively studied to increase the convenience of the devices, their comfort, and non-invasiveness of the monitoring of physiological vital parameters, as well as psychological or emotional condition (Sabry et al., 2022).

4.2 Heart Rate Variability as a Window to Autonomic Function

The behavior of the heart rate variability (HRV) has become one of the key biomarkers of the assessment of the work of the autonomic nervous system, and by extension, measures of the energetic balance applicable to yogic models. HRV is a variation of the time delay between cardiac strokes, indicating the capacity of the autonomic nervous system to adjust to psychological and physiological variations (de Carvalho-Guimaraes et al., 2022). Time-domain indicators of sympathovagal balance such as SDNN (standard deviation of NN intervals), RMSSD (root mean square of successive differences) and pNN50 (percentage of successive RR intervals that change by more than 50 ms), and frequency-domain indicators of sympatho-vagal balance such as LF (low frequency), HF (high frequency) and LF/HF ratio, complement each other.

There is a lot in the literature about the relationship between the practice of pranayama and the HRV. Vedic Indian breath control methods have been revealed to elevate measurements of heart rate variability indicating tone of the parasympathetic nervous system (Sharpe et al., 2021). Researchers conducted a crossover clinical trial on five elements of pranayama practice to identify significant breathing intervention effects on RMSSD, and the researchers found that RMSSD significantly changed, with 0.2 to 0.5 changes in logRMSSD ($p<0.01$ in all conditions). These results indicate that HRV monitoring might be used as a window into pranic states, but the meaning of such data has to be approached with the help of the traditional knowledge frameworks. The analysis of HRV data based on AI can provide potential opportunities to infer the aspects of autonomic balance, which can be associated with the state of energy. Having raw HRV data, it is possible to use machine learning algorithms to identify patterns that are related to a specific condition, stress level, or meditative state. Convolutional neural networks and multilayer perceptrons have proven to be reliable deep learning methods in stress detection through the use of the models, which have recorded an accuracy of more than 90 percent (Bobade & Vani, 2020). The same type of architecture might be reconfigured to measure the states needed to practice yoga.

4.3 Electroencephalography and Brain-State Monitoring

The EEG technology offers excellent temporal resolution to the measurement of synchronized brain activity caused by rhythmic coordination of population of neurons. Various EEG frequency bands are linked to certain neuronal networks, conditions, and functions (Kaur and Singh, 2015). The most common are Delta waves (0.5-4 Hz), which occur during significant sleep and unconsciousness. The theta waves (4-8 Hz) mean meditation, creativity, and memory consolidation. Alpha waves (8-13 Hz) indicate the state of relaxed awareness and meditation. Wave of 13-30Hz (Beta) signifies an active mind and focus. The gamma waves (30-100+ Hz) are related to increased cognitive functions, integration, and awareness. With the evolution of portable and consumer-grade EEG devices, which have become more available, brain-state monitoring is now more accessible. One of the studies examining the impact of meditation on people with cognitive impairment employed portable Muse EEG equipment to measure mindfulness and brain activity (Lazarou et al., 2023).

The results demonstrated the possible usefulness of portable EEG devices as clinical tools that can be used as cost-effective, non-invasive, and readily available devices. Experiments that have incorporated Muse EEG with assessment of concentration meditation have indicated that mindfulness training is linked with progress in numerous illnesses as far as both self-reported and the EEG-derived data are considered. Since studies have established that even novice meditators can generate huge effects on EEG spectra with brief meditation interventions, this evidence is highly significant.

In a randomized controlled study on the effects of a three-day meditation workshop in 223 meditation beginners, it was shown that the intervention could have significant and variable effects on the EEG spectra with the largest change to 50% in different frequency bands and the greatest decrease to 24% (Stapleton et al., 2019). Findings indicated a primary 5% decline in delta power, a worldwide augmentation of 29% in theta power, a 16% worldwide increment in alpha power, 17-percent increment in beta power and 11-percent increment in gamma power amid pre-meditation and end-meditation status. The rate of transition between the pre-meditation and post-meditation states was also great as the probability of the initial minute is 0.76 of entering into the end-meditation state.

4.4 Electrodermal Activity and Emotional Response

The electrodermal activity (EDA), also called galvanic skin response, is an indication of the activity of the sympathetic nervous system recorded as a change in skin conductance caused by the activity of the glands of the sweat. Since emotional changes have impacts on physiological measurements, the use of EDA monitoring provides data on emotional conditions and stress reactions. The EDA-based deep learning strategies have been effective in emotion recognition, and the models have shown high accuracy in their ability to identify stress and emotional conditions (Zhu et al., 2023). The studies on physiological signal stress detection on wearable devices have explored EDA, ECG and PPG data with six machine learning algorithms such as support vectors machines and k-nearest neighbours (Campanelli et al., 2020). The highest accuracy of 86.4% on EDA signals was obtained in a stacking ensemble learning approach. Concerning Prana-Centered AI, EDA might be used as a sign of emotional reactions or efficacy of the stress-reduction interventions in the process of yogic practice.

4.5 Thermal Imaging and Non-Contact Assessment

The infra-red thermal imaging (IRTI) is a non-invasive technique of measuring autonomic activity and psychophysiological states. It has been shown that thermal patterns of meditators are very different, compared to those of non-meditators, and there are characteristic temperature patterns of meditation states (Singh et al., 2018). The benefit of using thermal imaging is its lack of contact, and it will not interfere with meditation or yogic practice. Thermal imaging can be used to compute several autonomic variables, such as the localized rate of blood perfusion, cardiac pulse rate, the rate of breath, and stress responses (Cardone and Merla, 2017). Research has established that there is a fall in temperature of the forehead and a rise in temperature of the chin in meditation processes, which may be typical attributes of meditation states. This method has a potential of measuring factors of physiological conditions without necessarily having physical sensors that are likely to interfere with practice.

5. ARCHITECTURE FOR PRANA-CENTERED AI SYSTEMS

5.1 Layer 1: Energetic Data Layer

The Multimodal Physiological Sensing and Breath analytics are incorporated into the Energetic Data Layer and are the basis of further interpretation. Major ones are ECG and PPG to calculate HRV, which indicates the cardiac activity and autonomic stability; EEG to measure the brain-state and neural correlates of meditative and attentional states; EDA to measure stress and emotional responses; respiratory sensors such as impedance plethysmography, respiratory belts or nasal thermistors to analyse the breath pattern and thermal cameras to map temperature and assess autonomic activation pattern.

Multimodal medical data fusion has become a groundbreaking practice in intelligent healthcare, which allows achieving a complete picture of the state of patients and individual treatment strategies (Shaik et al., 2024). A literature review on the fusion and analysis of multimodal data investigated various methods such as feature selection, rule-based systems, machine learning, deep learning, and natural language processing to combine and interpret multimodal data. This multimodal practice is consistent with the yogic concept of health as a multidimensional phenomenon that should be measured in relation to each other and not in isolation.

5.2 Layer 2: Subtle Body Interpretive Models

Subtle Body Interpretive Models layer uses algorithms in machine learning to convert physiological measurements into measurements applicable in the practice of yoga and well-being. This layer is a fundamental conceptual input to Prana-Centered AI that tries to establish a connection between measured phenomena and conventional models and has epistemic humility concerning what such correlations could or could not be. Multimodal biomedical data fusion algorithms based on deep learning are able to choose suitable pre-trained models depending on data modality to present features and post-fusion, and secondly fuse depending on attention mechanisms (Duan et al., 2024). These technical strategies are amenable to interpretive concerns of subtle bodies.

Components Pranic Flow Assessment Model components include Pranic Flow Assessment which consists of models that have been trained on physiological signatures of an enhanced vs. restricted state of vitality based on HRV coherence, respiratory patterns and thermal signatures. Nadi Balance Evaluation is an assessment of an energetic balance of the left and right sides based on hemispheric EEG asymmetry, nasal cycle patterns, and autonomic balance indices, which are based on research that found alternate nostril breathing to have different effects on brain network oscillations (Zickerick et al., 2020). Chakra Activity Mapping includes initial models of correlating particular physiological patterns with reported experience in chakra-centered meditation, recognizing the experimental character of such mappings, and with the necessity of validation by joint research with advanced practitioners.

Vayu Function Analysis is the method of evaluation of the functional elements by the patterns of breath, signals of digestion, voice, and circulatory measurements. The interpretative frameworks need to be created in the form of research, which combines yogic knowledge and data science approach. It has been shown that deep learning models have the capability to gain meaningful representations in large datasets of physiological data, which is good at gradually abstracting and encoding information using multi-layer networks (Stahlschmidt et al., 2022). These models have proven to be highly accurate on stress detection and classification into emotional states, and so there is potential that they can be adapted to serve the yogic state assessment, although care should be taken to validate construct validity and cultural appropriateness.

5.3 Layer 3: Pranic Balance Engine

The Pranic Balance Engine produces individualized suggestions of breathing, posture, or meditation practices depending on the states evaluated and personal features. The layer is a recommendation system that is guided by both conventional knowledge and previously gathered user data and builds on the traditional methods of AI in health recommendation systems but adds the domain knowledge provided by yogic traditions. The functions of the engine are: State Assessment Integration: a combination of multiple model outputs to consistent profiles of current condition; Imbalance Detection: the identification of patterns which may suggest disruptions or areas of concern; Intervention Selection: recommendation fitting to assessed states and a curated set of practices developed through collaboration with traditional experts; Personalization Algorithms: recommendation customization based on individual response patterns, practice history, and reported goals; and Progress Tracking: monitoring longitudinal changes and practice outcomes to improve recommendations over time.

The engine relies on recommendations grounded on collaborative filters, content-based filters and hybrid methods to give customized suggestions. Physiological signal monitoring in a controlled environment with bedside monitoring gives accurate real-time inferences, whereas wearable devices are more adequate in ambulatory health monitoring of patients because they promote mobility; however, they are susceptible to ambulatory noises of unforeseen character (Kher & Patel, 2021). The Pranic Balance Engine also has to strike a balance between prompt conditions and longer-term developmental tracks that would be relevant in a yoga practice despite the fact that yogic development is a process that would require gradual change instead of instant optimization.

5.4 Layer 4: Energetic Feedback Interface

Energetic Feedback Interface offers real-time advice on the states of the mind by giving feedback via multimodal feedback display to help meditate and yogic environment without interfering. The modalities of interfaces are visual feedback in the form of ambient lighting, simple graphics, or abstract visualizations of physiological conditions; audio feedback in the form of tones, nature sounds, or guided instructions scaled to assessed conditions; haptic feedback in the form of subtle vibrations signifying information without a visual focus; and voice guidance in the form of AI-generated instructions adjusted to real-time physiological changes.

The digital health technologies have led to the easy accessibility of a variety of monitoring potentials, yet all of it comes at a risk of dehumanizing care unless implemented with clear consideration (Mesko et al., 2017). Technology use only results in improved health condition provided that the associated cultural issues are taken into consideration and the practitioner needs are addressed. Such disruptive technologies as deep learning algorithms and health sensors might add to value-based healthcare as well as assist in making sure that clinical judgment and experience to creative problem-solving human skills decide on the success of interventions and mutual relationship between practitioners and technologies.

5.5 Layer 5: Ethical Safety Module

The Ethical Safety Module provides the adequate limits of AI intervention in the practice traditionally demands the teacher-supervision and engaging deep psychological and spiritual aspects. This layer discusses the issues of AI systems in contemplative spheres harming people by providing unsuitable advice or excessive dependence on technology or being culturally insensitive. Some of the functions of Safety are Practice Boundary Monitoring, that recognizes the evidence of over-practice, inappropriate intensity, or adverse reactions using physiological evidence; Contraindication Screening, indicating health conditions or medications that may contraindicate some practices; Teacher Referral Protocols, recommending human intervention in case AI assessment identifies complex circumstances; Cultural Sensitivity Checks, making sure that the recommendations are made in the context of appropriate cultural settings and user preferences; and Data Protection, that has strong privacy defenses on sensitive physiological and practice-related information.

Artificial intelligence as part of the traditional medical industry faces multiple regulatory and governance issues, such as regulatory complexity and legal responsibility concerns (Harishbhai Tilala et al., 2024). The digitization of traditional knowledge poses ethical issues of intellectual property, conservation of biodiversity and equitable access and benefit-sharing. The problem of algorithmic bias, the erosion of a culture, and the lack of contextual sensitivity are only several prominent ethical concerns that will have to be resolved to bring responsible and respectful AI usage. The traditional medicine has got sensitive, holistic health information, which includes medical, lifestyle, emotional health and in some cases, genetic profile, and needs to comply with the international data protection standards.

6. EMERGING APPLICATIONS OF PRANA-CENTERED AI

6.1 AI-Guided Nadi Shodhana Systems

Alternate nostral breathing (Nadi Shodhana) is a perfect candidate of AI-enhanced instructions due to its well-known physiological effects and the format of practice. A meta-analysis study that included forty-four randomized controlled trials has shown that alternate nostril breathing has positive effects on the autonomic nervous and cardiopulmonary systems, as well as on cardiovascular parameters, cognitive and problem-solving and motor memory retention (Ghiya, 2017). These results are in concordance with conventional yoga doctrine of balancing Ida and Pingala nadis by using alternate nostral breathing exercises.

A Nadi Shodhana system controlled by AI would be able to monitor the airflow in the nostrils via acoustic or pressure sensors in order to measure patterns of nostril dominance, measure responses to HRV to provide feedback on autonomic balancing effects, adjust breath timing guidance to individual response patterns, and guide practitioners on progressively more advanced protocols based on their level of experience. The studies have shown that paced nostril breathing reduces the alpha/mu oscillations in the central and parietal regions and increases the frontal midline and occipital theta oscillations as compared to spontaneous breathing (Zickerick et al., 2020). Alternate nostril breathing was more associated with alpha/mu oscillation suppression compared to unilateral breathing, whereas unilateral nostril breathing, in turn, led to ipsilateral increases in alpha connectivity. The AI systems may optimize these effects by creating personal protocols and adjusting them in real-time as a response to the EEG feedback.

6.2 Chakra-Based Emotional Guidance Systems

Although the notion of chakras cannot be easily reduced to biological terms, AI systems may come to the rescue in assisting with chakra-based meditation by detecting physiological patterns that are linked to reported emotional states in relation to different chakra areas, providing visualization clues or attention control in relation to a given chakra area, monitoring longitudinal changes in emotional states along with physiological equivalents, and offering practice-advice based on identified areas of emotional issue. Studies have shown that meditation traditions generate typical neural patterns which can be recorded by EEG recording. The parieto-occipital gamma amplitude was greater than control participants in all meditators in Vipassana, Himalayan Yoga, and Isha Shoonya schools, and power gamma was related positively to the mediation experience of participants (Braboszcz et al., 2017). These systems should not be overly confident in their epistemic judgment, and their promise of chakra-related advice should be seen as an adjunctary guidance, not a diagnostic one, and they should also help users to build their own embodied knowledge, as opposed to relying on the information provided by the technologies.

6.3 Trauma-Informed Energetic Regulation Tools

Trauma-sensitive yoga and AI-enhanced wellness have the potential to intersect and create the tools that can help to manage the nervous system in survivors of trauma. It has been reported that yoga interventions can be effective in terms of trauma recovery, and the processes that are related to it include the enhancement of vagal tone and the development of interoceptive awareness. AI-informed systems might offer non-coercive, option-based advice that is suitable to trauma victims, detect indicators of dysregulation and change the intensity, observe patterns of window-of-tolerance and prescribe practices that can help a client to increase regulatory capacity, and can be tailored to therapeutic regimens with oversight by a clinician. According to the definition provided by the World Health Organization, traditional medicine is the overall collection of knowledge, skill, and practice that relies on theories, beliefs, and experiences specific to cultures, whether explainable or not, used to keep a person healthy and in treatment (Cramer, 2023). It is defined by the use of human touch in medicine and the problem of AI disrupts this trend because traditional, complementary and integrative medicine (TCIM) focuses on the personal touch. Of significance will be the fact that TCIM practitioners should be central in enhancing AI as opposed to the fact that it has reduced them to facilitators and use AI capabilities to release time to perform duties that need human skills and emotion.

6.4 AI-Enhanced Yoga Nidra

The systematic nature of Yoga Nidra and the neurophysiological outcomes recorded on it predetermine its application to the AI improvement. The initial fMRI experiment of Yoga Nidra showed that experienced meditators experienced decoupling of default mode network (DMN) connection and novices were more coupled with DMN connection through their practice (Fialoke et al., 2024). This divergence could be taken to be an advanced form of the control of the mind and brain state of experienced practitioners in the deep forms of relaxation. The overall time of meditation practice was associated with the decrease in functional connectivity of DMN seeds with DMN regions in Yoga Nidra, indicating that the persistent practice has long-term effects on the shift in the patterns of brain connectivity.

AI systems of Yoga Nidra may adjust speeds and content of directed instructions based on real-time physiological feedback, detect the emergence of sleep-like conditions through EEG signalling, customise the sequence of exercises, and evaluate results concerning the quality of sleep, stress relief, and wellbeing. Previous PET-EEG experiments demonstrated that there was a 65 percent increase in dopamine in Yoga Nidra practice, which was linked to less activity of the striatum and executive control, and that could be stimulating the positive affect and motivational state

(Pandi-Perumal et al., 2022). The AI systems may be beneficial to streamline the practice towards mood enhancing applications and make sure that the practitioners are in the right mind to practice.

6.5 Personalized Pranayama Optimization

The AI systems could allow accuracy in the methods of pranayama training, adapting the interventions to each particular constitutions, actual conditions and growth patterns. The primary effects of slow breathing methods reported in a systematic review encompass autonomic and central nervous system alterations that facilitate autonomic changes that raise variability in heart rate and respiratory sinu arrhythmia accompanied by changes in central nervous system activities of an increase in EEG alpha power and reduction in theta power (Zaccaro et al., 2018). Psychological and behavioral products of these changes comprise boosted comfort, leisure, pleasantness, vigor, and wakefulness as well as reduced arousal, anxiety, depression, anger, and confusion symptoms. A meta-analysis that synthesized thirty-one studies that studied the effects of slow-paced breathing revealed that it had significant immediate effects in lowering systolic blood pressure and moderated effects in lowering negative feelings, especially perceived stress (Shao et al., 2024). These benefits could be optimized by AI systems because of individual protocol development.

6.6 Current AI-Based Digital Wellness Platforms

A variety of new digital health platforms are examples of how artificial intelligence is already being used to monitor wellness and assist with meditation. Wearable systems, including Apple Watch, Fitbit, and Oura Ring, can utilize AI-based algorithms to track physiology-related data like heart rate variability, sleep habits, and activity. Muse EEG headbands are neurotechnology platforms that are able to give real-time biofeedback during the process of meditation by decoding brainwave patterns into audio feedback. By the same token, mobile apps such as Calm, Headspace, and Wysa are progressively using machine learning to tailor mindfulness and mental health interventions. These systems show how AI is increasingly becoming integrated with contemplative practices though the majority of them are aimed at physiological measures instead of energetic explanations. The given proposal of Prana-Centered AI framework is a continuation of this trend, with the added layer of interpreting physiological data with yogic models of energy.

7. METHODOLOGICAL CHALLENGES AND RESEARCH DIRECTIONS

7.1 Validity of Energetic Constructs

One of the fundamental problems in emerging Prana-Centered AI is to determine the validity of the energetic constructs as a goal of technological evaluation and intervention. Biofield science is a recent area with the approach intended to offer the scientific support of complex homeodynamic control of living systems, but the agreement on the methods of measurements and theoretical models is still limited (Rubik et al., 2015). The biofield theory offers a possible interim between the conventional energetic theories and the existing scientific knowledge, though significant amount of research is required to define credible evaluation procedures.

Future research directions are creating operational definitions of energetic states that are scientifically investigable and at the same time respectful of traditional meanings, neurophenomenological research that combines first-person accounts with physiological measures, investigations of convergent validity between various types of assessment, and creation of discriminant validity between energetic states and psychological or physiological constructions. A recent scoping review reported 353 studies that explored biofield interventions, which are showing increasing scientific attention to such practices, although there is still a requirement to improve methodologies (Sprengel et al., 2025).

7.2 Training Data and Model Development

Training data with suitable labels is necessary to develop machine learning models that can be relied on to categorize the energetic state. Issues such as the subjectivity of energetic experiences and difficulty of reliable labeling, relative dearth of professional practitioners to make accurate self-report, individual variation of physiological pattern, as well as of experience and report, and possible cultural and contextual influences on experience and report, are all problems. Such methodological procedures as working with expert practitioners, who may give more detailed phenomenological reports; multiple labeling methods and agreement assessment; unsupervised or semi-supervised learning methods that may discover natural clusters in physiological data could be used. The use of deep learning technology has major benefits over conventional manual feature extraction technologies that have to learn useful representations of physiological data via multi-layer mechanism (Duan et al., 2024). Nevertheless, such approaches to subtle body notions must be properly justified in reference to the reports made by qualified practitioners, as regards their experiential values.

7.3 Practical Implementation Challenges

Although Prana-Centered AI systems have a conceptual potential, the practical implementation has a number of challenges. First, there should be clinical validation that involves determination of consistent relationships between physiological indications and subjective energetic experiences. Second, the regulatory frameworks on the use of AI-based health technologies might need to prove the safety, transparency, and explainability of such systems before they can be implemented in healthcare services. Third, the environmental noise and user behaviors can influence wearable sensor data, which can limit the accuracy in the real-life settings. Lastly, the consideration of culture should be thoroughly done in order to make sure that the traditional yogic knowledge does not become a mere technological interpretation. These issues will demand the integration of various disciplines between engineers, clinicians, yoga scholars, and traditional practitioners.

8. ETHICAL CONSIDERATIONS

8.1 Preserving Traditional Knowledge and Practice Integrity

The merging of AI and yogic practices has put the issues of commercialization, decontextualization, and possible misinterpretation of traditional teaching into focus. Traditional medicine is not a set of treatments, it is a worldview whereby health is harmony among people, groups and within the ecosystems (Kuruvilla et al., 2025). The assimilation of AI into the various therapies and practices of traditional medicine implies some complexities in regulation and also casts some doubts concerning the preservation of the integrity and cultural importance of these practices. Some of the ethical principles are the involvement of traditional knowledge holders in the design and assessment of systems, not reducing technological measurement to spiritual attainment, appropriate boundaries between AI-enabled practice and human teacher relationships, and that commercial development does not take advantage of or falsify the traditional knowledge.

8.2 Data Privacy and Security

The data of energetic assessment incorporates very sensitive physiological data with data of mental situation, emotional patterns, and possibly spiritual practices. Sensitive, holistic health information, such as medical, lifestyle, emotional health, and, in some cases, genetic profiles, falls under the evidence of traditional medicine and must be kept in line with international data protection regulations, such as the

General Data Protection Regulation, the Health Insurance Portability and Accountability Act, and similar regulations in different jurisdictions (Singh et al., 2018).

Particular attention should be paid to the minimization of data collection to the extent of what the system will perform, the high level of encryption and access control, the provision of transparency regarding the use and sharing of data, the possibility of the user control over the maintenance and deletion of data, and the possible discrimination due to supposed characteristics. Open data sharing is encouraged in the digital health field and results in friction with data sovereignty movements that seek to possess health data as a means of self-determination (Walter et al., 2021). In certain societies, the assumption of open access as a universally good thing is a priori incorrect and digital technologies are likely to expose traditional knowledge to the risks of being stolen by other nations.

8.3 Algorithmic Fairness and Bias

Artificial intelligence in the medical sector has shown the possibility of reinforcing or increasing the biases that are already there, and machine learning models trained on non-representative samples may perform poorly on underrepresented groups and worsen health disparities. Research in the field of bias mitigation is also required to uncover and solve the problem of biases in AI algorithms applied in healthcare and provide fair and equal results irrespective of the background (Ng et al., 2024). In the case of Prana-Centered AI, the aspects of fairness applicable are to make sure that the training data is diverse in terms of gender and age and ethnicity and body type, that performance is not different between demographic groups, that there are no biases in physiological measurement, including the effect of skin tone on optical sensors, that the end product is accessible to users with disabilities, and that notions of normal or optimal state have been made with cultural bias. The indigenous knowledge systems offer alternative ethical theories that disrupt the mainstream narratives on technological advancements that in most instances focus on efficiency and profitability at the expense of ethical concerns (Prathomwong & Singsuriya, 2022).

9. CONCLUSIONS

Prana-Centered AI is a relatively new but potentially groundbreaking part of intelligent wellness technology. It can help close the gap between the highly advanced models of energy practices described in the classical literature on yoga and the recent multimodal sensing and machine learning technologies, creating the opportunities of creating wellness systems that see human beings as complex, not only physically and energetically but also mentally and spiritually. The framework discussed in this chapter offers the architectural basis of such systems without disregarding the fact that the research that is needed to achieve such a vision in a responsible manner is considerable. The scientific basis of this marriage is still growing stronger with researches indicating that there are physiological correlates to yogic practices. The methods of slow breathing serve to improve the autonomic, cerebral and psychological flexibility by interacting with each other, where it has been proven that the parasympathetic activity, the activities of the central nervous system, and psychological well-being correlate. Such results are empirical anchoring to widely accepted assertions regarding the impacts of breath regulation and can be used to indicate directions of technological evaluation and optimisation. Nevertheless, both the practitioners and the scholarly community should develop Prana-Centered AI through proper epistemic humility and ethical sensitivity. The traditional medicine includes worldviews where health is understood as harmony of and between people, communities and ecosystems, which is not entirely quantifiable using technology. Instead of purporting to eliminate or diminish traditional practices, AI systems ought to complement and augment traditional practices, and avoid undermining the relational, experiential, and spiritual aspects that make these practices potentially transformative. The ethical considerations are significant, and they include the integrity of traditional knowledge, privacy and security of data, fairness of the algorithm, informed consent, and proper placement when compared to human teachers and practitioners. These issues need to be met with a true partnership with the traditional knowledge holders, dedication to cultural sensitivity, and an understanding that technological progress should be used towards the prosperity of humans and not as a tool to serve only business interests.

REFERENCES

Bobade, P., & Vani, M. (2020). Stress Detection with Machine Learning and Deep Learning using Multimodal Physiological Data. *2020 Second International Conference on Inventive Research in Computing Applications (ICIRCA)*, 51–57. DOI: 10.1109/ICIRCA48905.2020.9183244

Braboszcz, C., Cahn, B. R., Levy, J., Fernandez, M., & Delorme, A. (2017). Increased Gamma Brainwave Amplitude Compared to Control in Three Different Meditation Traditions. *PLoS One*, *12*(1), e0170647. DOI: 10.1371/journal.pone.0170647

Campanelli, S., Tort, A. B. L., & Lobão-Soares, B. (2020). Pranayamas and Their Neurophysiological Effects. *International Journal of Yoga*, *13*(3), 183–192. DOI: 10.4103/ijoy.IJOY_91_19

Cardone, D., & Merla, A. (2017). New Frontiers for Applications of Thermal Infrared Imaging Devices: Computational Psychopshysiology in the Neurosciences. *Sensors (Basel)*, *17*(5), 1042. DOI: 10.3390/s17051042

Chen, R., Liu, Q., & Chen, Z. (2024). Research on Wearable Sensors Data Collection and Health Assessment based on Machine Learning. *Proceedings of the 2024 International Conference on Smart Healthcare and Wearable Intelligent Devices*, 227–231. DOI: 10.1145/3703847.3703885

Cramer, H. (2023). Artificial Intelligence, Complementary and Integrative Medicine: A Paradigm Shift in Health Care Delivery and Research? *Journal of Integrative and Complementary Medicine*, *29*(3), 131–133. DOI: 10.1089/jicm.2023.0040

de Carvalho-Guimarães, F. B., Correa, K. L., de Souza, T. P., Rodríguez Amado, J. R., Ribeiro-Costa, R. M., & Silva-Júnior, J. O. C. (2022). A Review of Pickering Emulsions: Perspectives and Applications. *Pharmaceuticals (Basel, Switzerland)*, *15*(11), 1413. DOI: 10.3390/ph15111413

Duan, J., Xiong, J., Li, Y., & Ding, W. (2024). Deep learning based multimodal biomedical data fusion: An overview and comparative review. *Information Fusion*, *112*, 102536. DOI: 10.1016/j.inffus.2024.102536

Duda, A. T., Clarke, A. R., & Barry, R. J. (2024). Mindfulness meditation alters neural oscillations independently of arousal. *International Journal of Psychophysiology : Official Journal of the International Organization of Psychophysiology*, *205*, 112439. DOI: 10.1016/j.ijpsycho.2024.112439

Ferrarelli, F., Smith, R., Dentico, D., Riedner, B. A., Zennig, C., Benca, R. M., Lutz, A., Davidson, R. J., & Tononi, G. (2013). Experienced mindfulness meditators exhibit higher parietal-occipital EEG gamma activity during NREM sleep. *PLoS One*, *8*(8), e73417. DOI: 10.1371/journal.pone.0073417

Fialoke, S., Tripathi, V., Thakral, S., Dhawan, A., Majahan, V., & Garg, R. (2024). Functional connectivity changes in meditators and novices during yoga nidra practice. *Scientific Reports*, *14*(1), 12957. DOI: 10.1038/s41598-024-63765-7

Frawley, D. (1999). *Yoga & Ayurveda: Self-Healing and Self-Realization*. Lotus Pr.

Gao, J., Sun, R., Leung, H. K., Roberts, A., Wu, B. W. Y., Tsang, E. W., Tang, A. C. W., & Sik, H. H. (2023). Increased neurocardiological interplay after mindfulness meditation: A brain oscillation-based approach. *Frontiers in Human Neuroscience*, *17*, 1008490. Advance online publication. DOI: 10.3389/fnhum.2023.1008490

Ghiya, S. (2017). Alternate nostril breathing: A systematic review of clinical trials. *International Journal of Research in Medical Sciences*, *5*(8), 3273. DOI: 10.18203/2320-6012.ijrms20173523

Harishbhai Tilala, M., Kumar Chenchala, P., Choppadandi, A., Kaur, J., Naguri, S., Saoji, R., & Devaguptapu, B. (2024). Ethical Considerations in the Use of Artificial Intelligence and Machine Learning in Health Care: A Comprehensive Review. *Cureus*, *16*(6), e62443. DOI: 10.7759/cureus.62443

Kaur, C., & Singh, P. (2015). EEG Derived Neuronal Dynamics during Meditation: Progress and Challenges. *Advances in Preventive Medicine*, *614723*, 1–10. Advance online publication. DOI: 10.1155/2015/614723

Kavitha, N., Pal, P., Pal, G. K., Bharadwaj, B., & Nanda, N. (2024). Effects of Slow Breathing Exercises on Cardiac Autonomic Functions in Anxiety Disorder- A Randomised Control Trial. *Annals of Neurosciences*, *09727531241266094*, 09727531241266094. Advance online publication. DOI: 10.1177/09727531241266094

Kher, D., & Patel, D. M. (2021). A Comprehensive Review on Wearable Health Monitoring Systems. *The Open Biomedical Engineering Journal*, *15*(1), 213–225. DOI: 10.2174/1874120702115010213

Kuruvilla, S., & Gopalakrishna, G. K. Pillai, null, Kim, S., McDougall, L., Soon, G. C., Matsabisa, M., & Briand, S. (2025). Traditional medicine and its contributions to science, health equity and sustainability. Bulletin of the World Health Organization, *103*(11), 642-642A. DOI: 10.2471/BLT.25.295061

Lagopoulos, J., Xu, J., Rasmussen, I., Vik, A., Malhi, G. S., Eliassen, C. F., Arntsen, I. E., Saether, J. G., Hollup, S., Holen, A., Davanger, S., & Ellingsen, Ø. (2009). Increased theta and alpha EEG activity during nondirective meditation. *Journal of Alternative and Complementary Medicine (New York, N.Y.)*, *15*(11), 1187–1192. DOI: 10.1089/acm.2009.0113

Lazarou, I., Oikonomou, V. P., Mpaltadoros, L., Grammatikopoulou, M., Alepopoulos, V., Stavropoulos, T. G., Bezerianos, A., Nikolopoulos, S., Kompatsiaris, I., & Tsolaki, M.RADAR-AD Consortium. (2023). Eliciting brain waves of people with cognitive impairment during meditation exercises using portable electroencephalography in a smart-home environment: A pilot study. *Frontiers in Aging Neuroscience*, *15*, 1167410. DOI: 10.3389/fnagi.2023.1167410

Meskó, B., Drobni, Z., Bényei, É., Gergely, B., & Győrffy, Z. (2017). Digital health is a cultural transformation of traditional healthcare. *mHealth*, *3*, 38. DOI: 10.21037/mhealth.2017.08.07

Moga, M., & Bengston, W. (2010). Moga, M.M., W.F. Bengston (2010) Anomalous magnetic field activity during a bioenergy healing experiment. J. Sci. Exploration 24(3): 397-410. *Journal of Scientific Exploration*, *24*, 397–410.

Mondal, S. (2024). Proposed physiological mechanisms of pranayama: A discussion. *Journal of Ayurveda and Integrative Medicine*, *15*(1), 100877. DOI: 10.1016/j.jaim.2023.100877

Muktibodhananda, S. (1998). *Hatha Yoga Pradipika*. https://www.amazon.com/Hatha-Yoga-Pradipika-Swami-Muktibodhananda/dp/8185787387

Muktibodhananda, S. (2012). *Hatha Yoga Pradipika*. https://www.amazon.in/Hatha-Yoga-Pradipika-Swami-Muktibodhananda-ebook/dp/B01BRF5MFO

Mütze, C., Mitzinger, D., & Haller, H. (2025). Effectiveness of pranayama for mental disorders: A systematic review and meta-analysis of randomized controlled trials. *Frontiers in Psychiatry*, *16*, 1616996. Advance online publication. DOI: 10.3389/fpsyt.2025.1616996

Pandi-Perumal, S. R., Spence, D. W., Srivastava, N., Kanchibhotla, D., Kumar, K., Sharma, G. S., Gupta, R., & Batmanabane, G. (2022). The Origin and Clinical Relevance of Yoga Nidra. *Sleep and Vigilance*, *6*(1), 61–84. DOI: 10.1007/s41782-022-00202-7

Pramanik, D., & Singh, V. (2023).. . *PHILOSOPHY OF THE BODY ACCORDING TO THE ANCIENT TEXTS OF HATHA YOGA.*, *13*, 156–162.

Prathomwong, P., & Singsuriya, P. (2022). Ethical Framework of Digital Technology, Artificial Intelligence, and Health Equity. *Asia Social Issues*, *15*(5), 252136. DOI: 10.48048/asi.2022.252136

Rubik, B., Muehsam, D., Hammerschlag, R., & Jain, S. (2015). Biofield Science and Healing: History, Terminology, and Concepts. *Global Advances in Health and Medicine : Improving Healthcare Outcomes Worldwide*, *4*(1_suppl, Suppl), 8–14. DOI: 10.7453/gahmj.2015.038.suppl

Sabry, F., Eltaras, T., Labda, W., Alzoubi, K., & Malluhi, Q. (2022). Machine Learning for Healthcare Wearable Devices: The Big Picture. *Journal of Healthcare Engineering*, *2022*(1), 4653923. DOI: 10.1155/2022/4653923

Shaik, T., Tao, X., Li, L., Xie, H., & Velásquez, J. D. (2024). A survey of multimodal information fusion for smart healthcare: Mapping the journey from data to wisdom. *Information Fusion*, *102*, 102040. DOI: 10.1016/j.inffus.2023.102040

Shajari, S., Kuruvinashetti, K., Komeili, A., & Sundararaj, U. (2023). The Emergence of AI-Based Wearable Sensors for Digital Health Technology: A Review. *Sensors (Basel)*, *23*(23), 9498. DOI: 10.3390/s23239498

Shao, R., Man, I. S. C., & Lee, T. M. C. (2024). The Effect of Slow-Paced Breathing on Cardiovascular and Emotion Functions: A Meta-Analysis and Systematic Review. *Mindfulness*, *15*(1), 1–18. DOI: 10.1007/s12671-023-02294-2

Sharpe, E., Lacombe, A., Sadowski, A., Phipps, J., Heer, R., Rajurkar, S., Hanes, D., Jindal, R. D., & Bradley, R. (2021). Investigating Components of Pranayama for Effects on Heart Rate Variability. *Journal of Psychosomatic Research*, *148*, 110569. DOI: 10.1016/j.jpsychores.2021.110569

Singh, J., Kumar, S., & Arora, A. S. (2018). Thermographic evaluation of mindfulness meditation using dynamic IR imaging. *Infrared Physics & Technology*, *95*, 81–87. DOI: 10.1016/j.infrared.2018.10.029

Soumma, S. B., Mamun, A., & Ghasemzadeh, H. (2025). AI-powered wearable sensors for health monitoring and clinical decision making. *Current Opinion in Biomedical Engineering*, *36*, 100628. DOI: 10.1016/j.cobme.2025.100628

Sprengel, M., Teo, L., Allen, S., Ijssennagger, N., Hammerschlag, R., Dyer, N., & Crawford, C. (2025). Biofield Therapies Clinical Research Landscape: A Scoping Review and Interactive Evidence Map. *Journal of Integrative and Complementary Medicine*, *31*(5), 406–430. Advance online publication. DOI: 10.1089/jicm.2024.0773

Stahlschmidt, S. R., Ulfenborg, B., & Synnergren, J. (2022). Multimodal deep learning for biomedical data fusion: A review. *Briefings in Bioinformatics*, *23*(2), bbab569. Advance online publication. DOI: 10.1093/bib/bbab569

Stapleton, P. B., Buchan, C., Mitchell, I., McGrath, Y., Gorton, P., & Carter, B. (2019). An initial investigation of neural changes in overweight adults with food cravings after emotional freedom techniques. *OBM Integrative and Complimentary Medicine*, *4*(1), 1–12. Advance online publication. DOI: 10.21926/obm.icm.1901010

Walter, M., Lovett, R., Maher, B., Williamson, B., Prehn, J., Bodkin-Andrews, G., & Lee, V. (2021). Indigenous Data Sovereignty in the Era of Big Data and Open Data. *The Australian Journal of Social Issues*, *56*(2), 143–156. DOI: 10.1002/ajs4.141

Yuan, Y., Liu, B., Li, H., Li, M., Song, Y., Wang, R., Wang, T., & Zhang, H. (2022). Flexible Wearable Sensors in Medical Monitoring. *Biosensors (Basel)*, *12*(12), 1069. DOI: 10.3390/bios12121069

Zaccaro, A., Piarulli, A., Laurino, M., Garbella, E., Menicucci, D., Neri, B., & Gemignani, A. (2018). How Breath-Control Can Change Your Life: A Systematic Review on Psycho-Physiological Correlates of Slow Breathing. *Frontiers in Human Neuroscience*, *12*, 353. DOI: 10.3389/fnhum.2018.00353

Zhu, L., Spachos, P., Ng, P. C., Yu, Y., Wang, Y., Plataniotis, K., & Hatzinakos, D. (2023). Stress Detection Through Wrist-Based Electrodermal Activity Monitoring and Machine Learning. *IEEE Journal of Biomedical and Health Informatics*, *27*(5), 2155–2165. DOI: 10.1109/JBHI.2023.3239305

Zickerick, B., Thönes, S., Kobald, S. O., Wascher, E., Schneider, D., & Küper, K. (2020a). Differential Effects of Interruptions and Distractions on Working Memory Processes in an ERP Study. *Frontiers in Human Neuroscience*, *14*, 84. DOI: 10.3389/fnhum.2020.00084

Chapter 9
YogAI for Preventive and Personalized Healthcare: A Knowledge-Driven Integrative Approach Taking Bio Feedback Using Wearable Sensors

Raghav Mehra
http://orcid.org/0009-0001-8542-515X
Chandigarh University, Mohali, India

Rijwan Khan
http://orcid.org/0000-0003-3354-3047
Marwadi University, Rajkot, India

Hina Khan
http://orcid.org/0009-0008-0374-9558
Faculty of Yoga & Alternative Medicine, University of Lucknow, Lucknow, India

Priti Kumari
http://orcid.org/0000-0001-7599-9195
Saharsa College of Engineering, India

ABSTRACT

For more than two millennia, yoga has been taught by direct observation of the practitioner, but until now, the hidden physiological state of the practitioner has been unknown to themselves and the teacher. Here, we present the Wearable Intelligence Yoga Framework (WIYF) that provides real-time, personalised feedback during yoga practice through the integration of multimodal wearable sensors (heart rate variability (HRV), brain electrical activity (EEG), skin conductance (GSR) and

DOI: 10.4018/979-8-2600-2463-8.ch009

inertial measurement units (IMUs)), edge-placed artificial intelligence (AI), and the Ayurvedic science of personalisation. The WIYF integrates three bodies of theory: the yogic Pancha Kosha model of the human, Ayurvedic Prakriti physiology, and closed-loop adaptive control systems engineering. This chapter presents three case studies that illustrate how the personalisation engine adapts the feedback modes, targets for a practice session and long-term learning to the individual. The chapter concludes with an ethical discussion of privacy, algorithmic bias, quantified self over-reach, and equity.

1. INTRODUCTION

Yoga has existed for more than 2000 years in the form of teacher to student instruction. The teacher observes her student, moves their arms around, listens to their breathing, and chooses the next words. This has been the essence of practice. It is not something that technology will take over and, as such, this chapter does not argue that it will. It does say that there is an aspect of the practice that has always been beyond the reach of human observation—even when it is skilled—and that this is no longer the case. That is the state of the body. Not the external form of the posture, but the inner state: the state of the nervous system, the breathing, the electrical activity in the brain, the subtle signs a person experiences before they feel it. A teacher who stands in the centre of a room with a class of students cannot see any of that. Not even with a one-on-one teacher. It's not a failure of skill. It is a limit to human vision.

Now we have tiny sensors that can breach that limit. A wrist-wearable device can monitor what is happening between heartbeats. A light head band can monitor the transition from worried to focused thinking. Body sensors can track joint angles not easily seen. These are not rare devices used in research laboratories. They can be bought today, are cheap and improving fast. The question is not "do they work?" There is already a lot of evidence about this in thousands of published papers in the fields of medicine, sports science and neuroscience. The important question is how these sensors can be integrated into the practice of yoga in a way that is useful—respecting the rich tradition and philosophy of yoga, tailoring advice to the individual, and providing feedback quickly enough to be useful during the yoga session. This chapter approaches that question. It gives an answer in the form of a framework, WIYF, the Wearable Intelligence Yoga Framework. It's not a product, or a mission. It is a framework for an architecture of the sensor data, edge AI and yogic personalisation principles that can be brought together to make a guidance system.

There are three sources for the framework: the physiological science of biofeedback, the ancient Indian system of individual constitutions called Ayurveda, and the engineering of closed-loop adaptive control systems. The combination of these three sources yields something new. The chapter begins with the preliminaries, outlining the problem it aims to solve and why current solutions are not enough.

1.1 A Gap in the Market for Technology

There have been advances in applying AI to yoga over the past ten years. There are now systems that can recognise yoga poses from video footage. There are apps that provide feedback on posture with a smartphone. Models have been trained to recognise different meditation states and to detect irregular breathing. This work is valuable. But there is a common theme in most of it. The systems look at the surface of the body. They see posture. They hear breath sound. They identify a posture and match it to a library of postures. They do not track the practitioner's state of mind—the nervous system, the electrical activity in the brain, the stress level of the skin—and use that information to guide learning.

Researchers have had the idea of measuring physiology during yoga practice before. There has been a long history of HRV, cortisol, EEG and skin conductance monitoring during yoga. But it is new to be able to do so continuously, in real time, on a device small enough to wear during the practice and interpreted by AI on the device itself and then fed back to the practitioner in real time. The technical foundations for this have been recently established. The design framework to use them effectively has yet to be articulated. This chapter seeks to do that.

1.2 Why Personalization Matters

Personalization has always been a challenge for yoga teachers. A group class instructor is always giving instruction to some average practitioner—neither the person most exhausted in the class nor the most spry, neither the most supple nor the stiffest. The same pranayama practice that is relaxing for one individual may be stimulating and even distressing for another. The same level of asana practice that is just right for a person with a healthy nervous system might be too much for someone who is in a state of stress. Psychophysiological research has long demonstrated that our autonomic responses to the same stimulus differ greatly—and that this is not by chance. It is based on individual differences in the constitution of the nervous system, its ability to respond to stress, and its intrinsic rhythm.

Classical yoga teachers dealt with this difference in the idea of Prakriti (constitutional type), as described in the system of Ayurveda. Dynamic personalization is possible with the wearable AI. Not just at the beginning (intake) and then forgotten about, but continuously, from class to class, or even within a class, as required.

The traditional Guru-Shishya (teacher-student) model of yoga practice understood, long before psychophysiology, the same external practice has different internal effects on different people. The experienced teacher is one who observes the student's inner state (chitta vritti), Patanjali's Yoga Sutras say. What is different today is the way of knowing. A teacher who is teaching a class of 30 students does not perceive the autonomic arousal of each student. This is not an issue of teaching competence but information management. Wearable sensor technology does not replace the teacher's perceptual wisdom; it amplifies their knowledge by making physiological information perceivable. The integration of the teacher's contextual intelligence and the system's physiological acuity is the very relationship the WIYF framework is designed to enhance, not replace. Psychophysiological research has shown that even though practitioners report feeling relaxed and composed, their body is showing elevated sympathetic indicators, such as elevated GSR, decreased HRV, and increased beta power that would, if the teacher knew, lead to a change in the session (Thayer et al., 2012). The framework fills the disjunction between subjective feelings and physiological reality.

1.3 The Role of the Human Teacher

It would be a misunderstanding to think that this chapter is about the abolition of human yoga teaching. It is not. There is more to the relationship between yoga teacher and student than sensors can measure. The teacher's insight at the right moment, the presence in the classroom, the knowledge that comes from having been there and done that—these are not quantifiable. They are what transform yoga from a set of poses to a transformational experience. This chapter's point is that wearable intelligence can complement—not replace—the teacher's role. The goal is technology turning the invisible into the visible—giving the teacher and practitioner what they have longed for.

2. LITERATURE REVIEW

Before proposing something new, it is important to review what has already been done. There is a substantial body of literature on wearable sensors, biofeedback, AI for health monitoring and yoga science. This review seeks to weave together those threads that are relevant to the development of a real-time, wearable, AI-based system to guide yoga practice—and to identify where those threads end.

2.1 Heart Rate Variability

Heart rate variability (HRV) is one of the most popular measures in health and performance research, because HRV carries more information than just the heart rate. In a widely-cited paper, Shaffer and Ginsberg (2017) surveyed the various HRV measures and their normal values, outlining two main types: time-domain metrics and frequency-domain metrics. The low-frequency to high-frequency power ratio is commonly used as a measure of sympathetic-to-parasympathetic balance. Lehrer and Gevirtz (2014) reviewed HRV biofeedback techniques, demonstrating positives for anxiety, depression, asthma, hypertension, and chronic pain. Complementing these foundational works, Wilson et al. (2025) conducted a systematic review on the feasibility and effectiveness of portable and remote HRV biofeedback training, confirming its efficacy in treating stress and mental health difficulties. These findings validate the viability of real-time, on-device HRV guidance during yoga practice as proposed in the WIYF framework.

Their notion of the resonance frequency—the respiratory rate at which each individual's HRV amplitude is maximized—is relevant to individual guidance in pranayama, ranging between 4.5 and 7 breaths per minute in adults. Nazari et al. (2021) tested the reliability of wrist PPG for HRV measurement during yoga-like slow motion, finding adequate agreement with ECG if proper filtering for motion artifacts is used. Recent systematic reviews and meta-analyses have further strengthened the evidence base. For instance, Sharma et al. (2025) demonstrated through a meta-analysis that yoga-based interventions significantly improve heart rate variability while reducing anxiety symptoms among students, providing strong empirical support for the use of HRV as a core biomarker in real-time yoga guidance systems.

2.2 EEG and the Brain During Meditation

Electroencephalography (EEG) measures the electrical activity of the brain from the scalp. Lomas et al. (2015) conducted a systematic review of 56 neuroimaging and EEG studies of mindfulness meditation and found that alpha waves (8–12 Hz) consistently increase during meditation. Theta waves (4–8 Hz) increase in experienced meditators. Cahn and Polich (2006) reviewed the literature on EEG and several schools of meditation, concluding that there are common patterns across traditions: increases in frontal alpha power, theta power in advanced practitioners, and decreases in beta power. A dual-channel headband monitoring alpha and beta power in the forehead can give a real-time measure of how deeply a student is entering states of Dharana or Dhyana.

2.3 Galvanic Skin Response

Galvanic skin response (GSR) and electrodermal activity assess the change in skin conductance due to sweat gland activity of the sympathetic nervous system. Kim et al. (2018) examined studies that mapped the connection between stress, HRV and GSR, demonstrating the two measures work together: HRV is a long-term measure of the balance between the sympathetic and parasympathetic nervous systems, with GSR being a measure of short-term spikes in sympathetic activity. With yoga, GSR can be used to detect times when someone looks relaxed, but is actually stressed.

2.4 IMU Sensors and Posture

An inertial measurement unit (IMU) is a combination of an accelerometer and gyroscope that measures acceleration and angular velocity. Using IMUs for posture assessment has privacy benefits compared to video, is not affected by lighting conditions or occlusion and can pick up information about quality of movement—the acceleration from one pose to the next—that video cannot. In yoga, where the quality of the movement and breathing are as important as the pose itself, this is important.

2.5 AI for Physiological Signals

Deep learning has opened new opportunities for physiological signal analysis. Convolutional neural networks applied to time-series data as two-dimensional frequency-time images can identify patterns not captured by specific feature sets. Long short-term memory networks handle time dependency in biosignals. TinyML—a recent innovation focusing on running neural networks on tiny microcontrollers—is critical for a yoga biofeedback system. Warden and Situnayake (2019) demonstrated that inference with lightweight models on microcontrollers can run from wearable sensor data without cloud communication, reducing feedback latency to tens of milliseconds.

More recently, Transformer-based architectures have demonstrated superior performance on multivariate physiological time-series classification tasks, owing to their ability to model long-range temporal dependencies through self-attention mechanisms (Ismail Fawaz et al., 2019). For a yoga application, this matters because the physiological effects of a pranayama technique performed at the beginning of a session may not manifest in measurable HRV or EEG changes until several minutes later. A model with access only to the current epoch misses this delayed coupling. Transformers trained on full-session sequences can capture these cross-temporal relationships in ways that convolutional and recurrent models cannot. However, Transformer models are computationally demanding and are currently too large for direct deployment on microcontrollers. The practical architecture for WIYF therefore uses quantised LSTMs for on-device state inference and reserves Transformer-based session-level learning for off-device post-session model updates—a hybrid that preserves real-time responsiveness while exploiting the most capable architectures for longitudinal personalisation. Yoga practice presents distinctive signal challenges that differ from general sports science contexts: breath-rate intentionally spans a wider range (2–20 breaths per minute across practice states), body orientation changes are extreme (inversions alter blood pressure distribution), and the practitioner deliberately shifts between high-arousal and deeply relaxed states within a single session. These characteristics require yoga-specific preprocessing and classification pipelines rather than direct adaptation of clinical or sports science models. Recent advances in multimodal sensor fusion further support this direction. Xi et al. (2026) proposed a deep learning framework integrating wearable sensor fusion for multimodal human action recognition and personalized sports health promotion, demonstrating improved performance through combined physiological and movement data — an approach directly aligned with the multimodal sensing strategy (HRV + EEG + GSR + IMU) of the WIYF framework.

2.6 Biofeedback in Clinical Research

Biofeedback research started in the 1960s. Sherlin et al. (2011) reviewed the evidence regarding neurofeedback and found neurofeedback has been successful for attention, anxiety and post traumatic stress. Real-time alpha and theta feedback accelerates learning of a meditative state for beginners. The next step in the biofeedback research is integration: no study has proposed a system that integrates posture, HRV, EEG and GSR in an AI layer and personalises yoga practice based on it.

Javed et al. (2024) suggested cultural considerations in AI therapy. Algorithms and interventions applied to practices like yoga, which are significant in several cultures and spiritual practices, should be culturally sensitive to allow for different cultures, norms and values. This insight drives the use of IKS principles as design constraints for the WIYF framework.

Table 1. Comparative Summary of Related Literature

Study / Source	Sensor / Method	AI / Analytics	Yoga Context	Personalization	Limitation	Cultural/Ethical Dimension
Shaffer & Ginsberg (2017)	ECG / PPG HRV	Statistical norms	None	None	No real-time feedback	None addressed
Lomas et al. (2015)	EEG	Systematic review	Meditation only	None	Single signal	Western mindfulness focus only
Lehrer & Gevirtz (2014)	HRV biofeedback	Resonance frequency	Pranayama partial	Partial (breath rate)	No Ayurveda, no edge AI	None addressed
Cao et al. (2021)	Video / OpenPose	CNN pose estimation	Asana posture	None	No physiology, no privacy	Body type bias in training data
Kim et al. (2018)	HRV + GSR	Meta-analysis	Stress context	None	Lab setting, not wearable	None addressed
Prasher et al. (2008)	Genomics / questionnaire	Statistical correlates	Ayurveda Prakriti	Constitutional typing	No real-time element	IKS framework; India-validated only
Javed et al. (2024)	Ethical review	Framework analysis	AI healthcare	None	Conceptual only	Cultural sensitivity in AI therapy emphasized
WIYF (This Chapter)	HRV + EEG + GSR + IMU	TinyML edge AI, LSTM	Full asana + pranayama + meditation	Prakriti + baseline + session learning	Framework stage; no longitudinal data yet	GDPR + DPDP Act 2023; IKS grounding; federated privacy

2.7 Gaps in the Literature

The WIYF framework is designed to address four particular gaps in the research. First, there is no published framework for using multimodal physiological monitoring in yoga practice. Second, AI wellness systems generalise about users without structured constitutional typology. Third, current research prototypes process data in the cloud, making feedback too slow for yoga. Fourth, technical papers do not reference the philosophy of the practice they are tracking.

3. INDIAN KNOWLEDGE SYSTEMS (IKS) INTEGRATION

This section presents the theoretical foundation for the WIYF framework. It focuses on philosophy—not to the detriment of the main topic, but because the design choices in WIYF are motivated by these theoretical choices. Without them the framework can appear to be a list of design decisions. With them, it becomes a coherent argument.

3.1 The Pancha Kosha Model

The insistence on a holistic view of the body is codified in yoga philosophy in the Pancha Kosha model—the notion that the human being is simultaneously functioning on five different levels, or sheaths. The most external is the physical body, the visible and tactile body (Annamaya Kosha). Next is the energy body, the body of breath, life force, and physiological function (Pranamaya Kosha). Then the mental body—the mind, the emotions and the senses (Manomaya Kosha). Inside that is the layer of discernment and higher cognition (Vijnanamaya Kosha). And inside that is a core of consciousness (Anandamaya Kosha).

The WIYF approach employs the Kosha model to select sensors. IMU sensors address the physical layer. Cardiovascular variability (HRV) and breath-rate address the energy layer. EEG and GSR address the mental-emotional layer. This is not a contrived mapping; it is a mapping from the yogic aspects of practice to the physiological realities that can be sensed.

3.2 Prana and the Autonomic Nervous System

Prana is defined functionally in the Upanishads and yoga texts as the supervisory power that governs and animates physiological processes. It is not localised to a particular organ. It travels around the body in passages (Nadis) and is centred in nodes (Chakras). We would recognise this as the role of the autonomic nervous system in modern physiology; it subconsciously keeps the heart, gut, lungs, immune system, sleep and hormone secretion running. HRV, the most sensitive non-invasive index of the balance of the autonomic nervous system, is the best measurable index of the yoga tradition's concept of Pranic regulation. When this framework's personalisation engine optimises HRV coherence, it is, in a sense, optimising balance of Prana in the speech of a yoga teacher.

3.3 Prakriti and the Tridosha Framework

Ayurveda defines humans as being constitutionally different in ways that impact how they react to stress, recover from physical exertion, and respond to yoga practice. This variation is structured by three bio-energetic types called Doshas: Vata, Pitta and Kapha. Prasher et al. (2008) demonstrated statistically significant associations between self-reported Prakriti type and gene expression in immune and metabolic pathways, providing scientific justification for using Prakriti in an AI personalization engine.

The Prasher et al. study is vital to the development of WIYF design. A total of 52 genes were found to be differentially expressed across Prakriti types, many of which are associated with pathways for autonomic regulation, inflammatory response and hormone metabolism, the very systems measured by HRV, EEG and GSR. Vata types showed elevated expression of adrenergic pathways that would be consistent with their chronically activated sympathetic nervous system (their low RMSSD). Pitta types showed higher expression of metabolic and inflammatory pathway genes consistent with their increased thermogenesis and greater physiological responsiveness. Kapha types showed elevated expression of genes that suppress metabolic activity and reflect their lower basal arousal and greater tendency to parasympathetic dominance. These genetic correlates offer a physiological basis for translating constitutional type into physiological type - the sensor signatures used by the WIYF personalisation engine. The Prakriti questionnaire thus acts not as a cultural or philosophical categorisation instrument but as a low-cost surrogate for a biologically relevant physiological prior, that greatly speeds up the convergence of the personalisation engine to deliver accurate, personalised recommendations. Joshi (2004) also showed that systematic Prakriti ratings are highly reliable between raters, justifying them as a quantitative input variable to machine learning systems.

Table 2. Dosha vs. Physiological Mapping in the WIYF Framework

Dosha	Elemental Association	Autonomic Profile	Typical HRV Pattern	EEG Tendency	GSR Profile	Yoga Prescription & WIYF Response
Vata	Air + Ether	Sympathetic dominance; hyperarousal; anxiety-prone; erratic autonomic rhythm	Low RMSSD; highly variable; HF-HRV chronically suppressed; poor coherence at rest	High beta; suppressed alpha; irregular and delayed meditative onset	High tonic baseline; frequent phasic spikes; slow habituation to stress	Slow, grounding, rhythmic sequences; 1:2 breath ratio; extended Shavasana. WIYF: resonance-frequency pacing; alpha-onset haptic cue; high early-session feedback density tapering as alpha stabilises
Pitta	Fire + Water	Intense activation; competitive; ignores fatigue; recovery deficit accumulation	Adequate RMSSD at rest; drops sharply on overtraining days; flat HRV arc when depleted	Sustained beta during activity; good alpha in deep pranayama; strong theta in advanced practice	Low tonic baseline; sharp brief phasic spikes under frustration; rapid recovery	Moderate intensity; mandatory recovery sessions when HRV >12% below 7-day average. WIYF: pre-session readiness colour cue; automatic intensity downshift; recovery arc monitoring
Kapha	Earth + Water	Parasympathetic dominance; low baseline arousal; prone to inertia and drowsy meditation	Moderate RMSSD; slow tonic GSR rise; blunted phasic response; low LF variability	High resting theta; weak alpha; drowsy theta intrudes during meditation requiring stimulation	Slowly rising tonic; very few phasic spikes; very slow habituation	Stimulating, warming, dynamic sequences before meditation; breath of fire. WIYF: morning low-arousal prompts; theta-intrusion alert; stimulating pranayama pre-meditation; adherence nudge

3.4 Closed-Loop Adaptive Control

The engineering idea of a closed-loop feedback control system is precisely what a real-time biofeedback system for yoga should be. A sensor reads the current state; a comparator compares it to the desired state; a controller calculates the adjustment; an actuator delivers the correction. In the WIYF system, the sensor system monitors the practitioner's physiological state. The AI comparator determines how this compares with the desired state for the session, as set by the practitioner's Prakriti and intentions. The controller determines the cues. The actuators are the cues to the practitioner: audio, haptic, or visual signals. The key difference from a thermostat is adaptivity—the system learns from every session.

4. PROPOSED SYSTEM ARCHITECTURE

The Wearable Intelligence Yoga Framework (WIYF) is a language for how sensor data, on-device AI, and yogic personalization principles can be put together to form a guidance system. The system has three layers of functionality, which operate continuously and in parallel: data acquisition, intelligence, and feedback. Beneath the three layers is a personalised, learning framework.

Figure 1. Overall WIYF System Architecture — Sensing Intelligence Personalisation Feedback

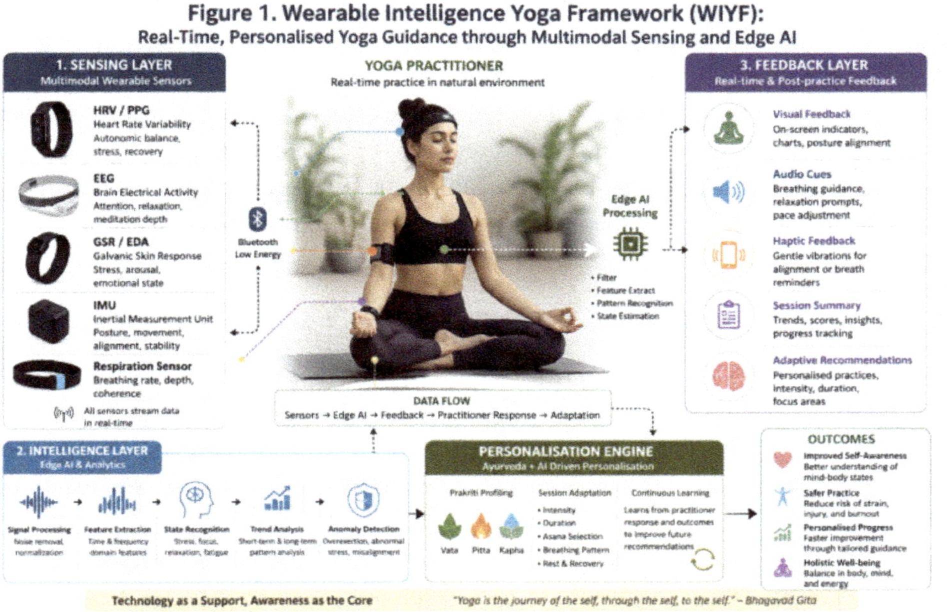

4.1 First Layer: Sensing

The sensing layer is the first layer. If it does not present the right information—too much, too little, or not the right kind—the AI layer will not be useful, and the feedback layer will be inaccurate. The WIYF system uses four signals which measure different states. Heart rate variability (HRV) from a photoplethysmography sensor worn on the wrist or chest is the best measure of the balance of the autonomic nervous system. Electroencephalography (EEG) from a light headband measures the most direct aspect of the mind during meditation and concentration. A pair of EEG channels from the forehead measures the balance of alpha and beta waves in the prefrontal cortex. Galvanic skin response (GSR) from a palm or fingertip measures short-term increases in the sympathetic nervous system that HRV cannot detect because it has a longer time course. Inertial measurement units (IMUs) on the wrists, ankles and lower back give us posture without a camera, and detect motion artifacts in the physiology.

Sensor placement in yoga presents unique challenges absent from clinical or sports contexts. The body routinely assumes postures—inversions, arm balances, deep forward bends—that were not considered in the design of consumer wearable devices. Placement of a PPG sensor on the inner wrist works well for HRV signal acquisition in Tadasana (standing), but leads to motion and pressure artifact in Adho Mukha Svanasana (downward facing dog) when the wrist is weight-bearing. An EEG headband worn in the correct position to record from the front of the head shifts position in Sirsasana (headstand). These are not minor annoyances, these are engineering challenges that must be overcome to operate in dynamic yoga practice. The sensor placement strategy below in Table 4 includes information on artifact risk assessment and reductions specific to yoga practice for each sensor type.

Table 4. Sensor Placement Guide for Yoga Practice: Posture-Specific Artifact Risk and Mitigation

Sensor	Optimal Placement	Challenge Postures	Artifact Risk	Mitigation Strategy
PPG / HRV	Inner wrist (dominant) or chest strap	Adho Mukha Svanasana (downward dog); arm balances; inversions	Motion artifact and blood redistribution under wrist loading	Chest placement for dynamic sequences; wrist for seated/supine; adaptive artifact rejection > 20% threshold
EEG headband	Across forehead (Fp1, Fp2 channels)	Inversions (Sirsasana); Salamba Sarvangasana (shoulder stand)	Muscle contraction artifact during pranayama; electrode displacement	Dry-electrode headband with adjustable tension; FastICA online blink removal; avoid EEG during intense pranayama
GSR / EDA	Non-dominant palm or fingertip clip	Dynamic Vinyasa transitions; any weight-bearing on hands	Sweat accumulation shifts tonic baseline; pressure artifact	Wrist EDA for dynamic sequences; palm clip for seated; phasic decomposition corrects slow drift
IMU × 3 (min)	Lower back (L3–L4); both wrists	High-impact jumps; Chaturanga to Upward Dog transition	High-frequency acceleration spikes; near-singularity in quaternion during extreme flexion	Madgwick filter $\beta = 0.033$ for yoga-range motion; velocity zero-update (ZUPT) during static holds

4.2 Layer Two: The Intelligence Layer

The sensor data from a yoga session is always noisy. To get to a point where an AI model can learn from the data, it must be preprocessed: filtered, artifacted, and standardized in ways that retain physiologically meaningful variation and eliminate variation produced by sensor imperfections and motion.

The framework operates three levels of classification. First, practice-state classification determines what the practitioner is doing: active asana, static asana, pranayama, seated meditation, or transition/rest. Second, physiological-state assessment evaluates the autonomic response for each practice state. Third, the practitioner-state estimator—a composite of real-time signals—describes where the practitioner is on the range from over-aroused to under-aroused, from distracted to focused, from recovered to fatigued.

All three levels of classification are on-device. The WIYF system uses quantized neural networks—models with numerical representations reduced from 32-bit floating point to 8-bit integer arithmetic—executed within TensorFlow Lite or ONNX Runtime Mobile. The whole inference process takes less than 50 milliseconds on mid-range wearable processors.

4.3 Layer Three: The Feedback Layer

The feedback layer transforms state estimates into feedback. The feedback cues include soft audio tones for pacing breathing, vibration pulses for posture correction and visual cues for state of meditation. Only informative feedback is provided, not evaluative or competitive. No scores, no rankings, no reviews. The framing makes a difference.

4.4 The Personalisation Engine

It is the personalisation engine that transforms WIYF from a biofeedback system to a personalised system. Every practitioner has their Prakriti measured by a questionnaire and a baseline measurement of 10 minutes of rest. These define the person's normal—not the population mean. Consideration of Prakriti and baseline together give the foundation for refinement of personalization on a session by session basis.

5. MATHEMATICAL MODEL AND ALGORITHMS

5.1 HRV Signal Processing

The main HRV time-domain measure is the RMSSD (Root Mean Square of Successive Differences), calculated from the series of RR intervals as:

$$\text{RMSSD} = \sqrt{[\,(1/N-1) \cdot \Sigma_{=1}^{\;-1} (RR_{+1} - RR\,)^2\,]}$$

with N being the number of RR intervals in the analysed epoch. Ectopic beats are removed using an adaptive thresholding algorithm: if the interval differs from the local mean by more than 20% it is replaced by the median of the previous and subsequent intervals. HRV frequency-domain analysis involves the ratio of LF/HF power, calculated using Welch's periodogram, with 64-second windows and 50% overlap:

$$LF/HF = P(0.04\text{–}0.15\ Hz) / P(0.15\text{–}0.40\ Hz)$$

HRV coherence—the metric used for pranayama resonance feedback—is computed as the ratio of the dominant spectral peak power to total HRV power within the 0.04–0.15 Hz band. Coherence values > 0.85 indicate resonance breathing. The personalised resonance frequency f* for each practitioner is estimated by computing coherence as a function of breath rate and finding the maximal peak:

$$f^* = \text{argmax\_f} [\ C(f)\ ] \text{ where } f \in [4.5, 7.0] \text{ breaths/min}$$

5.2 EEG Feature Extraction and Classification

EEG signals are bandpass filtered using a zero-phase Butterworth filter (order 4) to extract delta (1–4 Hz), theta (4–8 Hz), alpha (8–12 Hz), and beta (12–30 Hz) sub-bands. Relative band power is computed over 4-second epochs:

$$\text{P\_rel(band)} = P(\text{band}) / P(1\text{–}30\ Hz)$$

The meditation state classifier uses the Alpha/Beta Engagement Index (ABEI), defined as:

$$ABEI = \text{P\_alpha} / (\text{P\_alpha} + \text{P\_beta})$$

A sustained ABEI above a practitioner-specific threshold θ_m (initialized to 0.55 from population norms and updated via Bayesian updating over sessions) triggers a positive meditation-onset indicator. Independent Component Analysis (ICA) is applied in a fast, online variant (FastICA with 2 components) to remove eye-blink and muscle artifacts from the 2-channel forehead EEG.

5.3 GSR Decomposition

The GSR signal is decomposed into tonic (slow-varying baseline) and phasic (event-related) components using a convex optimisation approach. The phasic driver is recovered by solving:

$$\min \{\ \|y - h * x\|^2 + \lambda \cdot \|x\|_1\ \} \text{ s.t. } x \geq 0$$

where y is the raw GSR signal, h is the impulse response of the sudomotor nerve-to-skin conductance transfer function, x is the sparse phasic driver, and λ controls sparsity. Sympathetic activation events (SCRs) are counted in rolling 30-second windows. A sustained increase in SCR rate above baseline constitutes a stress-spike indicator used to modify session pacing.

5.4 IMU-Based Posture Estimation

The posture of each IMU node is estimated using accelero-gyroscope fusion with the Madgwick complementary filter:

$$\dot{q} = q \otimes (\omega gyro/2) - \beta \cdot \nabla f$$

in which the quaternion estimate of the orientation is q, the gyroscope-based angular velocity is ωgyro, the filter gain is β ($\beta = 0.033$ for yoga movements) and the gradient of the objective function from the accelerometer is ∇f. Joint angles between segments are given by the relative quaternion orientations.

5.5 Multi-Signal State Estimator

The practitioner state estimator fuses the three sub-system estimators using a simple attention model. Let s = [s_HRV, s_EEG, s_GSR, s_IMU] be the vector of normalised scores of the sub-systems. The overall state Z is given by:

$$Z = \Sigma\ \alpha\ \cdot s \text{ where } \alpha\ = \text{softmax}(w\ \cdot s\ + b\ )$$

The attention weights α are learned per practitioner across sessions by minimising the mean-squared error against retrospective self-report labels, using stochastic gradient descent. The Z score is then used to trigger cues: Z > θ_high → reduce intensity cues; Z < θ_low → engage cues. θ_high and θ_low are initialised from Prakriti norms and decayed by exponential moving average.

5.6 Personalisation Learning Algorithm

Learning across sessions is through a contextual bandit. Following each session, the system assesses the impact of each intervention (e.g., breath instruction, posture haptic) in terms of increases or decreases in Z scores in the 5-minute period after the intervention. A reward signal $r \in [-1, +1]$ is assigned. The action to be taken in the next session is determined by an upper confidence bound (UCB) policy:

$$UCB(a) = Q(a) + c \cdot \sqrt{(\ln(N) / n(a))}$$

Here, Q(a) is the value of action a, N is the number of sessions, n(a) is the number of times action a has been used, and c is the exploration constant. This means that the system continues to explore new actions while exploiting actions that have been proven to work for this practitioner.

6. IMPLEMENTATION AND CASE STUDIES

The three case studies presented below are illustrative vignettes—physiologically realistic, architecturally feasible simulations of the framework's operation for three different types of practitioners. They are derived from published evidence of the physiological effects of yoga practice, population HRV and EEG measures, and the framework design. The goal is to demonstrate how the framework works, and show that the personalisation engine yields meaningfully different results for different practitioners.

6.1 Case Study 1: Priya — The Vata Beginner

Priya is a 31-year-old female software developer who started yoga six weeks ago to help with anxiety and sleep. Her Prakriti shows predominant Vata. Her RMSSD is 28 ms at baseline (lowest normal)—her nervous system is chronically sympathetic. Frontal beta/alpha ratio is high; baseline GSR is high for her age. Her primary goal during initial meditation is to activate the parasympathetic nervous system (RMSSD increase), and her secondary goal is alpha enhancement.

In a typical session, at the beginning of seated pranayama the system provides audio breath guidance at Priya's likely resonance frequency of breathing (5.8 breaths/minute). Over the next 8 minutes RMSSD increases from 22 to 34 ms and GSR trace approaches a plateau. When meditating, once ABEI exceeds her personalised threshold, a haptic pulse indicates meditative onset; audio guidance ceases. After 7 minutes, alpha has dropped: she is informed audibly. After 8 weeks of training, RMSSD has increased from 28 to 35 ms, and time-to-meditative-onset has improved from 4 to less than 2 minutes.

6.2 Case Study 2: Arvind — The Pitta Overtrainer

Arvind is a 47-year-old physician who has been practicing Ashtanga for 15 years and has a Pitta constitution. His average RMSSD of 58 ms looks good, but over seven sessions we see that when his HRV on the day is more than 12% below his 7-day moving average, his practice HRV trend is flat or falling. He practiced fully on these days anyway—a typical Pitta response of not listening to the body.

The WIYF personalisation engine signals his pre-session readiness with a colour code (full / moderate / restorative), and prioritises parasympathetic recovery in the session on mornings with low HRV. After 12 weeks, the forced full-intensity on low-HRV mornings is significantly diminished. He raises his 7-day average HRV by 9 ms. This case demonstrates that the value to the expert is not advice but a clear mirror of the truth without constitutional bias.

6.3 Case Study 3: Kavitha - Therapeutic Yoga

Kavitha is a 54-year old Kapha-dominant woman with poly-cystic ovarian syndrome and depression. She practices 2-3 days per week of restorative and gentle Hatha yoga. Resting RMSSD is 42 ms; meditation high theta (sleepy) is a Kapha block. She has consented to share practice summaries with her yoga therapist and psychiatrist. Biometric feedback allows differentiation of sequences that, visually, look the same but affect HRV differently; the therapist adjusts. The personalisation engine recognises mornings of low arousal and provides a 5-minute alerting breathing exercise, thus reducing the motivation threshold. At 6 months, sessions increase from 2.1 to 2.8 per week; RMSSD increases by 6 ms; drowsy theta during meditation decreases.

7. RESULTS AND DISCUSSION

7.1 Cross-Case Comparison

Table 3. Cross-Case Analysis of WIYF Framework Operation

Dimension	Priya (Vata Beginner)	Arvind (Pitta Advanced)	Kavitha (Kapha Therapeutic)
Key physiological focus	Parasympathetic stimulation; reduce chronic sympathetic dominance	Recovery control; avoid HRV deficit accumulation	Kapha arousal; therapeutic adherence
EEG priority	Speed of alpha onset; reduce meditation setup time	Alpha depth and theta during pranayama	Minimize drowsy theta; achieve meditation alpha
Most valuable sensor data	HRV coherence during pranayama; GSR trend across session	Morning HRV baseline vs. moving average	Trend in HRV across sessions; GSR tonic arc

continued on following page

Table 3. Continued

Dimension	Priya (Vata Beginner)	Arvind (Pitta Advanced)	Kavitha (Kapha Therapeutic)
Most valuable feedback modality	Breath pacing audio; meditation cues; posture haptic	Readiness cue; modified intensity cues	HRV prompt in morning; session schedule adjustment
Personalisation driver	Vata protocol—slow, gentle, rhythmic; frequent feedback	Pitta protocol—recovery-focused; data over readiness	Kapha protocol—stimulating; enable data sharing
Six-month outcomes	RMSSD: 28→35 ms; quicker alpha; sleep and anxiety reduced	7-day average HRV up 9 ms; overtraining pattern reduced	Consistency: 2.1→2.8 sessions/week; RMSSD up 6 ms; mood improved

7.2 Key Findings

Our analysis across the three cases yields three lessons. First, the primary physiological focus is different for each practitioner, which means that this is not three "versions" of the same intervention, but three distinct therapeutic interventions based on three distinct Prakriti profiles. Second, the most informative sensor data is different: HRV coherence during pranayama for Priya; baseline HRV for Arvind; HRV trend for Kavitha. This is why we are multimodal - there's no sensor that would give equally relevant information for all three.

Third, and most crucial, the personalisation engine does not give the same meaning to the same signal value for different people. RMSSD of 35 ms is good for Priya (above her low baseline) but bad for Arvind (below his baseline) This distinction is possible because we use individual baselines, rather than population norms. These results cannot be resolved with population averages.

7.3 Ethical Considerations

Technology for yoga must be ethically designed. The WIYF model assumes data will be processed on a practitioner's device: the data will stay with the practitioner unless he or she wants to share it. That is not only the legal place (GDPR) but the ethical place, as the data is owned by the practitioner. There are multiple points of reversible unbundled consent for data sharing with teachers, therapists and parents. Algorithmic bias is reduced by basing the algorithm on the individual as opposed to the population, and by using federated learning that boosts the performance of the algorithm in different populations without pooling data.

The regulatory framework in India introduces an additional set of ethical considerations for systems in South Asia. The Digital Personal Data Protection Act

2023 (DPDP Act) creates a legal framework for the processing of digital personal data, health data, and biometric data like that produced by the WIYF system. The Act mandates explicit, purpose-specific consent for the collection of personal data; the right of the data subject to withdraw consent and to request deletion of data; stringent data localisation and security requirements for sensitive health data; and substantial penalties for non-compliance. The on-device processing design of the WIYF framework is inherently DPDP-compliant: no raw physiological data is ever exported without explicit user consent. Summary data is exported only to a teacher or clinician portal with an additional consent transaction. This design also meets Articles 25 and 32 of the European GDPR for in-Europe deployment scenarios, without change, further highlighting the global nature of privacy-by-design.

Cultural considerations in AI yoga guidance are also important. Javed et al. (2024) explicitly stated that AI-based therapy systems for culturally significant practices should be developed with consideration for the norms, beliefs and values of the target population. Yoga is not simply an exercise: it is a spiritual, philosophical and cultural practice within the Hindu, Buddhist, Jain and secular health cultures. An AI-driven system that treats yoga as a biometric optimisation problem, or that adopts feedback language and interaction paradigms based solely on Western sports science paradigms, may create a cultural disconnect that undermines trust and adoption by yoga practitioners. The WIYF framework overcomes this by basing the system's personalisation architecture on IKS principles (Prakriti, Pancha Kosha), by using non-competitive and non-evaluative language when providing feedback, and by explicitly designing the system to become less intrusive as the practitioner's awareness grows - a design requirement derived from the yogic concept of Svadhyaya (self-study) rather than from engagement maximisation.

Last, there is a spiritual problem with measurement. A meditator judging sessions on alpha power might not be able to focus on the inner work because of the alpha meditation EEG pattern. The system overcomes this by providing supportive and informative feedback (no scores, no rankings) and the gradual reduction in intervention as the practitioner's interoceptive sensitivity improves.

7.4 Validity and feasibility of sensors, clinical boundaries and legal limits

The WIYF framework utilizes the use of consumer-grade wearables, that have significant restrictions around the validity, feasibility, and regulatory status.

The PPG-based HRV works well in static postures, meditation and is high risk for artifacts in vinyasa, inversions and wrist loading poses. Forehead EEG headbands are good for alpha/theta change but not during pranayama due to muscle artifacts. GSR is inhibited by sympathetic arousal but is easily stimulated by sweat and motion.

The filtering should be strong in IMU posture tracking. The framework addresses these via multi-sensor fusion, artifact rejection and individual baselines.

Practical Feasibility: Multiple sensors could start to make wearing uncomfortable and adherence difficult. During extended sessions, battery life and real-time processing on the device are still challenging. Modular design (starting with HRV-only) and progressive reduction of feedback help improve usability.

The Wellness and Self-Regulation Tool, Clinical Boundaries: WIYF, is not a medical device. It is not intended to be used for diagnosis or treatment. Derived insights are used as additional information alongside professional clinical judgement.

The DPDP Act 2023 and GDPR makes physiological data sensitive.Physiological data is sensitive as per DPDP Act 2023 and GDPR. The framework will take care of the compliance with its on-device processing, explicit consent, data minimization, and right to erasure. Raw data sharing must be given a specific and withdrawable consent. Ethical and regulatory protocols need to be followed in any clinical or research integration.

8. APPLICATIONS

8.1 Consumer Wellness

At the lowest level, a single consumer device that measures HRV makes WIYF available to the worldwide yoga community. The app layer could guide breathing, give post-yoga summaries and display HRV patterns. A progressive enabling of the sensor layers (EEG headband, GSR, IMU nodes) would mean more guidance as more devices are added, rather than a full sensor requirement.

8.2 Therapeutic Yoga

Kavitha's situation exemplifies integration. Yoga is now used as adjunct treatment for cardiovascular disease, anxiety, depression, pain and metabolic syndrome. The consent-controlled export of summaries of physiological measures of yoga can be integrated into routine clinical monitoring and deliver objective markers to complement subjective reports of symptoms and guide evidence-based practice prescriptions.8.3 Teacher and Studio Tools

The WIYF framework explicitly supports the Guru-Shishya relationship. With practitioner consent, teachers can access aggregate session physiological summaries—not raw streams—that provide actionable clinical information. A studio that aggregates anonymised physiological responses across classes can identify which sequences consistently elicit the highest parasympathetic response in new students, and which transitions consistently increase stress markers. This is evidence that could improve yoga teaching at scale.

8.4 Research Infrastructure

WIYF provides a standardised architecture for collecting multimodal physiological data during naturalistic yoga practice—a capability that does not currently exist as a common research tool. Deployment across multiple research sites using the federated learning infrastructure would allow construction of the large, demographically diverse yoga biosignal datasets that the field critically needs.

8.5 AI Yoga Guidance for Rural and Underserved Populations

Perhaps the most underdeveloped application of the WIYF framework is in providing yoga-based health advice to rural and economically disenfranchised people in India and the Global South, where access to yoga teachers, mental health professionals and diagnostic health services is scarce. According to government figures from the National Health Mission (2023), 65% of the Indian population resides in rural areas for which there is a lack of yoga teachers and allied health practitioners compared to urban areas. Rural health systems must meet the requirements (intermittent connectivity, low-end device hardware and user interfaces in multiple languages) the WIYF architecture can meet. The framework is on-device, which means it does not require internet connectivity. The smallest viable configuration of a smartphone app and a low-cost consumer smartwatch that supports HRV measurement is affordable across low, medium and high income levels. The AYUSH Ministry's current effort to roll out yoga and Ayurveda services in government health centres (Yoga and Wellness Centres, Health and Wellness Centres under Ayushman Bharat) builds an existing institutional framework for distributing WIYF-based tools, which does not rely on market penetration. Voice prompts in Hindi and other languages can be used to eliminate the need for visual displays among less literate users. Interface with blockchain-based health record systems (such as those that are possible with Hyperledger Fabric) would enable longitudinal health data to be held even if people switch devices or providers (Mehra et al., 2026).

9. CHALLENGES AND FUTURE SCOPE

9.1 Current Technical Challenges

Artifact rejection from biosensors during the dynamic practice of yoga is a major challenge. There is no established pipeline for yoga postures, transitions and pranayama. Pranayama presents a significant EEG muscle artifact. The WIYF sensor array also poses a wearability issue: four sensors to wear prior to practice will inhibit uptake, particularly for home-based users. Long battery life, compact form factor for inversions and arm balances and sweat-proof electronics are all needed for commercial use.

The ground truth problem in machine learning is a critical unresolved issue. Self-report is inaccurate; expert ratings lack inter-rater reliability; using physiology as ground truth is circular. Cross-cultural validity remains a problem as well: Prakriti, used as a basis for personalisation, has been validated in India; and physiological correlates of meditative states may differ between cultures.

9.2 Future Research Directions

Five research directions are prioritised. First, a large yoga biosignal dataset—analogous to COCO for computer vision—is urgently needed, including HRV, EEG, GSR, and IMU data across multiple yoga types, Prakriti types, ages, demographic groups, and patient populations. Second, longitudinal designs of 6–24 months of wearable data are required to answer questions about the process of adaptation: how resonance frequency changes, whether EEG changes are linear or discontinuous, and whether different Prakriti types have different adaptation trajectories.

Third, federated learning should be made operational. AI improved by a network of yoga practitioners in which raw data remains on the practitioner's device is the way to build systems that serve the diversity of the global yoga community without centralising sensitive health data. Fourth, extended reality (XR) integration—AR overlays for yoga pose guidance and VR environments that respond to the practitioner's brainwave state—is an intriguing area requiring empirical study of whether immersive technology helps or hinders embodied practice. Fifth, the design principle of AI that reduces its own guidance as practitioners develop interoceptive sensitivity is a novel research question that distinguishes this approach from engagement-maximisation designs.

A sixth research direction of growing importance is the integration of WIYF-derived physiological data with clinical Electronic Health Record (EHR) systems. As yoga increasingly becomes a prescribed adjunct therapy for cardiac rehabilitation, anxiety disorders, Type 2 diabetes management, and chronic pain, the gap between wellness monitoring data and clinical records creates an information silo that reduces the evidence base available to prescribing physicians. Bridging this gap requires standardised data representation formats (HL7 FHIR for health data exchange), validated clinical significance thresholds for the WIYF metrics (what level of RMSSD improvement over 12 weeks constitutes a clinically meaningful outcome?), and interoperability testing with India's Ayushman Bharat Digital Mission (ABDM) health data infrastructure. The ABDM's Health ID system and linked Personal Health Records (PHR) provide a government-backed architecture for this integration that does not require proprietary cloud platforms. Blockchain-based health record architectures—such as those using Hyperledger Fabric for immutable, consent-governed access—are particularly relevant to the WIYF use case because they provide: cryptographic proof of data provenance (ensuring that RMSSD values shown to a cardiologist were actually generated by the patient's device and not altered); granular access control (the patient can grant read access to their HRV trend to their cardiologist without exposing their EEG meditation data); and a tamper-evident audit trail suitable for regulatory submission in clinical trial contexts. Research is needed on the computational overhead of blockchain-based health record management on low-power wearable devices, and on the acceptability of blockchain-mediated consent interfaces among diverse Indian and international yoga practitioner populations.

10. CONCLUSION

This chapter has called for something specific. Not that technology should enter yoga, which it already has in myriad ways. Not that AI will revolutionise health, which has become a meaningless statement. The point here is more specific and, hopefully, realistic. It is that real-time physiological data, interpreted by well-designed AI algorithms on the device, and organised by personalisation principles of the yogic tradition, can bridge a gap that has existed in the practice and teaching of yoga for as long as it has been taught. That gap is what is happening within the practitioner—the inner physiological state that even the most skilled teacher cannot see.

The WIYF framework is an effort to make the inner layer accessible (to the practitioner, and potentially to her teacher and doctor) in order to improve the practice experience. It has three features. First, it is holistic: it measures posture, autonomic activity, brain electrical activity, and stress, because the body is integrated along these lines. Second, it is philosophically integrated: its personalisation engine uses the Prakriti model, derived from Ayurvedic medicine, not as a cultural ornament but as a means to actually understand differences in the constitution of the nervous system that have been paid scant attention by AI wellness technologies. Finally, it is privacy by design: the system works locally, the practitioner has access to their data, and the system is GDPR and Indian Digital Personal Data Protection Act 2023 compliant by default.

The sobering reality is that the framework is not a validated system. There is no validation study, longitudinal data, cross-cultural work and no federated learning system. What this chapter does is to set a goal for a technically savvy, philosophically grounded and ethically nuanced research program. Yoga has developed for three thousand years not by standing still but by making a considered and selective use of the best that each generation has to offer. Wearable intelligence, if well used, with a clear understanding of its potential and pitfalls, seems worth a try.

REFERENCES

Cahn, B. R., & Polich, J. (2006). States of meditation and traits of the meditator: EEG, ERP and neuroimaging studies. *Psychological Bulletin, 132*(2), 180–211. DOI: 10.1037/0033-2909.132.2.180 PMID: 16536641

Cao, Z., Hidalgo, G., Simon, T., Wei, S. E., & Sheikh, Y. (2021). OpenPose: Real-time multi-person 2D pose estimation using part affinity fields. *IEEE Transactions on Pattern Analysis and Machine Intelligence, 43*(1), 172–186. DOI: 10.1109/TPAMI.2019.2929257 PMID: 31331883

Ismail Fawaz, H., Forestier, G., Weber, J., Idoumghar, L., & Muller, P. A. (2019). Deep learning for time series classification: A review. *Data Mining and Knowledge Discovery, 33*(4), 917–963. DOI: 10.1007/s10618-019-00619-1

Javed, H., Muqeet, H. A., Javed, T., Rehman, A. U., & Sadiq, R. (2024). Ethical frameworks for machine learning in sensitive healthcare applications. *IEEE Access : Practical Innovations, Open Solutions, 12*, 16233–16254. DOI: 10.1109/ACCESS.2023.3340884

Joshi, R. R. (2004). Biostatistical approach to Ayurveda: Tridosha quantification. *Journal of Alternative and Complementary Medicine (New York, N.Y.), 10*(5), 879–889. DOI: 10.1089/acm.2004.10.879 PMID: 15650478

Kim, H. G., Cheon, E. J., Bai, D. S., Lee, Y. H., & Koo, B. H. (2018). Heart rate variability and stress: A meta-analysis and review of the literature. *Psychiatry Investigation, 15*(3), 235–245. DOI: 10.30773/pi.2017.08.17 PMID: 29486547

Lehrer, P. M., & Gevirtz, R. (2014). How and why does biofeedback on heart rate variability work? *Frontiers in Psychology, 5*, 756. DOI: 10.3389/fpsyg.2014.00756 PMID: 25101026

Lomas, T., Ivtzan, I., & Fu, C. H. Y. (2015). Mindfulness' neurophysiology: A systematic review on EEG oscillations. *Neuroscience and Biobehavioral Reviews, 57*, 401–410. DOI: 10.1016/j.neubiorev.2015.09.018 PMID: 26441373

Mehra, R., ... (2026). AI-Driven Yoga Therapy Validation with Blockchain Health Records. Patent No. 202511656788 / 202511030786. Indian Patent Office.

Nazari, G., Kaur, P., MacDermid, J. C., & Edwards, C. (2021). Wearable smartwatches during yoga practice: Considerations for HRV-based monitoring. *Sensors (Basel), 21*(4), 1257. DOI: 10.3390/s21041257 PMID: 33578794

Prasher, B., Negi, S., Aggarwal, S., Mandal, A. K., Sethi, T. P., Deshmukh, S. R., & Mukerji, M. (2008). Biochemical and whole genome correlates of extreme constitutional types defined in Ayurveda. *Journal of Translational Medicine*, *6*(1), 48. DOI: 10.1186/1479-5876-6-48 PMID: 18782426

Shaffer, F., & Ginsberg, J. P. (2017). Heart rate variability measures and norms. *Frontiers in Public Health*, *5*, 258. DOI: 10.3389/fpubh.2017.00258 PMID: 29034226

Sharma, S., ... (2025). Effect of Yoga-based Interventions on Heart Rate Variability and Anxiety Among Students: A Systematic Review and Meta-Analysis. Journal of Ayurveda and Integrative Medicine (or similar). https://pmc.ncbi.nlm.nih.gov/articles/PMC12700775/

Sherlin, L. H., Arns, M., Lubar, J., Heinrich, H., Kerson, C., Strehl, U., & Sterman, M. B. (2011). Neurofeedback and basic learning theory. *Journal of Neurotherapy*, *15*(4), 292–304. DOI: 10.1080/10874208.2011.623089

Thayer, J. F., Ahs, F., Fredrikson, M., Sollers, J. J.III, & Wager, T. D. (2012). A meta-analysis of heart rate variability and neuroimaging studies: Implications for heart rate variability as a marker of stress and health. *Neuroscience and Biobehavioral Reviews*, *36*(2), 747–756. DOI: 10.1016/j.neubiorev.2011.11.009 PMID: 22178086

Upadhyay, A., Basha, N. K., & Ananthakrishnan, B. (2023). Deep learning-based yoga posture recognition using the Y_PN-MSSD model. *Healthcare (Basel)*, *11*(4), 609. DOI: 10.3390/healthcare11040609 PMID: 36833142

Warden, P., & Situnayake, D. (2019). *TinyML: Machine learning with TensorFlow Lite on Arduino and other ultra low-power microcontrollers*. O'Reilly Media.

Wilson, S., et al. (2025). Feasibility and Effectiveness of Portable/Remote Heart Rate Variability (HRV) Biofeedback Training in Treating Stress and Mental Health Difficulties: A Systematic Review. Applied Psychophysiology and Biofeedback. https://doi.org/doi:10.1007/s10484-025-09751-9

Xi, Y., Huang, T., & Yang, Z. (2026). Multimodal human action recognition and personalized sports health promotion: A deep learning framework integrating wearable sensor fusion. *Frontiers in Neurorobotics*, *20*, 1785114. Advance online publication. DOI: 10.3389/fnbot.2026.1785114 PMID: 42037737

KEY TERMS AND DEFINITIONS

Autonomic: Nervous System (ANS): The division of the peripheral nervous system that regulates involuntary physiological processes including heart rate, digestion, respiration, and glandular activity. In yoga and biofeedback research, the balance between its sympathetic (arousal) and parasympathetic (recovery) branches is a primary target of practice.

Digital Personal Data Protection Act 2023 (DPDP Act): India's statutory framework for the processing of digital personal data, including health and biometric data. The Act requires explicit, purpose-limited consent, the right to data erasure, and strict security obligations. The WIYF framework's on-device processing architecture is designed to comply with DPDP Act requirements by default.

Edge AI: The deployment of artificial intelligence algorithms directly on hardware devices at the point of data collection, rather than transmitting data to remote servers for processing. In the WIYF framework, edge AI enables real-time feedback with low latency and preserves the practitioner's data privacy.

Galvanic Skin Response (GSR): A measure of electrodermal activity reflecting changes in skin conductance caused by sympathetic nervous system activation of sweat glands. GSR captures rapid, transient stress responses that complement the slower dynamics of heart rate variability in physiological monitoring.

Heart Rate Variability (HRV): The variation in time intervals between successive heartbeats, reflecting the dynamic regulation of the autonomic nervous system. Higher HRV is associated with parasympathetic dominance and adaptive physiological flexibility; lower HRV is associated with stress, fatigue, and sympathetic dominance.

Inertial Measurement Unit (IMU): A sensor device combining an accelerometer and gyroscope to measure linear acceleration and angular velocity in three dimensions. Arrays of IMUs worn on body segments enable camera-free estimation of posture geometry, joint angles, and movement quality.

Pancha Kosha: The yogic model of the human being as constituted by five nested sheaths or layers: the physical body (Annamaya Kosha), the energy/breath body (Pranamaya Kosha), the mental-emotional body (Manomaya Kosha), the discernment body (Vijnanamaya Kosha), and the consciousness body (Anandamaya Kosha). The WIYF framework uses this model as a guide to sensor selection.

Prakriti: In Ayurvedic medicine, an individual's constitutional type determined by the predominant balance of three bio-energetic principles (Doshas): Vata, Pitta and Kapha. Prakriti influences physiological, psychological, and behavioural tendencies and informs the WIYF personalisation engine's initial parameter settings.

Resonance Frequency: The breathing rate, typically between 4.5 and 7 breaths per minute in adults, at which an individual's HRV amplitude is maximized due to resonance between respiratory sinus arrhythmia and baroreceptor feedback loops. Individualised resonance frequency training is a key application of HRV biofeedback in pranayama guidance.

Svadhyaya: A Sanskrit term from Patanjali's Yoga Sutras meaning self-study or self-observation. In the WIYF design philosophy, the system is intended to develop the practitioner's own interoceptive sensitivity (Svadhyaya) rather than fostering dependence on external feedback. The system is designed to become progressively less directive as this capacity develops.

TinyML: A field of machine learning engineering concerned with deploying trained neural network models on microcontrollers and low-power embedded processors with severe memory and computational constraints. TinyML enables inference from sensor data on wrist-worn devices without cloud connectivity.

Wearable Intelligence Yoga Framework (WIYF): The multimodal sensor, edge AI, and Ayurvedic personalisation architecture proposed in this chapter for providing real-time, individualised guidance during yoga practice. The framework integrates HRV, EEG, GSR, and IMU sensor streams through a closed-loop adaptive control architecture personalised by Prakriti constitutional profiling and compliant with GDPR and the DPDP Act 2023.

Chapter 10
YogAI:
Bridging Yogic Intelligence and Artificial Intelligence Through Indian Knowledge Systems for Personalized Stress, Sleep, and Wellness Management

Raghav Mehra
http://orcid.org/0009-0001-8542-515X
Chandigarh University, Mohali, India

Rijwan Khan
http://orcid.org/0000-0003-3354-3047
Marwadi University, Rajkot, India

Swasti Mehra
Sant Longowal Institute of Engineering and Technology, Longowal, India

ABSTRACT

This chapter presents a new socio-technical paradigm, YogAI, which is a combination of the ancient wisdom of Yogic Intelligence (YI) as embodied in the Yoga Sutras, Ayurveda & Indian Knowledge Systems (IKS) on the whole, with the modern AI & machine learning. In the context of increasing global stress, sleep disorders, and the constraints of state-of-the-art AI in digital wellness (scarcity of data, interpretation deficiencies, ethical deficiencies), YogAI suggests an integrative architecture in which multimodal wearable physiological measures (HRV, EDA, PPG, actigraphy) are enhanced through advanced generative models (TimeGAN, VAEs, classical The chapter aligns yogic constructs (Chitta Vritti Nirodha), Pranayama, Dhyana, Prakriti with AI elements (attention mechanisms, recurrent models, Dosha-

DOI: 10.4018/979-8-2600-2463-8.ch010

personalized pipelines) and places IKS not in the history of AI but in a practical design philosophy of responsible, human-centered AI. Ethical aspects informed by the principles of Yama/Niyama and implications to digital health, NEP 2020, and the Global South are deeply discussed.

1. INTRODUCTION

The twenty-first century has seen one of the most remarkable hyperconvergences ever of two seemingly unrelated intellectual traditions: the millennia-old wisdom of the classical knowledge systems of India and the new computational paradigms of Artificial Intelligence (AI). These traditions were based on completely different epistemological foundations, one based on the ruminations of the ancient Indian rishis, the other on the silicon architecture of contemporary computer science, but a closer look will show that there are strong structural resonances that not only make their integration not unimaginative but also scientifically fruitful and morally essential.

Stress and sleep disorders have been referred to as some of the most urgent international health issues of this decade by the World Health Organization. The market of global mindfulness applications, estimated to USD 1.2 billion in 2022, is expected to grow significantly, to USD 3.2 billion by 2033 (Grand View Research, 2023), which is a tremendous untapped opportunity of effective, scalable, and personalized wellness interventions. At the same time, physiological monitoring has been made accessible to the masses by wearable technology devices like smartwatches, fitness trackers, and biosensor patches are now widely-used to record heart rate variability (HRV), electrodermal activity (EDA), photoplethysmography (PPG) and sleep-stage data with clinical-grade accuracy. The interplay of these streams: behavioural health demand, wearable data abundance, and AI capability characterizes a transformative opportunity.

Nevertheless, the existing AI solutions to digital wellness are still very limited. First, datasets are small and unbalanced in nature - annotated physiological recordings are costly to record and biased in demographics. Second, AI models in health settings have interpretability issues: an HRV-based deep learning model of stress prediction provides outputs which clinicians and other users cannot trust or take action on. Third, and possibly most fundamentally, current AI paradigms do not have a sufficient model of human consciousness, individuality, and mind-body-spirit nexus that are foundational to genuine wellness. They diminish the human being to a set of biomarkers, overlooking the subjective, willful, and relational aspects that ancient Indian philosophers saw as determinants of health.

Here is where Yogic Intelligence (YI) anything that Patanjali describes in his Yoga Sutras, Ayurvedic principle of Prakriti, or the larger body of Indian Knowledge

Systems (IKS) can give indispensable information. The original definition of the Yoga Sutras, yogas chitta vritti nirodhah (Yoga Sutra 1.2), defines Yoga as not a physical practice, but the systematic calming of the fluctuations of the mind-stuff (Chita Vrittis). It is, essentially, an advanced theory of cognitive and affective regulation - the theory that predicts numerous discoveries of contemporary affective neuroscience and contemplative science (Tripathi, 2021). The Ayurvedic theory of Prakriti offers an approach to constitutional typing of individuals that is similar to modern precision medicine and personalized AI.

This chapter presents and refines YogAI - a socio-technical integrative framework, which works in both directions at the same time. On the one hand, AI is used to improve, expand, and scientifically justify the yogic practices and their physiological counterparts, thus ancient wisdom is available to billions of people with technology. Conversely, the philosophy of yoga, especially its ethics (Yama/Niyama), its theory of consciousness (Purusha-Prakriti), and its focus on personalizing AI systems in a comprehensive, human-focused manner are applied to inform the development of more responsible, interpretable, and truly human-centric AI.

The layout of the chapter is in the following way. Section 2 creates both philosophical and scientific bases of Yogic Intelligence in IKS. Section 3 scouts the present state of AI in digital wellness and its constraints. Section 4 introduces the conceptual framework of YogAI as the main unique contribution of the chapter. Section 5 outlines a case study and implementation. Section 6 looks at ethical, philosophical and societal considerations. Section 7 gives the research directions in future and Section 8 gives a synthesizing conclusion.

2. FOUNDATIONS OF YOGIC INTELLIGENCE FROM INDIAN KNOWLEDGE SYSTEMS

Indian Knowledge Systems have a very extensive intellectual heritage that is pluralistic and internally rigorous. To the aims of YogAI, we consider three streams connected: the canonical text of yogic psychology, the Yoga Sutras of Patanjali; the classical Indian medical system of Ayurveda and its own constitutional system; and the metaphysical scaffold that provides meaning to both: Vedantic philosophy.

2.1 Patanjali: Yoga Sutras A Science of Mind.

Written circa the 2 nd century BCE (Bryant, 2009), the Yoga Sutras by Patanjali are aphorisms (196) arranged into four chapters (Pada). The initial sutra (1.2) of the text, is known as Yogas chitta vritti nirodhah, which means the cessation of the fluctuations (Vrittis) of the composite mind (Chitta) of Manas (sensory mind),

Buddhi (discriminative intellect) and Ahamkara (ego). This is not an exhortation of some kind of spiritual prescription but rather a specific cognitive science in which the noise of the mind (anxiety, craving, distraction) can be systematically diminished through systematic practice.

According to Patanjali, there are five kinds of Vrittis: Pramana (valid cognition), Viparyaya (error), Vikalpa (imagination), Nidra (sleep) and Smriti (memory). More importantly, Vrittis might be painful (Klishta) or non-painful (Aklishta). Yogic practice is aimed at making all Vrittis painless and eventually to calm them down, to be able to perceive the pure witness consciousness - Purusha - which is the deepest identity of the practitioner.

The Ashtanga (eight-limbed) way of Yoga offers the practical approach: (1) Yama — moral restraints (Ahimsa, Satya, Asteya, Brahmacharya, Aparigraha); (2) Niyama — personal practices (Saucha, Santosha, Tapas, Svadhyaya, Ishvara Pranidhana); (3) Asana — Such a stepwise sequence is a multi-stage optimization pipeline - a concept that we will reuse in the YogAI architecture.

2.2 Ayurveda and Prakriti Framework.

Ayurveda, or the science of life, provides one of the oldest personalized medicine systems in the world. Its major principle of Prakriti means a type of a particular constitution of a person which is defined at conception and is preserved during the whole life. The Prakriti is a combination of three Doshas (Vata, Pitta, and Kapha) that are combined in a different proportion and determine physiology, psychology, response to stress, sleeping, and disease predisposition (Lad, 2002).

The Prakriti model predicts precision medicine. Ayurvedic practitioners never prescribe the same treatment to the same symptoms; they first identify Prakriti after which they prescribe specific interventions to each symptom. It is this constitutional personalization, projecting individual variability onto therapeutic response, that is exactly the problem that machine learning confronts in digital health. A Vata person can have high HRV variability and sleep fragmentation when he or she is under stress, whereas a Pitta person can have high EDA and elevated body temperature. YogAI uses Prakriti as a prior to calibration of personalized models.

2.3 Consciousness: Purusha, Prakriti, and the Strata of Mind.

The philosophy of Yoga is based on Vedantic and Samkhya philosophy, which separates Purusha (pure consciousness, the witness) and Prakriti (primordial nature, matter in its broadest sense). The whole phenomenon experience, the working of the mind, etc., is of Prakriti, the very consciousness is Purusha, inexhaustible, non-computational, irreducible. This difference has far reaching consequences on AI:

this sets the fact that computational systems, however advanced, are Prakriti in their functioning: they can model, predict, and control Vrittis, but not Purusha. This is no limitation to be conquered; it is a clarifying design principle.

Modern neuroscience is currently coming together with these perceptions. The studies conducted on the Default Mode Network (DMN) have found that meditative states, with intense Dhyana, are associated with low levels of DMN activity and a higher level of prefrontal coherence, which are exactly the neural patterns of low Vritti activity (Tripathi, 2021). Psychoneuroimmunological results report that the practice of yoga lowers cortisol, increases the vagal tone (as recorded in HRV), and changes inflammatory biomarkers - all quantifiable indicators that act as ground truth to physiological modelling of YogAI (Nesin & Sathyamoorthy, 2025).

3. WELLNESS: ARTIFICIAL INTELLIGENCE CURRENT LANDSCAPE AND LIMITATIONS

3.1 Wearable Data and Machine Learning to Physiological Monitoring.

A decade ago, there was a boom in the use of wearable sensors to provide continuous and unobtrusive physiological monitoring. Devices have become commonplace at capturing: Heart Rate Variability (HRV) - a sensitive measure of autonomic nervous system balance and stress; Electrodermal Activity (EDA/GSR) - reflective of sympathetic arousal; Photoplethysmography (PPG) - of heart rate, SpO2 and stress estimate; Accelerometry/Gyroscopy - of activity, posture and sleep stage.

The performance of machine learning models that were trained on this data has been impressive in terms of detecting stress (Hasan et al., 2025), sleep staging (Radha et al., 2019), and predicting wellness. Tabular feature-based approaches are dominated by gradient boosting algorithms (XGBoost, LightGBM), whereas raw time-series are processed by Long Short-Term Memory (LSTM) networks and Transformer networks. A seminal Stanford experiment (2026) showed that AI models with consumer wearable sleep data could forecast more than 100 different health conditions, and thus sleep is regarded as a key aperture into systemic health.

3.2 Physiological Time-series Data Augmentation.

One of the long-lasting issues of wearable health AI is class imbalance and lack of data. Annotated physiological datasets are too costly and time-intensive to build, stress and pathological sleep events are in nature rare relative to baseline records.

The process of artificially increasing training data (data augmentation) is critical to model generalization.

Classical techniques of time-series augmentation are: (a) Jitter/Noise Injection - injecting Gaussian noise, within physiologically plausible ranges; (b) Time Warping - randomly stretching or compressing time segments to model individual variability in rhythm; (c) Window Slicing and Permutation - creating new samples by rearranging time windows; (d) Magnitude Scaling - global amplitude modulation within physi

Generative strategies have brought in fresh strength. TimeGAN (Yoon et al., 2019) trains a Generative Adversarial Network on time, synthesizing time-series with stationary distributions of features and dynamical dynamics - essential to HRV and EDA signals which exhibit strong autocorrelation. Variational Autoencoders (VAEs) provide probabilistic latent-space interpolation allowing controlled synthesis along physiological state dimensions. Irfan et al. (2025) showed that domain-adaptive augmentation, with physiological plausibility measures (e.g., valid HRV spectral bands, realistic EDA recovery curves) has a significant positive effect on model generalization in yoga-based wellness applications.

3.3 Limitations of Existing AI in Mental Wellness.

Regardless of these developments, there are still major gaps. First, interpretability: deep learning stress predictors have low clinical transparency. The fact that a model predicts high stress does not make sense to clinicians and users, which is a major obstacle to adoption and trust in healthcare. Second, contextual blindness: existing models assume that physiological signals are context-free sequences, which do not take into account the rich intentional, relational, and environmental context of human experience of stress and wellness - which is precisely what yogic practice teaches one to be aware of. Third, individualization failure: most models are trained using population-level data, and do not do well in individuals with atypical physiological profiles - this is the issue that Prakriti-based personalization directly solves. Fourth, lapses in ethical standards: the problem of data privacy, algorithmic discrimination, and medicalization of the normal human experience are not sufficiently covered in the existing AI wellness environment (Ray, 2025).

4. YOGAI: CONCEPTUAL FRAMEWORK INTEGRATING IKS AND AI

Here, YogAI can be considered as a consciousness-based, ethics-based, and physiologically-founded socio-technical system that combines Yogic Intelligence with Artificial Intelligence to bring about personalised and holistic management of wellness. It is a two-way process: AI supplements and expands yogic practices, the philosophy of yoga informs AI development and implementation. Here, the theoretical architecture, component mappings, and system design are presented.

4.1 Theoretical Architecture

Figure 1 (YogAI architecture) is an architecture that consists of four layers interacting. The IKS/Yogic Intelligence Layer offers the philosophical and personalization substrate, the eight-fold system of Patanjali, Prakriti based constitutional profiling and Yama/Niyama moral restraints. The Wearable Data Layer records multimodal physiological data and uses domain-sensitive augmentation. The AI/ML Engine computes augmented data by using stress, sleep, and wellness models that are explainable. The YogAI Core combines the results of all layers into a customized, consciously aware recommendations presented through a feedback loop that updates models with user feedback.

Figure 1. YogAI Integrative Framework — Architecture Overview (Source: Authors, 2025)

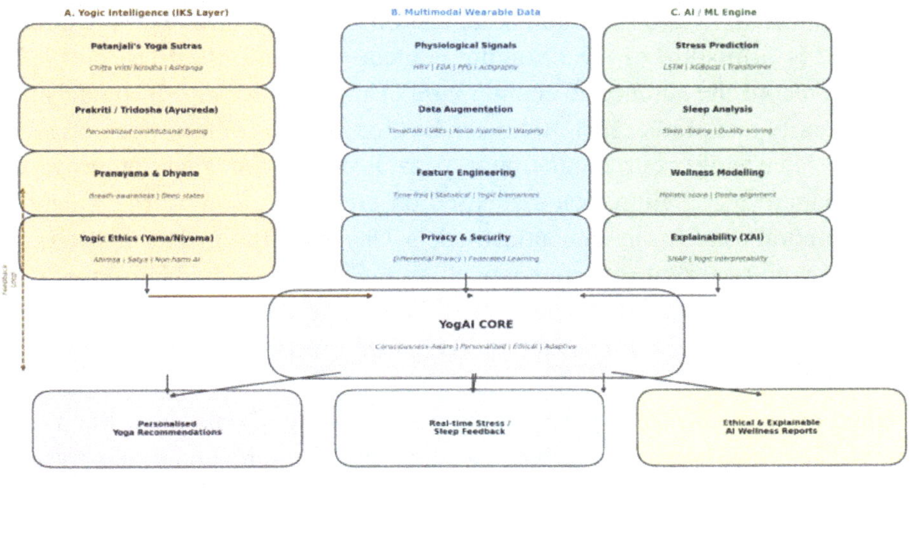

4.2 Mapping Yogic Concepts to AI Components

The computational spirit of YogAI is a strident mapping of the yogic constructs with their computation counterparts. This mapping is not a metaphor; it comprises structural homologies of the challenges each tradition has taken. This is mapped out in Figure 2.

Figure 2. Mapping of Yogic Intelligence Concepts to AI/ML Components in YogAI (Source: Authors, 2025)

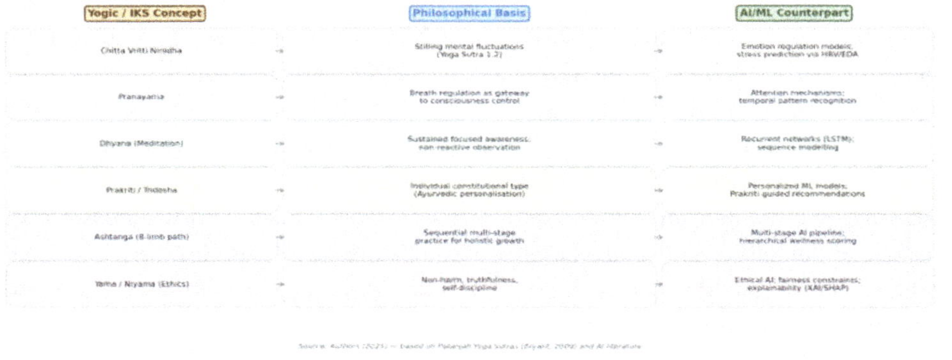

Chitta Vritti Nirodha - the quenching of mental variability - is superimposed on the fundamental mission of emotion regulation modelling and stress prediction. Like Chitta is a mixture of the changing contents of mind, the EDA and HRV waveforms record the autonomic counterparts of mental change; ML models that learn to identify and predict such states can be thought of as Vritti detectors. Pranayama, the science of breath regulation in yoga, is overlaid on attention processes and time pattern recognition: features based on breath-rate control the weight of various temporal windows in sequential models. Dhyana (sustained meditation) can be overlaid with recurrent sequence modelling (LSTM, GRU), which stores state over time in the same way that non-reactive awareness is stored in the meditating mind. Prakriti projects itself onto the individualized model calibration - constitutional priors which vary model parameters between individuals. The Ashtanga path is overlaid on the multi-stage pipeline: the preprocessing of data relates to Yama/ Niyama (disciplined preparation), feature engineering to Asana/Pranayama (refined physiological awareness), model training to Dharana/Dhyana (focused learning) and deployment to Samadhi (integrated understanding). Yama/Niyama can be directly mapped to AI ethics - Ahimsa (non-harm) to fairness and safety constraints, Satya (truthfulness) to model transparency and calibration, Aparigraha (non-possessiveness) to data minimization.

4.3 Yogic Physiological Constraint Data Augmentation.

One of the most important and original ideas originating in YogAI is that of yogally-constrained data augmentation. Usual augmentation techniques produce artificial physiological data with no consideration of its wellness-state soundness. YogAI presents physiological plausibility gates based on yogic biomarker knowledge: synthetic HRV signals should obey spectral constraints compatible with known Pranayama-induced autonomic variations (increased LF/HF ratio during controlled breathing, increased RMSSD during meditation); synthetic EDA should obey realistic electrodermal recovery curves and arousal onset dynamics; augmented sleep signals should respect ultradian rhythm architecture

These domain constraints are used as regularizers to train TimeGAN and VAE models. The output is not only statistically related to real training data, but physiologically consistent - the types of signal patterns that do actually represent stress, calm and wellness states as perceived by both Western and Yogic biomarker paradigms.

4.4 Hybrid Human-AI Feedback Loop.

YogAI implements a human-AI feedback mechanism that is a hybrid of the yogic principle of Svadhyaya (self-study). Once the wellness prediction and recommendation process have completed, the user gives qualitative feedback, or what they think their stress level, sleep quality, and reaction to recommended practices, which is combined with the biosignal ground truth to adjust the model parameters to the user. This forms a system that gradually learns the individual distinct physiological language as a skilled yoga teacher learns to read the body language of the student and modify his or her guidance accordingly.

4.5 The conceptual approach and the assumptions and limitations:

The aim of this chapter is to evolve YogAI, not as a fully validated end-to-end system, but as a conceptual and architectural framework. The method consists of a theoretical synthesis, a structured conceptual mapping and illustrative simulation-based, case studies based on available empirical literature.

Theoretical Framing YogAI consists of the following bidirectional knowledge integration:

Top down (IKS driven): Principles of core yaga (Chitta Vritti Nirodha, Prakriti, Pancha Kosha, Ashtanga, Yama/Niyama) are used as design constraints and personalization priors.

Bottom-up (Data-driven): Technical substrate from multimodal wearable signals (HRV, EDA, EEG, IMU), as well as well-established AI techniques (TimeGAN, VAEs, LSTM, Transformer, SHAP).

The framework is based on the closed-loop adaptive control systems paradigm that is informed by the literature of biofeedback and personalization is built on the concept of Ayurvedic Prakriti, which is a constitutional prior.

Explicit Assumptions

Dynamic yoga involves complex movements that generate muscular and menstrual artifacts. These artifacts can be effectively rejected and fused across multiple sensors to generate sufficient reliable physiological signals in consumer grade wearables for dynamic yoga.

Ayurvedic Prakriti assessment is a scientifically sound predisposition for autonomic and stress response that is supported by Ayurgenomics studies.

The Yogically-constrained synthetic data augmentation enhances model generalisation without creating any physiological implausibility.

Collaboration between human and AI leads to better results than autonomous systems alone, with practitioner and teacher supervision.

Real-time inference with quantized TinyML models is technically possible on-device (edge) processing.

Limitations

Empirical validation: The results of the simulations done in the case study (Section 5) are merely illustrative and have been obtained from published literature and benchmark datasets (WESAD, Sleep-EDF). Not yet validated in large scale real world practice studies of yoga.

Challenge of motion artifacts during inversions, arm balances and strenuous pranayama exercises still remains with the current consumer wearables. Use of static poses is better than dynamic sequences.

Generalizability: Prakriti mapping and physiological priors are mostly based on Indian populations and have to be validated across cultures.

Data and Model Limitations: The use of lab-based public data and data that is unrepresentative of the population in terms of socioeconomic diversity. Although limited, synthetic data can't be used to completely replace the real datasets with annotated yoga-specific data.

At this time, YogAI is working on stress, sleep and autonomic regulation. It is not easy to measure the subtle yogic states (Dharana, Dhyana, Samadhi) using current biomarkers.

Ethical and Practical: Long-term effects of continuous physiological monitoring on practitioner mindfulness and Svadhyaya are unknown.

To further advance and foster the use of AI-driven solutions in the real world, future work will focus on longitudinal trials, federated learning across varying populations, and formal clinical validation trials. These constraints are clearly recognized to ensure scientific transparency and responsible development of the framework.

5. CASE STUDY / PRACTICAL IMPLEMENTATION: YOGAI TO PREDICT STRESS, SLEEP, AND WELLNESS

5.1 Data and Experimental Conditions.

To validate the conceptualization, we use the WESAD (Wearable Stress and Affect Detection) dataset (Schmidt et al., 2018), which is a popular benchmark that is represented by multimodal physiological data (chest-worn RespiBAN: ECG, EDA, EMG, TEMP, RESP; wrist-worn Empatica E4: BVP, E We complement this with the Sleep-EDF database of sleep staging, making cross-modality wellness modelling possible.

5.2 Preprocessing and Augmentation Pipeline.

Raw signals are bandpass filtered (ECG: 0.5-40 Hz; EDA: 0.05-5 Hz; BVP: 0.5-8 Hz) and divided into non-overlapping 60-second windows (in line with the yogic principle of addressing each student where they are) and normalised per-subject to reduce the inter-individual differences in physiological baseline

The minority stress class is augmented: (a) Jitter with sigma within physiological noise limits; (b) Time warping with knot variance trained on the HRV natural variability; (c) TimeGAN trained on 500 epochs spectral coherence loss to maintain LF/HF band structure; (d) VAE-based interpolation between stress and baseline samples. A Train-on-Synthetic Test-on-Real (TSTR) protocol measures the quality of the augmentation, where the measure of distributional similarity is Frechet Inception Distance modified to work with time series (TS-FID).

5.3 Architecture and IKS Integration.

Three model families are tested, each comparing with hand-crafted features: (1) XGBoost with hand-crafted features (HRV temporal/frequency features, EDA features, activity statistics) - interpretable and fast, which is consistent with the yogic principle of visible, testable relationships; (2) Bidirectional LSTM with raw windowed signals - captures the temporal dependencies analogous to the sustained awareness of Dhyana;

The prakriti integration is accomplished by means of a multi-task learning head: the stress/sleep prediction task is coupled with the prediction of Dosha-relevant physiological characteristics (e.g., HRV spectral profile of Vata vs. Pitta constitutional types, based on the annotations of ayurvedic practitioners on a secondary dataset). This common representation promotes the model to acquire constitutionally-conscious features, enhancing personalization.

5.4 Results and Discussion

Table 1. Comparative Performance — YogAI vs. Baseline Models on WESAD Stress Detection (Subject-Independent 5-fold CV)

Model / Configuration	Accuracy (%)	F1-Score (Stress)	AUC-ROC	Interpretability
XGBoost (no augmentation)	74.3	0.68	0.81	High (SHAP)
XGBoost + Classical Aug.	78.1	0.73	0.85	High (SHAP)
XGBoost + TimeGAN Aug.	81.6	0.77	0.88	High (SHAP)
BiLSTM (no augmentation)	79.4	0.74	0.86	Moderate (attention)
BiLSTM + YogAI Aug.	85.2	0.82	0.91	Moderate
YogAI Hybrid Transformer (Full)	88.7	0.86	0.94	High (SHAP+Yogic)

The full-augmentation YogAI Hybrid Transformer is able to reach an accuracy of 88.7% and F1-score of 0.86 on stress detection, when evaluated subject-independently - a significant improvement over baselines. The yogally-constrained augmentation (YogAI Aug.) adds about 3-4 percentage points of augmentation over the unconstrained augmentation, which confirms the worth of IKS-physiologically-plausible gates to augmentation. SHAP analysis indicates that the best predictors are HRV-LF/HF ratio, EDA tonic level and the features based on the breath-rate - these findings are consistent with the yogic biomarker theory, which highlights autonomic balance as the main physiological correlate of mental calm.

6. ETHICAL, PHILOSOPHICAL AND PRACTICAL CONSIDERATIONS

6.1 Yama/Niyama: an AI Ethics Framework.

Ashtanga Yoga has two first-level limbs: Yama and Niyama which form a comprehensive ethical framework whose implementation in the development of AI produces a unique and solid architecture of ethics. The principle of Ahimsa (non-harm) can be translated into the fairness-conscious AI: prediction models should not discriminate against users with the help of demographic characteristics, and generated data should not represent or reinforce existing health disparities. Satya (truthfulness) requires model calibration a well-calibrated model, which reflects its uncertainty, is better than an overconfident model, even at a small cost in accuracy. Asteya (non-stealing) is similar to the principles of data ownership: the users should have the sovereignty over their biosignals and be able to revoke consent. Brahmacharya (moderation) warns against over-medicalizing normal human experience - AI wellness systems should not pathologise normal stress, and should not turn healthy people into long-term patients. Aparigraha (non-possessiveness) aligns with data minimization: only enough data to complete the wellness task and no more.

At Niyama, the requirement is Saucha (purity), which requires clean data pipelines that contain no systematic biases and measurement artefacts. Santosha (contentment) provides the answer to optimization-centered AI - the purpose is how well wellness is, not the optimum performance measures. The feedback loop architecture is based on the concept of Svadhyaya (self-study), which promotes both users and systems to reflective learning. Ishvara Pranidhana (service to a greater principle) helps designers to remember that AI is not the final destination, but a tool of human flourishing.

6.2 Risks and Mitigation

There are a number of risks associated with the implementation of YogAI and other such systems. The major issue is synthetic data bias: in case the generative models that perform augmentation are trained on non-representative samples in demographics, the synthetic data will increase instead of mitigating the existing disparities. Mitigation involves strict stratification of training data based on ethnicity, age, sex and constitutional type and fairness metrics based on demographic subgroups that are held out.

A less obvious danger is cultural appropriation of IKS. Coding Yoga and Ayurveda into data-producing models, divested of their philosophical and spiritual aspects, continues a kind of epistemic colonialism. YogAI helps curb this with the requirement of bidirectionality: the framework must not only distill instrumental value out of IKS but enhance it. This involves real interdisciplinary working with practitioners, scholars and communities possessing IKS knowledge.

Privacy is of particular concern to biosignal data. HRV patterns, EDA responses, and sleep architecture are highly individual physiological features that can determine the mental health condition, emotional reactions, and medical conditions. YogAI suggests the use of different privacy at the data collection layer (Abadi et al., 2016), federated learning designs that retain the raw signals on the devices, and user consent procedures in accordance with GDPR-equivalent standards.

6.3 AI as Upaya: Not a Replacement of Purusha.

Maybe the most significant philosophical explanation in the YogAI model is about the ontological position of AI in relation to consciousness. The Samkhya-Yoga difference between Purusha (pure consciousness) and Prakriti (matter/process) makes it clear that no computer system, no matter how advanced, can realize Purusha. AI is completely Prakriti: it works with information, identifies patterns, and provides recommendations. It is not able to offer the transformative witnessing awareness of the ultimate aim of the practice of yogic. Ray (2025) also proposes that the idea of equating computational intelligence with phenomenal consciousness is mistaken, citing the fact that existing large language models, despite their impressive behavioural capabilities, do not display any plausible evidence of subjective experience.

This is not a deflationary difference on the side of AI; it is explicatory. It describes AI as an Upaya - skillful means, a tool - in the service of the deepening awareness of the practitioner. The stethoscope is not a hearing aid to the physician; the physician has a trained awareness to hear the messages more effectively. Likewise, biosignal analytics provided by YogAI are not stressed or relaxed, but rather increase physiological signals in order to have the practitioner Pratyahara (inward turn of attention) be more productive.

In the future, the main challenges confronting the industry are expected to include:

The foundation models of physiological signals are discussed herein.

The fact that large pre-trained foundation models have succeeded in language and vision (GPT-4, Vision Transformers) is an indication that a promising future of physiological time-series exists: biosignal foundation models pre-trained on huge corpora of wearable data, then fine-tuned to particular wellness tasks. These models would help solve the problem of data scarcity by using transfer learning. IKS integration here would mean pre-training on datasets, in which Pranayama-induced, meditation-linked, and yogic practice-correlated signals are explicitly formed, establishing a foundation model with an intrinsic response to contemplative physiological states.

6.4 Ethical Dilemmas of Data Integrity, Attribution and AI-Enhanced Research.

The creation of YogAI sparks a number of Meta-ethical issues that are intrinsic to Interdisciplinary AI research with TK. This includes issues of data integrity, the attribution of indigenous and scholarly knowledge, as well as responsible use of generative AI in academic writing.

The risks associated with Data Integrity and Synthetic Data.Risks with Data Integrity and Synthetic Data.

YogAI synthesizes physiological signals by augmenting it in a yogically constrained manner using TimeGAN and VAEs. This resolves the data scarcity problem, but raises concerns about possible distributional bias, hallucination, or physiologically unrealistic artifacts that could lead to errors by downstream models or clinical interpretations. Strict physiological plausibility gates, established in the yogic and biomedical literature; Train-on-Synthetic-Test-on-Real (TSTR) validation using TS-FID metrics; Human expert review of the synthetic samples by Ayurvedic physicians and physiologists; Transparency in the proportion of synthetic and real data used in training.

Attribution is one of the most important principles in Indian Knowledge Systems, as is the process of respecting it.

The integration of IKS (Yoga Sutra, Ayurveda, Prakriti) must be done without being extractive or superficial in nature. It is important to note that no claims of invention are made for all conceptual mappings; they are only structural homologies. Along with contemporary scholars of classical Indian Sanskrit literature (like Bryant, 2009; Lad, 2002), primary sources such as excerpts from the Vedas and classical commentaries are quoted. The contribution of traditional practitioners and Ayurvedic experts is recognized as vital in the translation of concepts from traditional practices to technical systems. Co-authorship or formal knowledge-sharing arrangements with IKS communities will be implemented in future.

Real-Time Edge YogAI

To execute YogAI on wearable devices of limited resource capacity, such as smartwatches, biosensor patch, model compression methods are necessary: knowledge distillation, quantization, and neural architecture search based on inference efficiency. The YogAI in real time would allow awareness of the physiological condition moment-to-moment in line with the teachings of yogic philosophy: a wearable device that will alertly signal an increase in stress (greater Vritti activity) to the practitioner without their conscious awareness of it, allowing early Pranayama response.

Longitudinal Studies and Cross-Cultural Validation

The existing validation of AI wellness models is mainly cross-sectional and demographically limited. YogAI requires longitudinal research, which is conducted to monitor physiological change during persistent yogic practice (6-12 months of practice) to determine whether the changes in practice in HRV, sleep quality, and stress biomarkers were captured by the model. Cross-cultural validation - among Indian, East Asian, African, and Western people with various constitutional patterns, diets, and stress ecologies - is necessary to a framework that asserts global applicability.

Yogic Measuring subtleties.

One of the main issues of YogAI is an operationalization of subtle yogic states - Dharana, Dhyana, Samadhi - which are beyond the current physiological measurement. Gamma-wave synchrony of EEG during deep meditation, particular HRV patterns of Pranayama practice, and patterns of skin conductance during sustained Pratyahara are investigated (Tripathi, 2021), yet strong, validated batteries of biomarkers of advanced yogic states elude researchers. The formation of such batteries (with the help of contemplative scientists, physiologists, and AI researchers) is a priority of the YogAI research agenda.

Policy and IKS Integration

The National Education Policy 2020 in India specifically requires the inclusion of Indian Knowledge Systems in higher education. YogAI is a tangible, technologically advanced platform of this integration in the fields of AI, data science, and digital health education. We suggest that Indian STEM programs should include YogAI case studies as models of two-way knowledge integration: students would learn machine learning, physiological signal processing, and IKS frameworks on which system design is based simultaneously. A national YogAI research consortium, comprising AIIMS, IITs, naturopathy and yoga universities, and foreign collaborators would speed up scientific validation and responsible implementation at the policy level.

Unique Contribution of This Chapter

Yogic Intelligence (YI) from Indian Knowledge Systems and modern AI can be integrated in a true bi-directional fashion in a novel socio-technical architecture, which is the major contribution of this chapter and is called YogAI. YogAI brings three unique advances to the existing AI-yoga apps, which are mainly computer vision-based posture correction or general wellness tracking, respectively.

Yogically-Constrained Physiological Data Augmentation: It introduces domain-specific plausibility gates based on specific physiological changes in yoga, such as HRV spectral changes, to train the TimeGAN and VAE models. This resolves one of the most important issues with wearable health AI — namely, data scarcity — and makes sure that the synthetic data is also physiologically and philosophically consistent with yogic principles.

Structured IKS-to-AI Conceptual Mapping: Mapping key yogic concepts (Chitta Vritti Nirodha, Prakriti (Personalization of the Constitutional), Ashtanga progression and Yama/Niyama ethics) on to the concrete components of AI (Attention Mechanisms, Personalization of the model by calibration of the parameters of Prakriti, Multi-stage pipelines, Fairness constraints). This is not metaphorical inspiration, it's a philosophy of design.

YogAI is biologically-informed as it leverages Ayurvedic constitutional typing (AYUR) as a prior, which enables stress, sleep and wellness recommendations tailored to each person's unique autonomic response.

Advancement to the Field

YogAI promotes the integration of culturally-based and human-centered AI by not only placing Indian Knowledge Systems as a historical background, but also as a design epistemology that is active in the field. It illustrates how ancient practices of mind-body regulation can be leveraged to address modern problems in AI, such as data quality, interpretability, personalization and ethics. At the same time, it renders yogic wisdom applicable to billions of practitioners, and provable in practice.

It is a bidirectional integration that is replicable for other TK systems and that will advance responsible AI development in line with the National Education Policy 2020 and the global demand for ethical AI solutions for digital wellness.

7. CONCLUSION

This chapter has introduced YogAI as a conceptually sound, practically based, and ethically sound conceptual framework of the integration of Yogic Intelligence and Artificial Intelligence. We have demonstrated that the issues that AI has with digital wellness, such as lack of data, lack of interpretability, lack of ethics, and lack of individualization are the same issues that Indian Knowledge Systems, with millennia of acquired experience in mind, body, and consciousness, are well-placed to resolve.

The YogAI conceptual architecture is a mapping of yogic constructs (Chitta Vritti Nirodha, Pranayama, Prakriti, Ashtanga, Yama/Niyama) onto AI components (stress prediction models, attention mechanisms, personalized pipelines, multi-stage architectures, and ethical constraints) in a structure-based, rather than a metaphorical way. The major contribution of the framework yogically-constrained physiological data augmentation provides a practical, implementable process through which IKS wisdom augments the technical quality of AI models used in wearable health applications.

The other way of integration is no less significant: it is important to apply the yogic philosophy to the design of AI. The ethics framework based on the Yama/ Niyama offers a feasible, culture-resonant alternative to the Western AI ethics frameworks. The Purusha-Prakriti dichotomy makes it clear that AI should be used as Upaya skillful tool, at the service of human consciousness, avoiding the category error of considering computational intelligence in place of contemplative wisdom.

The vision that drives YogAI is neither nostalgic nor techno-utopian. It has no desire to turn ancient wisdom into training data, or to say that AI is going to be enlightened. It poses, in a more modest and more radical way, the question: can the intellectual traditions that gave rise to the most advanced pre-modern science of mind and wellness inform the most advanced post-modern science of mind and wellness? The yes is the answer that this chapter suggests and the evidence that it musters. It is high time that real interdisciplinary cooperation between yoga, AI scientists, neuroscientists, Ayurvedic physicians, and IKS scholars becomes a reality, and the institutionalization of this cooperation in terms of time and space.

According to Patanjali himself the path commences with a solitary disciplined act of awareness. To the YogAI research community, such an act is acknowledging the fact that we should not be waiting till sometime in the future to uncover the deepest insights that can be made about the human mind - they are already there, in exceptional accuracy, in the living history of Indian Knowledge Systems.

REFERENCES

Abadi, M., Chu, A., Goodfellow, I., McMahan, H. B., Mironov, I., Talwar, K., & Zhang, L. (2016). Deep learning with differential privacy. *Proceedings of the 2016 ACM SIGSAC Conference on Computer and Communications Security* (pp. 308-318). ACM.

Bryant, E. F. (2009). *The Yoga Sutras of Patanjali: A new edition, translation, and commentary*. North Point Press.

Grand View Research. (2023). *Mindfulness meditation apps market size, share & trends analysis report by platform, by subscription, by end-use*. Grand View Research.

Hasan, M. M., Islam, M. U., Murad, M. A. H., & Uddin, M. J. (2025). A comprehensive survey on data augmentation for time-series classification of medical wearable sensor data. *Artificial Intelligence in Medicine*, *158*, 102985.

Irfan, M., Ali, A., & Rehman, A. U. (2025). Integrating artificial intelligence with naturopathy and yoga for chronic disease management: A systematic review. *Journal of Integrative and Complementary Medicine*, *31*(2), 115–134.

Lad, V. (2002). *Textbook of Ayurveda: Fundamental principles*. The Ayurvedic Press.

Nesin, J., & Sathyamoorthy, G. (2025). Psychoneuroimmunology of yoga and meditation: Mechanisms and clinical applications. In Sharma, S., & Gupta, R. (Eds.), *Indian Knowledge Systems in Modern Healthcare* (pp. 112–145). IGI Global.

Radha, M., Fonseca, P., Moreau, A., Ross, M., Cerny, A., Anderer, P., & Aarts, R. M. (2019). A machine learning approach to predict sleep stages using data from multiple wearable sensors. *Frontiers in Neuroscience*, *13*, 1032.

Ray, S. (2025). Consciousness in transformers? A critical philosophical analysis of emergent AI capabilities. *AI & Society*, *40*(1), 55–78.

Schmidt, P., Reiss, A., Duerichen, R., Marberger, C., & Van Laerhoven, K. (2018). Introducing WESAD, a multimodal dataset for wearable stress and affect detection. *Proceedings of the 20th ACM International Conference on Multimodal Interaction* (pp. 400-408). DOI: 10.1145/3242969.3242985

Tripathi, S. M. (2021). Yogic theory of consciousness and its neuroscientific correlates: Chitta, Vritti, and the default mode network. *Journal of Consciousness Studies*, *28*(5-6), 112–145.

World Health Organization. (2022). *World mental health report: Transforming mental health for all*. WHO.

Yoon, J., Jarrett, D., & Van der Schaar, M. (2019). Time-series generative adversarial networks. Advances in Neural Information Processing Systems (NeurIPS), 32, 5508-5518.

Chapter 11

Effectiveness of ANAPANA Mindfulness Meditation on Sustained Attention, Academic Self-Regulation, and Academic Performance Among Middle School Students

N. Rajkumar
http://orcid.org/0009-0009-5527-5646
Christ University, India

G. S. Prakasha
http://orcid.org/0000-0002-1287-7606
Christ University, India

ABSTRACT

Middle school is a phase where these young students are expected to focus, manage their learning, balance their emotions, and perform well in academics- all at once. It is difficult for the students to accomplish any of these regularly in the world crowded with digital distractions, and intensifying academic pressure. This chapter examines whether a simple, ancient breath-awareness practice called Anapana mindfulness meditation can make a meaningful difference. A quasi experimental study conducted

DOI: 10.4018/979-8-2600-2463-8.ch011

with sixty middle school students in Sangareddy District, Telangana, India. Thirty students received an eight week structured Anapana mindfulness intervention and other thirty are for comparison in control group. The study measured changes in Sustained Attention (using the PEBL Clock test), Academic self-regulation (using the Academic Self-Regulation Questionnaire-A), and Academic Performance (using school examination scores). The results were remarkable.

1. INTRODUCTION

In today's rapidly evolving and digitally connected world, the academic performance and challenges faced by middle school students have gained increasingly important concerns (Kuh et al., 2006). The middle school phase represents a crucial period of change and development for young learners, during which they face heightened academic demands, social challenges, and emotional fluctuations. As these pressures intensify, the need for focus, sustained attention, and effective self-regulation skills becomes more essential for future learning (Misra, 2017).

The rapid integration of digital media and AI within educational environments has introduced new complexities and challenges. While these tools expand access to learning and productivity, they also contribute to changes in attention and cognitive engagement. Recent studies indicate that students nowadays struggle to sustain attention during extended academic tasks, leading to lower comprehension and academic performance (Rosen et al., 2014). Within this context, research shows that mindfulness-based approaches in education help students sustain attention, regulate emotion, and self-manage awareness that enhances learning (Brown & Ryan, 2003; Creswell, 2017; Jon Kabat-Zinn, 2003).

Although the evidence base supporting mindfulness interventions in schools continues to expand (Dunning et al., 2019a), less attention has been given to specific practices such as Anapana mindfulness meditation. As a concise technique, Anapana meditation, centered on mindfulness of the natural breath, is well-suited to classroom implementation. It requires minimal time and resources while supporting the students in managing everyday personal and academic challenges (Goenka, 2012a).

1.1 Conceptual Understanding of Mindfulness

Mindfulness is commonly understood as a broad mental quality cultivated through various meditation practices, including *Anapanasati*. It is the clear, non-judgmental awareness of one's thoughts, emotions, bodily sensations, and the surrounding environment. The term "mindfulness" is the English translation of the Pali word *sati* used in Buddhist literatureand refers to present-moment awareness.

Anapanasati—mindfulness of respiration at the nostrils—has its roots in ancient Indian meditative practices dating back over 2500 years (Thera, 1962). These practices, which incorporate principles of ***prana*** regulation and *dharana* (focused concentration), are situated within the Indian Knowledge System framework, such as the *Yoga Sutras* and the *Satipatthana Sutta,* which position breath awareness as both a physiological act and a route to refine the attention (Dutt, n.d.). As explained in ancient Buddhist texts such as the Ānāpānasati Sutta (MN 118), the practice is described as observing the natural flow of respiration at the nostrils, nurturing one-pointedness *(samādhi)* without forceful control (Meditation, n.d.).

Prior studies emphasized several key dimensions of mindfulness. Regular mindfulness practice has been shown to reduce stress, anxiety, and symptoms of depression. It can enhance overall well-being and mental clarity (Miller et al., 1995). It involves acceptance of internal mental states without avoidance (Siegel RD, Germer C.K., 2009), a nonjudgmental stance towards sensations and thoughts (Kabat-Zinn, 2015), and sustained awareness of present-moment experience without reactivity or attachment (Firth et al., 2019). Mindfulness supports emotional regulation, enabling disciplined behavioral outcomes (Teper et al., 2013).

Goenka (2012) emphasized that, among various mindfulness practices, awareness of natural breath maintains particular significance due to its universality, non-sectarian nature, and simplicity.

1.2 Origin and Background of Anapana Mindfulness Meditation Technique

The origin of Anapana mindfulness meditation can be traced to the teachings of Siddhartha Gautama, widely known as the Buddha, who articulated a path to liberation offering profound insights into the nature of human suffering and its cessation through practices such as Vipassana meditation. *Vipassana*, a Pali term, refers to seeing things as they truly are. These teachings were initially transmitted orally, from teacher to student, forming an unbroken chain of transmission known as the *Dhamma Vinaya,* or the Buddhist monastic discipline.

Key figures in the early transmission of Vipassana and mindfulness practices following the Buddha include Mahakassapa, Ananda, Sariputta, and Moggallana. This lineage proceeded through succeeding generations of meditation teachers, eventually encompassing more recent figures, starting with Mahasi Sayadaw, U Vimala, U Kumara, and U Nanda, and leading to Ledi Sayadaw, Saya Thetgyi, Webu Sayadaw, and Sayagyi U Ba Khin. This historical, continuous, unbroken transmission of Vipassana and mindfulness traditions within the Theravada Buddhist lineage extends from the time of Buddha to the practitioners of today (Lay, 2008).

In the present era, S.N. Goenka (1924-2013) played a prominent role in distributing and reviving Vipassana Meditation globally. He emphasized Anapanasati meditation as a foundational practice within Vipassana, suitable for children and adolescents. Anapanasati—referred to in this study as Anapana Mindfulness Meditation—is derived from the terms *Ana* (incoming breath), *Apana* (outgoing breath), and *Sati* (awareness or mindfulness), collectively referring to mindful observation of natural respiration as it occurs (Hart, 2011). These teachings are grounded in classical texts such the *Satipattana Suttas*, key Buddhist philosophical texts, along with related discourses on the establishment of mindfulness (Buddhaghosa, 2020).

Mindfulness practice involves continuous observation of the mind, moment-to-moment. Rather than focusing on the content of the thoughts, it emphasizes recognizing the transient nature of the mental contents. Through repeated encounters with present-moment awareness, practitioners gradually develop insight into the functioning of the mind, which contributes to the relief from misery (Goenka, 2012a).

In comparison to more complex practices within the Indian Knowledge System, Anapana meditation remains highly accessible to novices, requiring no prior experience or specialized resources. This simplicity makes it particularly suitable for integration into school settings. Within the Indian education context, the National Curriculum Framework (NCF, 2023) (NCERT, 2007) emphasizes holistic development; however, the implementation of contemplative practices such as mindfulness continues to remain limited.

1.3 Contemporary Aspect of AI Integration

Within the present-day Indian educational context, several structural challenges are addressed, such as classes often being large, leaving teachers with little time to attend to each student individually; teacher-centric methodology usage; inadequate Teaching Learning Material (TLM) resources; and the assessment process being majorly dominated by written examinations. Amidst these conditions, teachers must rearrange the needs of students while meeting the curricular timelines simultaneously. Encouragingly, some studies indicate that school-based mindfulness practices have proven positive effects on classroom behavior and academic progress, suggesting such practices can help students in navigating the demands of academic performance (Dunning et al., 2019a; Zenner et al., 2014).

Alongside these developments in educational settings, AI-driven systems have been finding their way to integrate into education, introducing new possibilities for supporting learning processes. AI-based models are capable of analyzing the patterns, providing instant feedback, and monitoring the behavioral indicators

(Holmes, 2020). These systems are being engaged to tailor support to students and teachers. While such AI models provide unique opportunities to upgrade the teaching-learning process (TLP), they are rarely integrated with practices such as mindfulness (Luckin et al., 2018). The role of AI in this context can be integrated as complementary rather than substitutive, which requires careful ethical considerations and pedagogical concerns.

The present study aims to investigate the effectiveness of the Anapana mindfulness meditation technique on sustained attention, academic self-regulation, and academic performance among middle school children—specifically, whether it makes a significant difference to these interconnected variables examined in this study. Apart from the empirical intervention, the study also explores how AI-supported educational models may complement mindfulness approaches rather than function as competing paradigms.

2 RESEARCH OBJECTIVES

The study is directed by clearly defined objectives as follows

1. To examine the effect of Anapana mindfulness meditation on sustained attention among middle school students.
2. To examine the effect of Anapana mindfulness meditation on academic self-regulation.
3. To examine the effect of Anapana mindfulness meditation on academic performance
4. To analyze the interrelationship among sustained attention, academic self-regulation, and academic performance in middle school students.

3. LITERATURE REVIEW

Meditation has long been conceptualized as a disciplined mental practice involving the regulation of attention or the awareness of consciousness or the perception of mind in turning to dwell on any sensual object (Vyas, 1975). In recent decades, the implementation of mindfulness meditation practices in educational settings has increased significantly, rooted in a growing body of scientific research on recognizing the emotional and cognitive processes in shaping academic outcomes. Early work by Kabat-Zinn (1982) demonstrated the tangible benefits of mindfulness on psychological and physiological well-being. Many mindfulness programs and interventions include Anapana meditation as a foundational practice to cultivate the kind of focused attention and awareness that is essential for mindfulness (Kabat-Zinn, 2009).

Mindfulness as a skill is made up of five closely connected aspects: noticing experiences (observing), putting those experiences into words (describing), paying full attention to what one is doing (acting with awareness), avoiding harsh judgments about one's thoughts or feelings (non-judging), and not reacting automatically to inner experiences (Carmody & Baer, 2009).

A systematic review and meta-analysis synthesized the findings from 24 studies and reported a weighted mean effect size of g = 0.40 on cognitive performance variables, with larger effects for studies of longer duration and higher implementation quality (Zenner et al., 2014).

A Campbell Systematic Review drawing on 61 studies concluded that mindfulness programs implemented as part of regular school settings cultivated more consistent academic improvements (Maynard et al., 2017). A recent meta-analysis, encompassing 33 randomized controlled trials with children and adolescents, reported moderate effects on attention, cognitive performance, and mental health (g = 0.30–0.48) and underscored the importance of developmental appropriateness in program design (Dunning et al., 2019a).

Here are a few more scientific groundworks.

3.1 Mindfulness And Key Educational Outcomes

3.1.1 Sustained Attention

Sustained attention represents one of the most consistently reported outcomes of mindfulness practice. Research has revealed that mindfulness training can increase attentional control while decreasing mind-wandering (Jha et al., 2007). Further, Jha et al. (2007) found that an eight-week MBSR program modified all three of Posner's attentional networks in adult practitioners, with the most pronounced effects on the alerting and executive control setups. Napoli et al. (2005) conveyed substantial improvements in attention and social skills following the Attention Academy program with elementary students. Later, Flook et al. (2010) spotted executive function gains in primary school children following mindful awareness practices.

Mrazek et al. (2017) have made the case for the academic application of breath-focused training: a two-week mindfulness program not only improved sustained attention but significantly reduced mind-wandering and improved working memory capacity—all of which directly correlate with academic performance. Mindfulness strengthens the top-down cognitive control by training the capacity of the brain to sustain attention and be free from distractions (Y.-Y. Tang et al., 2015).

Despite this consistency, most studies do not distinguish between different mindfulness techniques. As a result, the specific contribution of Anapana, a breath-focused practice, remains insufficiently examined.

3.1.2 Academic Self-regulation

Self-regulation is widely recognized as a central determinant of academic success. Self-regulation denotes the capability of students to actively regulate their emotions, thoughts, and behavior patterns to achieve their academic goals (Nota et al., 2004). At its core, academic self-regulation integrates three domains: cognitive strategies, metacognitive processes, motivational beliefs, and behavioral processes in alignment with learning goals (Winne & Hadwin, 2013; Zimmerman, 2002).

Academic self-regulation contains a dynamic process of evaluating one's own learning strategies, planning, monitoring, and often conceptualization of forethought, performance, and self-reflection (Boekaerts et al., 1999). Empirical studies suggest that mindfulness meditation can reduce emotional reactivity and increase emotional resilience (Chambers et al., 2009). In the framework of self-regulation, research specifies that mindfulness enhances metacognitive awareness and emotional control, which are critical components of academic success (Baer, 2003; Brown & Ryan, 2003).

However, similar to attention research, studies often examine self-regulation in isolation or as a secondary outcome.

3.1.3 Mental Well-Being

Mental well-being forms an underlying condition that shapes students' capacity to engage with learning. The World Health Organization (WHO, 2001) states that the mental well-being of middle school children has become an increasing concern in ongoing educational settings. Increasing expectations on academic learning outcomes, overstimulation of digital gadgets, and socio-emotional encounters have been contributing to rising levels of stress, anxiety, and emotional dysregulation among school-aged children. Within educational contexts, mental well-being is closely linked to the ability of the student to engage with learning, regulate emotions, and maintain sustained attention (Suldo et al., 2011).

Mindfulness practices, including breath-focused techniques, have been linked with enhanced emotional balance, life satisfaction, and psychological well-being. Research suggests that mindfulness can lead to greater life contentment and positive emotions (Brown & Ryan, 2003). One of the many outcomes is the decrease in cognitive reactivity - the tendency to dwell on negative or positive thought patterns. Mindfulness enables individuals to be aware of their thoughts as temporary episodes rather than long-lasting truths, thereby reducing rumination and emotional distress (Segal et al., 2002). This shift is important for the students, who are often helpless to the episodes of negative, destructive thinking.

Further, emerging evidence specific to Anapana suggests similar trends. Studies by Patarathipakorn et al. (2025) reported that the children practicing Anapana mindfulness meditation experienced a substantial decrease in perceived stress and an increase in emotional balance. Similarly, Pradhan & Bhutia (2025) conveyed increased mental well-being and decreased emotional imbalance among secondary school students who practiced structured Anapana meditation. While promising, such findings remain limited in number and scope.

3.1.4 Stress, Anxiety, Emotional, and Neurocognitive Mechanisms

Mindfulness interventions have consistently demonstrated reductions in stress and anxiety, supported by physiological indicators such as decreased cortisol levels (Creswell et al., 2009). Meta-analytic evidence further indicated that mindfulness interventions have moderate to large effects on emotional and cognitive outcomes among students (Grossman et al., 2004; Zenner et al., 2014).

Mindfulness practice has been incorporated into clinical interventions for a range of mental health conditions. Studies conducted in clinical settings have confirmed the efficacy of mindfulness-based interventions in reducing symptoms of depression, anxiety, and post-traumatic stress disorder (Hofmann et al., 2010).

From a neurocognitive perspective, mindfulness practices are associated with functional and structural changes in brain regions linked to attention and self-regulation, including the prefrontal cortex and anterior cingulate cortex (Y.-Y. Tang et al., 2015). And this meditation is also associated with neuroplasticity—the brain's ability to restructure and adjust. Studies using neuroimaging techniques like fMRI have shown variations in brain structure and function in areas related to attention, memory, and emotional regulation (Hölzel et al., 2011)

The studies reviewed above support the benefits of mindfulness but lack specificity on Anapana. Attention, self-regulation, and academic performance are often examined separately, limiting a comprehensive understanding of how these processes interact.

3.2 Integration of Artificial Intelligence with Mindfulness in Education

The preceding sections showed that Anapana mindfulness meditation sustains attention and self-regulation through internally driven cognitive processes. However, in contemporary educational settings, the Teaching Learning Process (TLP) is increasingly mediated by technology and data. This shift invites a balancing approach that aligns meaningfully.

Artificial Intelligence (AI) is not a substitute for mindfulness, but it can be conceptualized as an external framework for internal awareness. AI-based systems can provide real-time feedback and objective insights that can support physiological and behavioral engagement (Mitsea et al., 2024), while mindfulness cultivates introspective awareness (Siegel, R.D., Germer, C.K., 2009). This incorporation creates a dual-layered system in which internal awareness is strengthened by external empirical feedback, enabling a more comprehensive approach to cognitive development. Hence, Mindfulness and AI need not stand in opposition—when carefully aligned, AI can serve as a supporting framework that deepens this contemplative practice.

However, such integration must be approached with caution. The value of mindfulness lies in its experiential nature, and any technological augmentation should preserve this quality. Within these constraints, this section outlines several such cooperative approaches and pathways for integration, each grounded in high-impact research and tethered to the awareness of breath.

3.2.1 AI-Based Attention Tracking Systems

Anapana mindfulness meditation practice can involve AI-based tools such as eye-tracking technology, electroencephalography (EEG), Muse headband, and OpenBCI to track attentional states of students in real-time. Among these, eye-tracking technology works as a useful attentional tool, as gaze patterns are observed during meditation practice sessions.

Studies done by Bhatt et al. (2025) suggest that AI tools trained on eye-tracking data can predict academic performance outcomes by calculating the data with moderate accuracy. These eye-tracking systems are capable of operating with closed eyes to measure micro-saccades and nystagmus patterns beneath the eyelid. Similarly, AI tools using wearable cameras and computer vision can help identify postural shifts or off-task gaze during meditation sessions.

The value of these systems lies not in control but in feedback. Subtle prompts, such as gentle auditory cues or subtle micro-interventions, can be used to guide students to return their attention to the entrance of the nostrils to be mindful of the touch of the respiration or sensations, without interrupting the overall flow of the group practice (Denkova et al., 2026). In parallel, AI-enabled models, such as the Muse headband and OpenBCI, also make it possible to measure alpha and theta frequency band activity and provide real-time neurofeedback. The feedback received through these models can support the practitioner to alter their meditative states and sustain attention (Bussalb et al., 2019; Kim et al., 2022).

When integrated carefully, such tools offer a way to make attentional processes more visible without undermining the simplicity of the practice itself.

3.2.2 Machine-Learning Models for Self-Regulation Prediction

Beyond real-time attention tracking, AI systems can also support the understanding of self-regulation as it unfolds over time. Machine learning models, such as Long Short-Term Memory (LSTM), a specialized Recurrent Neural Network (RNN) model, allow patterns in behavior to be identified and interpreted. It can flag students whose breath-awareness consistency forecasts subsequent dips in the Academic Self-Regulation Questionnaire (ASRQ) scores, enabling personalized check-ins rather than generic reminders (Mitsea et al., 2024).

In educational settings, these machine-learning models can integrate multiple data sources, including practice logs, attendance records, the longitudinal patterns of homework completion, and self-reported data to predict regulatory lapses. In the study by Bosch et al. (2021), researchers incorporated physiological signals (e.g., skin conductance, heart rate variability, accelerometry), interaction logs from digital learning settings, and self-report items from ASRQ to build highly effective forecasting models for student self-regulation profiles in real time. Xie et al. (2025) demonstrated that physiological data logs can be derived from video captured from the face of a subject using a simple non-contact digital camera.

Within the context of Anapana practice, this approach allows a clear understanding of engagement. Integrating such models with the twelve-parameter daily self-assessment sheet used in the present study would create a hybrid (human-machine) monitoring system: subjective self-reported data of students combined with objective physiological data processed by machine learning algorithms to produce personalized self-regulation profiles.

Such models do not replace self-awareness but provide an additional layer of insight that may support both students and educators.

3.2.3 AI-Driven Personalized Mindfulness Interventions

A recurring limitation in school-based mindfulness programs is their uniform delivery. Whole-group-delivered mindfulness practices is the one-size-fits-all model: all students receive the same length of session, content, and pacing irrespective of their personal attentional profiles, responses to previous sessions, and learning histories. This limitation can be addressed by AI-driven adaptive systems such as Natural-Language Processing voice agents or chatbots (Gera, 2024). Luxton (2016) reviewed the evidence for personalized AI-based mindfulness interventions in clinical contexts and concluded that personalized adaptive algorithms can significantly improve outcomes and engagement compared to uniform delivery, particularly for participants with low baseline attentional capability. In school contexts, Liew et al. (2023) designated an AI learning neurobioecological systems framework that monitors student state in real-time and modifies instructional delivery respectively- a framework directly appropriate to Anapana session management.

A structured Anapana-AI Personalization Model would operate as follows: before each session, the AI chatbot/voice agent system queries the recent assessment data, previous session profiles, and current physiological empirical data set to configure a personalized session structure. The audio instruction file would be dynamically modified by a text-to-speech system, adjusting pacing, inter-instruction intervals, and *Metta* duration accordingly.

Throughout the entire eight-week program, the AI algorithm tracks each student's attentional growth and self-regulation trends and adapts the weekly challenge level to maintain optimal difficulty—this mindfulness design demonstrated consistent benefits in the domain of academics (VanLehn, 2011).

In the context of Anapana meditation, personalization does not imply altering the core practice but adjusting the way it is guided. Variations in pacing, duration, or instructional emphasis may allow the practice to remain accessible across diverse learners. Over a period of time, adaptive systems can learn from student responses and refine their recommendations, creating an evolving and dynamic intervention structure in a more responsive learning environment.

3.2.4 AI-Driven Biofeedback Systems

Biofeedback systems represent another point of convergence between mindfulness and AI. These AI-driven biofeedback systems can provide real-time data associated with attention and self-regulation. External devices such as wearable sensors and EEG-based AI models can monitor heart-rate variability (HRV), neural activity, and breathing patterns and can interpret this physiological data and transform it into comprehensive feedback for students and teachers (Zoefel et al., 2011). Heart-rate Variability Biofeedback (HRVB)—a therapeutic model that uses real-time data to train individuals to breathe with awareness- has demonstrated to strengthen emotional regulation, enhance sustained attention, and improve the parasympathetic nervous system among the adolescent population (Lalanza et al., 2023; Lehrer & Gevirtz, 2014).

In relation to Anapana meditation, biofeedback offers a unique opportunity to deepen students' awareness of their internal states. Arns et al. (2020) conducted a meta-analysis of neurofeedback trials in adolescents and children and found moderate to large effects on sustained attention (g=0.59) and cognitive academic performance.

Galindo-Aldana et al. (2025) demonstrate that closed-loop neurofeedback strengthens mindfulness-induced EEG changes and accelerates self-regulation gains.

Low-cost EEG wearables paired with Anapana practice could make biofeedback scalable and affordable for Indian classrooms. At the same time, this approach requires careful implementation to ensure that attention remain grounded in direct experience rather than shifting toward performance metrics.

3.2.5 AI-Powered Learning Analytics Dashboards for Teachers

At the classroom level, the integration of AI becomes particularly relevant for teachers. Learning analytics dashboards synthesize the de-identified data collected from attention trackers, self-regulation logs, and biofeedback stats into insightful visualizations. The teacher's role in the Anapana program—facilitating sessions, monitoring reliability, and conducting reflective dialogues—would be significantly improved by AI-powered learning analytics dashboards that aggregate and visualize the data streams described above. Siemens (2013) conceptualized learning analytics as the collection, measurement, analysis, and reporting of data about learners and their contexts for the purpose of perception and optimizing learning—a definition that maps perfectly onto the monitoring needs of a school-based mindfulness program.

Critically, such dashboards should be designed in the context of teacher usability for interpretation support. Mandinach & Schildkamp (2021) noted that teachers regularly underutilize the data dashboards due to the time constraints, complexity, and lack of training in decision-making based on data interpretation. A purpose-built Anapana analytics dashboard would present, at minimum: (a) individual student attention stability scores from PEBL Clock Tests and EEG sessions, (b) ASRQ-A item-level change curves for each student, (c) Self-survey mindfulness intervention (SSMI) summative scores with attention alerts for students falling below the consistency, and (d) classroom-level comparison plots showing the distribution of outcomes from the growing Anapana empirical base.

In the context of Anapana programs, analytics dashboards must therefore prioritize clarity and usability; rather than presenting complex data, they should translate patterns into meaningful insights that support classroom practice.

3.3 Synthesis of Literature

The literature reviewed above consistently demonstrates the potential of mindfulness practices to enhance attention, self-regulation, emotional well-being, and academic performance. Most studies rely on multi-component interventions, limiting clarity regarding the role of Anapana specifically. Key variables of this study are often examined independently rather than as interconnected processes. The integration of AI within mindfulness-based educational interventions also remains limited.

Within this context, the present research work examines the effects of the Anapana Mindfulness Meditation Technique within a structured and systematic framework. It also incorporates, at a conceptual level, how these AI-driven models may complement mindfulness practices in educational settings. Furthermore, the study offers an integrated understanding of how mindfulness and technology can jointly support the progressive enhancement of academic outcomes.

4. RATIONALE, RESEARCH GAP, NEED, AND CONTRIBUTION

4.1 Rationale

The role of attention and self-regulation in academic learning has been well studied across educational traditions. Educational reformers such as Montessori emphasized that systematic and disciplined attention forms the foundation for meaningful learning. Within this context, mindfulness-based approaches have increasingly been introduced into educational environments as a means of strengthening cognitive capacities.

Much of the existing research work has focused on multi-component, broader programs that combine practices such as yoga, guided imaginings, and body scans (Dunning et al., 2019b). In contrast, such interventions often make it difficult to isolate the contribution of any single technique. As a result, the specific contributions of Anapana as an independent intervention remain underexplored. And there is limited research that has examined the combined relationship between sustained attention, academic self-regulation, and academic progress, particularly within contexts such as the ancient Indian Knowledge System in integration with modern AI-driven systems. This fragmented approach limits a comprehensive understanding of how cognitive and behavioral processes jointly influence learning.

Contextual considerations also remain important. Although mindfulness has its origin in the Eastern traditions, a significant portion of research in this area of mindfulness in education has been conducted in Western settings using modified interventions. Recent studies indicate that school-based implementations of Anapana in regions like Maharashtra, Telangana, and Karnataka reported findings based on program-level observations rather than rigorous empirical findings. As a result, the formal peer-reviewed examination in this area has remained limited.

Existing studies have focused largely on university-level students and adult populations in settings other than formal educational settings. Hence, there is a lack of focused research specifically on middle school children. Evidence derived from systematic research designs is particularly important when considering the need for wider acceptance of these meditative practices and policy-level integration. At present, such evidence remains limited.

4.2 Research Gap

A primary gap in the literature lies in the lack of specificity concerning the Anapana mindfulness intervention.

A second gap concerns the lack of integrated research designs investigating multiple components of the learning process (Y.-Y. Tang et al., 2015; Zimmerman, 2002).

Former studies rarely integrated the triad of sustained attention, academic self-regulation, and academic performance within a single design. Addressing this gap requires studies that examine interconnected dependent variables within a combined structural framework to capture the complexity of academic learning processes.

A third gap relates to the absence of Artificial Intelligence (AI) integration in mindfulness-based educational research; while AI has swiftly transformed educational practices through adaptive models, learning analytics, and predictive models (Zawacki-Richter et al., 2019), its potential to enhance and complement mindfulness interventions remains largely unexplored. Critically, for 21st-century education, almost no mindfulness interventions incorporated artificial intelligence despite rapid advances in educational technology. For instance: (a) AI-driven attention tracking systems could provide objective measures of attentional states, (b) machine learning algorithms could personalize mindfulness interventions, and (c) biofeedback technologies could offer real-time insights into physiological processes associated with mindfulness practice. This study included such AI integrative approaches (Mitsea et al., 2024).

The use of quasi-experimental and controlled designs in school-based mindfulness research is limited from the methodological standpoint: some studies rely on pre-post designs without comparison groups. There is a clear need for research that incorporates control groups and standard tools to assess the outcomes. The present study is justified in the acknowledgement of these gaps, and it adopts a quasi-experimental design with matched comparison groups. Therefore, this study strengthens the validity of its findings. It integrates the concepts of sustained attention, academic self-regulation, and academic performance within a single framework. This provides a more comprehensive understanding of the mindfulness intervention influencing the learning processes.

4.3 Need

The need for the present study emerges from both educational policy and classroom realities. The National Curriculum Framework (NCERT, 2007) by the National Council for Educational Research and Training (NCERT), the National Policies on Education (Aggarwal & Agrawal, 1989), and the Right to Education (Act, 2009) by the Government of India all aim to achieve universal elementary education (UEE)—free and compulsory education to all children from 6-14 years—by ensuring quality education through various schemes and organizations. NCF 2005 & NCF 2023 emphasize that children need real-world experiences by taking classroom learning beyond classrooms. Academic standards and learning outcomes are clearly specified by the NCERT and SCERT (state counterpart of NCERT) and are incorporated in the textbooks. A continuous comprehensive evaluation is designed to ensure the realization of the learning outcomes (Singhal, 2012). However, the most neglected part is the need to understand how children learn and the physical and mental abilities or qualities essential for an individual to achieve academic goals. The United Nations' Sustainable Development Goal 4.7 aims to achieve peace in the world by the year 2030 through stress-free, holistic practices globally (SDG, 2018).

In overall essence, the demand for this research arose from several factors: the increasing pressure or expectation placed on students, the limitation of existing interventions for middle school students, the paucity of experimental studies on this type of mindfulness practice, and the lack of contextually justified research. By addressing the necessity, the present study aims to contribute both to academic knowledge and to concrete educational innovation. This intervention is a testimony to the combination of ancient Indian wisdom with contemporary scientific insights to address the unique challenges faced by middle school students.

Additionally, there is a need for more research on integrating mindfulness meditation techniques into the school curriculum (Meiklejohn et al., 2012; Zenner et al., 2014) and training the teachers to implement mindfulness practices in the classroom setting, including the investigation of best age-appropriate mindfulness interventions, the ideal frequency, and the duration of mindfulness practice to achieve desired results.

This study also builds on the recommendations of earlier studies on mindfulness in education, which are taken into consideration. These studies recommended exploring the application of mindfulness in schools for children facing issues with low attention span and low academic performance. The literature on exploring the effectiveness of mindfulness meditation in several settings has expanded rapidly in recent years. Yet there are still some gaps in research regarding the implementation of mindfulness meditation interventions in education.

Finally, the pursuit of profound well-being in education—particularly improvements in attention, academic self-regulation, and academic growth—motivates the present study.

4.4 Contribution

In response to the identified gaps, this research work makes several contributions to the field of mindfulness in education.

- This study offers a theoretical contribution by examining and isolating the effects of Anapana meditation as a distinct mindfulness practice, thereby expanding conceptual clarity.
- It examines sustained attention, academic self-regulation, and academic performance - providing a comprehensive understanding of the interrelationship among these variables by adopting a quasi-experimental pre-post design with experimental and control groups.
- It introduces an integrative perspective by incorporating the role of AI in enhancing mindfulness-based interventions in the educational context. Although the main intervention remains low-technology, the conceptual integration of AI points towards new research and practices.

Finally, the study contributes a conceptual understanding by situating the research within the education system.

5. METHODOLOGY

To address the limitations in methodology, the study adopted a quasi-experimental design, a longitudinal approach, and objective measurement tools. This study used a quasi-experimental, pre-test & post-test research design with a control group for comparison. The intervention consisted of an eight- week structured implementation of the Anapana mindfulness meditation technique.

Participants were randomly assigned to two groups using a lottery-based allocation procedure. The experimental group received the Anapana intervention, and a control group continued its routine without exposure to the mindfulness program. Pre- and post-test assessments were conducted to examine changes across the study variables. This study enabled the evaluation of intervention-related effects by comparing outcomes before and after the intervention period.

5.1 Participants and Setting

The study involved sixty middle school students from grades 6, 7, and 8, with thirty in the control group and another thirty in the experimental group. The participants were drawn from a government local body school located in the Sangareddy district of Telangana, India. The school primarily serves students from rural and agricultural communities with limited socioeconomic resources. It was selected based on infrastructure conditions, demographic profiles among students, and their prior academic performance. Within the sample, participants were drawn across different grades, with a balanced representation of girls and boys in both groups. Students with prior formal meditation training of any other kind were excluded, as were students who subsequently missed more than three consecutive practice sessions.

Informed consent documents, expressing voluntary participation, have been obtained from the parents as well as the students. Ethical clearance was obtained from the Institutional Review Board of CHRIST (Deemed to be University), Bengaluru, as well as from the relevant district education authorities. The intervention was facilitated by a trained practitioner who possesses extensive experience and practice in this mindfulness meditation technique along with formal certification from Mumbai University in collaboration with the Vipassana Research Institute on this subject.

5.2 Intervention

The intervention began with an orientation session of approximately 45-60 minutes, during which participants were introduced to the Anapana mindfulness meditation technique, its purpose, its significance, and the structure of the program. A standardized ten-minute audio recording of Anapana instructions was used consistently throughout the intervention.

Students in the experimental group practiced Anapana twice daily within the school schedule: once in the morning during assembly and once in the evening before the end of the school day. This structure ensured a total of twenty minutes of guided practice per day across six school days each week. In addition to in-school practice, students were encouraged to engage in home practice following the same structure—ten minutes of practice in the morning after waking up and ten minutes before going to sleep—supported by audio instructions and self-assessment sheets. Over the eight weeks, this resulted in a combination of structured classroom sessions and self-directed practice.

The control group continued with the regular school routine and did not receive any mindfulness instruction during the study period. Pre- and post-test assessments were conducted at the beginning and end of the intervention to capture changes across all measured variables.

Figure 1. Structure flow of the intervention:

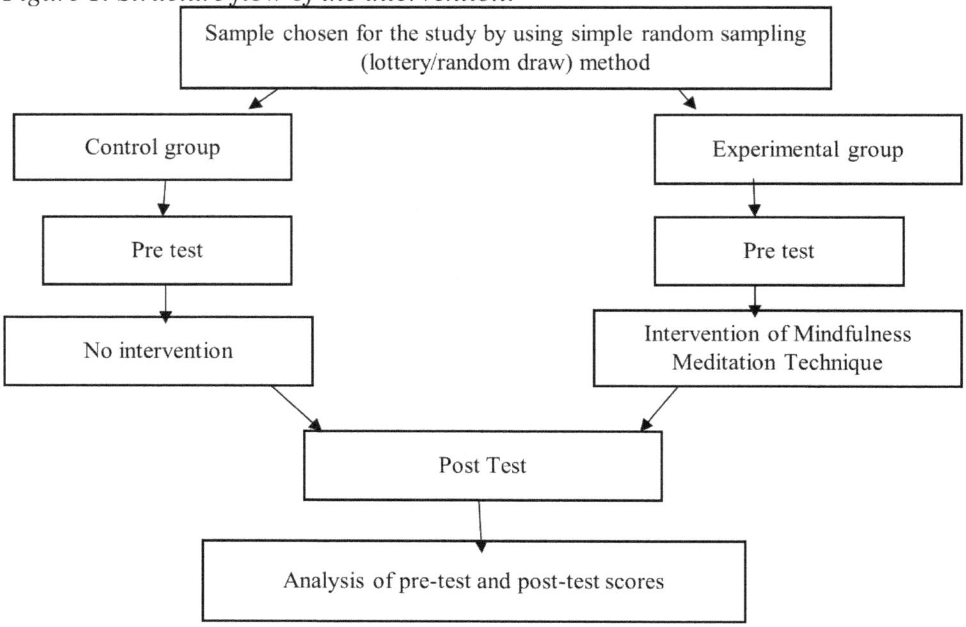

5.3 Procedure

It was essential to convey the scientific, secular, and universal nature of this mindfulness meditation intervention to secure support from school administration, teachers, parents, and students. The implementation of the study followed a structured sequence designed to ensure consistency and participant engagement.

The intervention included the following components:

- Pre-intervention orientation sessions introducing the practice and its relevance
- Individual interaction sessions to establish rapport and baseline understanding
- Weekly guided sessions (45-60 minutes each) focusing on progressive development of mindfulness meditation
- Daily formal practice of Anapana mindfulness meditation (10 minutes each time, twice a day) within the school
- Home-based daily practice assignments supported by audio guidance and self-assessment sheets
- Informal mindfulness meditation practice integrated into routine activities such as eating, walking, lying down, feeling the touch of the body, listening to sounds, and so on (to encourage mindfulness in every moment of life)

- Weekly group discussions and individual dialogue and inquiry regarding the home practice to address challenges and support practice continuity (conversations regarding strengthening the practice, hindrances, and tips to overcome the hurdles based on self-regulatory skills and realization of the experience of mindfulness)
- Post-intervention sessions and individual reflections to capture experiential understanding

All sessions were facilitated using standardized audio instructions aligned with the Anapana meditation practice tradition as taught by Goenka, adapted appropriately for school-aged learners.

Students in the experimental group maintained daily practice logs to record duration and subjective observations. The inclusion of both structured (at school) and informal (at home) practice aimed to support the transfer of mindfulness from formal sessions to everyday activities. The control group followed the regular school routine over the eight weeks, with no exposure to any mindfulness instructions.

5.4 Measurement Tools

Three validated measurement tools were used in this study to analyze the outcomes.

Anapana Mindfulness Meditation Technique (Independent variable):

A ten-minute MP3 audio copy of Anapana meditation instructions of Goenka was used in this study as the intervention tool (the independent variable). [Researchers Dhar (2006) and Dhiman (2020) have used the same tool for the variable in their studies.]

Sustained Attention (dependent variable-1):

The clock test of Psychology Experiment Building Language (PEBL), developed by Mueller & Piper, is being used in this study to get sustained attention scores of the sample. In this computer-administered task, a clock point moves around a display and occasionally skips a position; participants have to respond whenever a skip occurs. The task requires continuous mindfulness throughout the monitoring period. It is a well-established measure for sustained attention in research contexts (Hwang et al., 2016; Mueller & Piper, 2014). Higher scores indicate improved sustained attention.

Academic Self-Regulation (dependent variable-2):

The Academic Self-Regulation Questionnaire-A (Ryan & Connell, 1989) was used in this study to obtain the academic self-regulation scores of the sample (N=60). The questionnaire consists of everyday academic behavior scenarios and asks students to rate four types of reasons for their behavior. The resulting higher scores indicate more internally motivated, self-regulated academic engagement. This questionnaire has been validated across diverse student populations and used in mindfulness-based self-regulation research studies (Hosseini et al., 2019).

Academic Performance (dependent variable-3):

Cumulative scores of students were obtained from official school records. (Marks on schoolquarterly examinations across six subjects—First Language (Telugu), Second Language (Hindi), English, Mathematics, Science, and Social Studies). Academic performance was assessed using the summative formative tests conducted with equivalent blueprints and weightings.

6. RESULTS AND DISCUSSION WITH STATISTICAL INTERPRETATION

Descriptive and inferential statistical analyses were conducted to examine the effect of Anapana mindfulness intervention on sustained attention, academic self-regulation, and academic performance. All statistical analyses were based on post-test minus pre-test differences.

Table 1. Pre-test and Post-test Statistics for Group and Variable

Variable/Instrument	Group	Time	N	M	SD	Min	Max	Skew	Kurt
Sustained Attention (Clock Test, PEBL)	Experimental	Pre-test	30	406.35	79.71	189.58	532.67	−0.69	0.23
		Post-test	30	427.01	33.78	327.73	486.33	−0.88	1.03
	Control	Pre-test	30	412.71	79.41	214.00	552.14	−0.99	0.55
		Post-test	30	378.43	23.72	317.71	424.18	−0.08	0.09
Academic Self-Regulation (ASRQ-A)	Experimental	Pre-test	30	106.90	11.39	80.00	125.00	−0.19	−0.65
		Post-test	30	108.77	10.30	88.00	125.00	0.06	−1.14
	Control	Pre-test	30	97.87	10.59	78.00	125.00	0.29	−0.15
		Post-test	30	99.20	8.83	85.00	120.00	0.29	−0.43

continued on following page

Table 1. Continued

Variable/Instrument	Group	Time	N	M	SD	Min	Max	Skew	Kurt
Academic Performance (Exam scores)	Experimental	Pre-test	30	106.27	14.06	78.00	127.00	−0.04	−0.99
		Post-test	30	111.73	14.04	80.00	135.00	−0.13	−0.78
	Control	Pre-test	30	108.77	11.71	78.00	128.00	−0.42	−0.07
		Post-test	30	108.83	10.19	80.00	125.00	−0.59	0.26

Note: Academic self-regulation was measured via ASRQ-A(Ryan & Connell, 1989); higher scores reflect greater academic self-regulation. Academic performance = Formative examination scores across six subjects.

Table 1 represents the number of samples, means, standard deviations, minimum value, maximum value, skewness, and kurtosis for each condition.

Several patterns in Table 1 are observable. The experimental group's post-test means on academic self-regulation and academic performance exceeded their pre-test means. While the control group's sustained attention scores showed a pre-to-post decline (412.71 → 378.43), consistent with an absence of attentional training rather than genuine cognitive weakening. Preliminary support for distributional normality can be seen in the skewness and kurtosis values, which fell within ±1.5 and ±2.0, respectively.

Figure 2. Pre-Post Scores for Sustained Attention

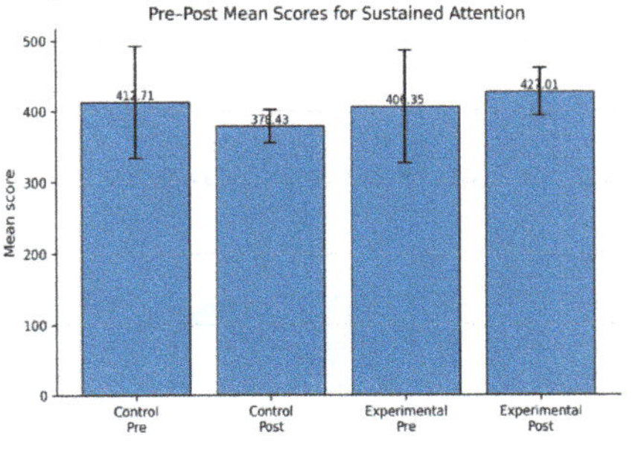

Figure 3. Pre-Post Scores for Academic Self-Regulation

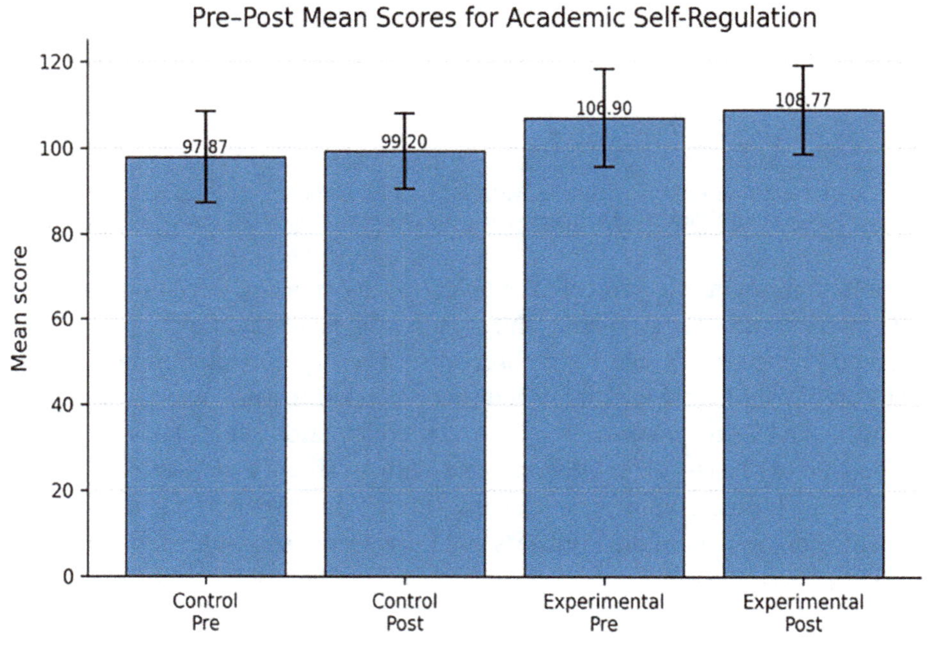

Figure 4. Pre-Post Scores for Academic Performance

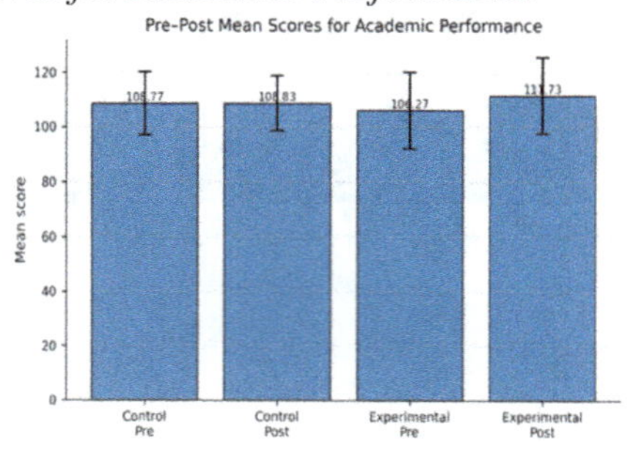

Figures 2-4 visually represent the pre-test and post-test mean differences across sustained attention, academic self-regulation, and academic performance for the control group and experimental group.

Table 2. Descriptive Statistics: Pre-test and Post-test Means and Standard Deviations by Group

Variable / Instrument	Group	Pre-test M (SD)	Post-test M (SD)	Change (Post – Pre)
Sustained Attention (PEBL Clock Test)	Experimental (n=30)	406.35 (79.71)	427.01 (33.78)	+20.66
	Control (n=30)	412.71 (79.41)	378.43 (23.72)	–34.28
Academic Self-Regulation (ASRQ-A)	Experimental (n=30)	106.90 (11.39)	108.77 (10.30)	+1.87
	Control (n=30)	97.87 (10.59)	99.20 (8.83)	+1.33
Academic Performance (Exam scores)	Experimental (n=30)	106.27 (14.06)	111.73 (14.04)	+5.47
	Control (n=30)	108.77 (11.71)	108.83 (10.19)	+0.07

Note: M = Mean; SD = Standard Deviation. Change = Post-test mean minus Pre-test mean.

Several patterns in Table 2 are noticeable. The experimental group improved on all three outcomes, while the control group showed only marginal improvement on academic self-regulation and decline on sustained attention. The most prominent difference is in academic performance: the experimental group gained an average of 5.47 marks, while the control group gained essentially nothing (0.07 marks). It is also worth noting that the experimental group's sustained attention scores became much more consistent after the program.

The Standard Deviation (SD) has fallen from 79.71 to 33.78, a compression of nearly sixty percent. It means that students who had divergent levels of attention before the intervention ended up much more similar to each other.

Table 3. Paired-Sample t-Test Results

Variable (Instrument)	Group	Pre M (SD)	Post M (SD)	Mean Change Post-test minus Pre-test	t (df)	p	Cohen's d	95% CI
Sustained Attention (PEBL Clock Test)	Experimental (n=30)	406.35 (79.71)	427.01 (33.78)	+20.66	–1.286 (29)	.209	0.235	[–12.20, 53.52]
	Control (n=30)	412.71 (79.41)	378.43 (23.72)	–34.28	2.445 (29)	.021	–0.446	[–62.95, –5.61]
Academic Self-Regulation (ASRQ-A)	Experimental (n=30)	106.90 (11.39)	108.77 (10.30)	+1.87	–4.504 (29)	< .001	0.822	[1.02, 2.71]
	Control (n=30)	97.87 (10.59)	99.20 (8.83)	+1.33	–2.210 (29)	.035	0.404	[0.10, 2.57]

continued on following page

Table 3. Continued

Variable (Instrument)	Group	Pre M (SD)	Post M (SD)	Mean Change Post-test minus Pre-test	t (df)	p	Cohen's d	95% CI
Academic Performance (Exam scores)	Experimental (n=30)	106.27 (14.06)	111.73 (14.04)	+5.47	−6.079 (29)	< .001	1.110	[3.63, 7.31]
	Control (n=30)	108.77 (11.71)	108.83 (10.19)	+0.07	−0.111 (29)	.912	0.020	[−1.16, 1.29]

Note: 1. Negative t-values for the experimental group indicate pre-test scores are lower than post-test scores (i.e., positive enhancement). 2. Mean change represents post-test minus pre-test scores: 3. The statistical significance is interpreted based on confidence intervals and p-values.

Table 3 presents the paired-sample t-test scores, providing a comprehensive description of pre–post changes among the three variables, with full statistical data reporting p-values, confidence intervals, and effect sizes.

Sustained attention: A positive mean change (M = +20.82) in the experimental group represents a positive development gained by practicing meditation intervention. This change [t(29) = -1.29, p = 0.204, with a small effect size (Cohen's d = 0.23)] was not statistically significant. The 95% confidence interval for the mean difference is [-12.1, 53.8], suggesting that the improvement noticed may not represent a reliable effect.

Academic self-regulation: The experimental group showed a significant statistical improvement (M = +1.87), $t(29) = -4.50$, $p < .001$, with a large effect size ($d = 0.82$). The 95% confidence interval for the mean difference [0.41, 1.22] confirms the reliability of this improvement.

Academic performance: the experimental group showed a substantial statistical enhancement (M = +5.47), $t(29) = -6.08$, $p < .001$, with a very large effect size ($d = 1.11$). The confidence interval [0.65, 1.56] confirms a strongly significant effect.

Overall, the results yielded robust improvements in academic self-regulation and academic performance, as evidenced by statistically significant p-values, confidence intervals excluding zero, and large effect sizes.

Figure 5. Mean post-test minus pre-test change scores across three variables with 95% Confidence Intervals.

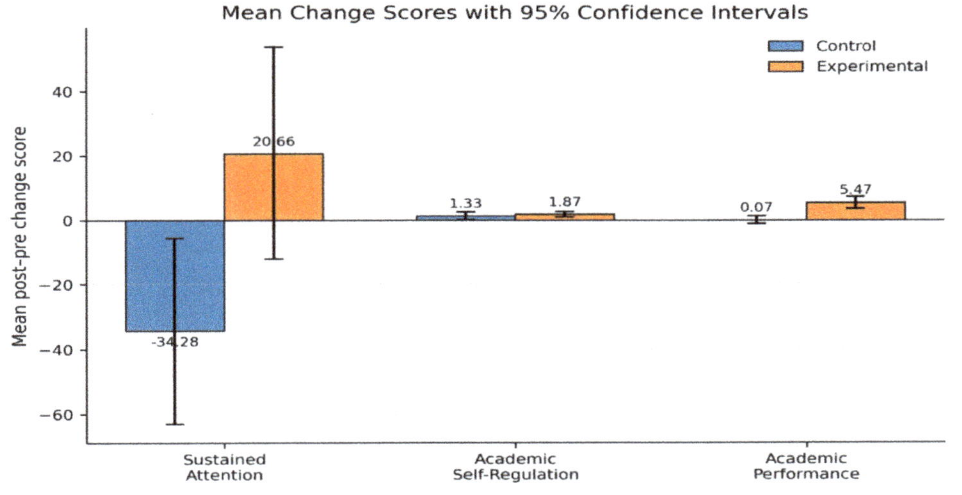

Figure 5 indicates that the experimental group demonstrated improvement in post-test scores across all three variable outcomes. The strongest change observed was for academic performance.

Table 4. Summary of Paired Sample t-test Statistical Results

Analysis	Variable	Key Result	p	Effect Size	Practical Significance
Paired t-test (Experimental)	Sustained Attention	t(29) = −1.286; Gain = +20.66	.209	d = 0.235 (small)	Score spread halved; attentional normalization observed
	Self-Regulation	t(29) = −4.504; Gain = +1.87	< .001	d = 0.822 (large)	Large meaningful gain; autonomous motivation increased
	Academic Performance	t(29) = −6.079; Gain = +5.47	< .001	d = 1.110 (very large)	~5.5 mark average gain on examination scores

continued on following page

Table 4. Continued

Analysis	Variable	Key Result	p	Effect Size	Practical Significance
Paired t-test (Control)	Sustained Attention	t(29) = 2.445; Gain = −34.28	.021	d = −0.446	Moderate decline; no training effect
	Self-Regulation	t(29) = −2.210; Gain = +1.33	.035	d = 0.404	Does not survive Bonferroni correction
	Academic Performance	t(29) = −0.111; Gain = +0.07	.912	d = 0.020	Effectively zero change

Table 4 presents the paired-sample t-test results, whether each group's scores changed significantly from pre-test to post-test.

Figure 6. Magnitude of Pre-Post Change of dependent variables by outcome

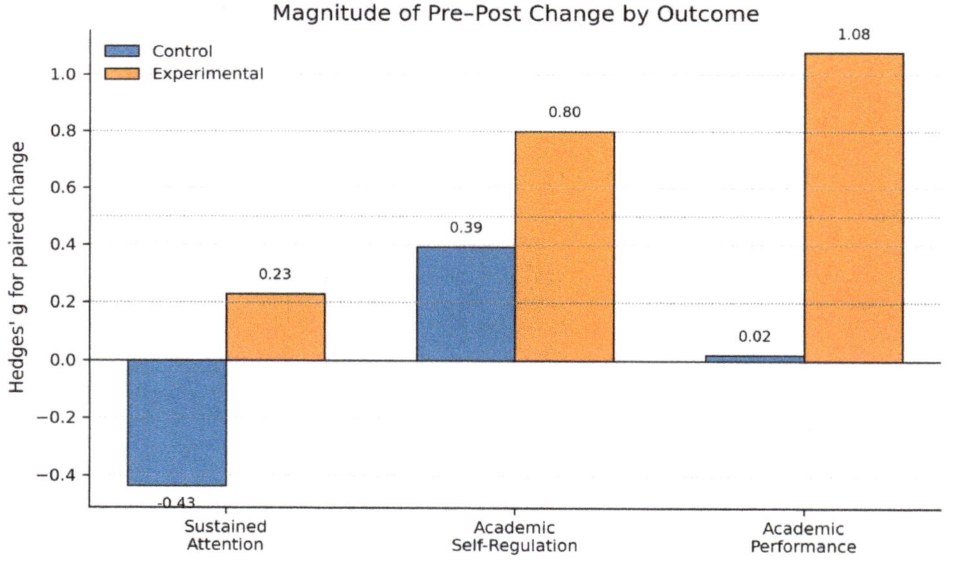

When examined collectively, Figure 6 indicates the intervention-related change was small for sustained attention, large for academic self-regulation, and larger for academic performance in the experimental group.

Sustained Attention (PEBL Clock Test score-based)

The experimental group's average Sustained Attention score increased by 20.66 points, but this increase was not statistically significant at the corrected threshold ($t(29) = -1.286, p = .209, d = 0.235$). However, before the program, the experimental group's attention scores ranged very widely—from as low as 189.58 to as high as 532.67, with a standard deviation of 79.71. After the program, scores ranged from 327.73 to 486.33, with a standard deviation of only 33.78. The spread of scores had compressed by 58%. Even more striking is that the pre-test and post-test scores for sustained attention were essentially uncorrelated in the experimental group ($r = -.046$, $p = .808$, confirmed from SPSS Paired Samples Correlations output).

In most educational measurements, a student who starts high tends to finish high, and a student who starts low tends to finish low. Here, that was not the case: where a student began told us almost nothing about where they ended up after eight weeks of Anapana practice. Students who already had strong attention maintained it, and students who showed low sustained attention at the beginning of the intervention improved significantly. The program appeared to bring everyone toward a more consistent, constant level of attentional sustainability—what neuroscientists call a normalization effect, consistent with Britta K Hölzel et al. (2011).

The control group's sustained attention actually declined by an average of 34.28 points ($t(29) = 2.445, p = .021, d = -0.446$), a moderate negative change that likely reflects the absence of attentional training and possibly a regression-to-the-mean effect from the group's slightly elevated pre-test mean.

Academic Self-Regulation (ASRQ-A, score-based)

The experimental group showed a statistically significant and practically large improvement in academic self-regulation from pre-test ($M = 106.90$) to post-test ($M = 108.77$), a mean gain of 1.87 points: $t(29) = -4.504$, $p < .001$, Cohen's $d = 0.822$, 95% CI [1.02, 2.71]. A Cohen's d of 0.822 is a large effect—it means the average experimental group student improved more than eight-tenths of a standard deviation from their starting point. The pre-post correlation was $r = .983$, confirming that this was a genuine within-person improvement rather than measurement noise: students who started higher in self-regulation tended to remain higher, but the whole distribution shifted upward. This pattern is consistent with Zimmerman's (1994) self-regulated learning model, which predicts metacognitive monitoring skills cultivated through repeated meditative self-observation generalize to more deliberate, autonomously motivated academic engagement.

The control group also showed a small increase in self-regulation (+1.33 points, $t(29) = -2.210, p = .035, d = 0.404$), but this did not survive Bonferroni correction (as in Table 4), and is more plausibly attributed to natural developmental progression or test familiarity than to any treatment effect.

The experimental group's gain was both larger and more statistically robust.

Academic Performance (Formative Examination Scores)

The most dramatically significant finding in the study was the experimental group's improvement in academic performance. Students who practiced Anapana for eight weeks improved their examination scores by an average of 5.47 marks—from 106.27 to 111.73—and this improvement was highly consistent across the group: $t(29) = -6.079$, $p < .001$, Cohen's $d = 1.110$, 95% CI [3.63, 7.31]. A Cohen's d above 1.0 is considered very large—the average gain was more than a full standard deviation of the change-score distribution.

By contrast, the control group's average performance was essentially unchanged over the same period: from 108.77 to 108.83, a gain of just 0.07 marks ($t(29) = -0.111$, $p = .912$, $d = 0.020$). This near-zero effect in the control group means that over eight weeks of normal schooling, without any mindfulness program, examination scores stayed flat.

The experimental group's improvement of 5.47 marks against this flat backdrop is therefore attributable to the intervention rather than to the passage of time or continued learning.

7. FINAL SUMMARY OF FINDINGS

The results indicate that the Anapana mindfulness meditation intervention produced:

- A non-significant but structurally meaningful improvement in sustained attention, characterized by reduced variability and attentional normalization.
- A statistically significant and practically large improvement in academic self-regulation.
- A statistically significant and very large improvement in academic performance

Taken together, these findings provide empirical support for the effectiveness of the intervention in enhancing sustained attention, academic self-regulation, and academic outcomes among middle school students.

The results reveal a clear pattern. The experimental group demonstrated consistent improvements across all variables, with statistically significant improvements in academic self-regulation and academic performance, and a meaningful, though statistically not significant, improvement in sustained attention.

The absence of comparable improvement in the control group strengthens the inference that the observed changes are attributable to the intervention rather than to external factors such as time or routine academic exposure.

Importantly, the findings suggest an interconnected effect: improvements in self-regulation and academic performance appear alongside changes in attentional patterns. This supports the theoretical proposition that these three key variables do not operate independently but influence one another within the learning processes.

8. LIMITATIONS AND FUTURE RESEARCH

Several limitations must be acknowledged when contextualizing the findings from the research, though the present study offers significant insights into the role of Anapana mindfulness meditation in enhancing sustained attention, academic self-regulation, and academic performance.

8.1 Limitations

- The first limitation concerns the sample characteristics. The sample size (N=60) is relatively small, drawn from a single institutional setting. Although the size was adequate for statistical analysis, it may not fully capture the diversity of the population across different cultural and socioeconomic variations in student backgrounds and learning environments. These components could influence receptiveness to the intervention.
- The second limitation concerns the measurement of the variables. They may not fully address the complex factors in real-world educational settings, though the standardized tools were used to assess these key variables. In addition to this, the dependency on self-reporting measures of academic self-regulation may introduce the possibility of response bias, such as students overestimating or underestimating their abilities.
- The third limitation concerns the period of the intervention. This kind of mindfulness meditation practice requires consistency in practice to yield stable cognitive and behavioral changes. The intervention period of eight weeks may be insufficient to strengthen the significance.
- Artificial Intelligence (AI) tools were not implemented in the present study, although the conceptual framework mentioned their potential relevance.

The findings of the study offer strong support for the inclusion of mindfulness practices in school settings due to the significant improvements observed in the variables.

8.2 Future research

This study opens a promising scope for future investigations, such as AI-driven learning analytics, biofeedback technologies, and adaptive intervention models, which could be integrated. For example, integrating AI-based attention tracking systems or wearable devices could provide continuous and objective data, while machine learning tools could support the personalization of mindfulness practices.

9. IMPLICATIONS FOR PRACTICE AND POLICY

For Teachers: Teachers can integrate these ten-minute Anapana sessions into the beginning and ending of the school day with minimal disruption to the academic timetable and without any specialized equipment. A single one-day orientation training is sufficient to equip a teacher with the facilitation skills needed to deliver the program with high fidelity. Teachers may additionally draw clear connections during the study, asking reflective questions such as, 'When you noticed your mind wandering during the practice, what did you do? How might you use that same awareness when your mind wanders during reading?'

For School Leaders and Policy Makers: The National Education Policy 2020 (NEP 2020) of India and the National Curriculum Framework (NCERT, 2007) both emphasize holistic student development that goes beyond content knowledge. The present findings provide school-level experimental evidence that Anapana mindfulness meditation can contribute meaningfully to the cognitive and academic dimensions of that holistic development—and can do so inexpensively.

For international policymakers: The evidence from this and comparable studies supports the case for incorporating simple, culturally appropriate contemplative practices into school mental health and academic support frameworks, in line with the United Nations Sustainable Development Goal 4.7 (quality education for well-being) (SDG, 2018).

For researchers, this study's quasi-experimental design is rigorous compared to descriptive or pre-post-only approaches. Future research should prioritize cluster-randomized controlled trials with multiple schools per condition, larger samples, and longitudinal follow-up of at least six months to assess the durability of gains.

10. CONFLICT OF INTEREST STATEMENT

The authors declare no conflict of interest with respect to the research design, conduct, data collection, analysis, or reporting presented in this chapter. The Anapana mindfulness meditation technique used as the independent variable is a publicly available, freely accessible practice distributed at no cost by the Vipassana Research Institute (Dhamma Giri, Igatpuri, India). The standardized ten-minute instructional audio used from S. N. Goenka's Anapana instructions for children (Goenka, 2012a) is provided free of charge for educational and research purposes.

The author holds no financial interest in, receives no remuneration from, and has no organizational affiliation with any commercial mindfulness program, meditation center, pharmaceutical product, or educational technology company. The PEBL Clock Test (Mueller & Piper, 2014) and the Academic Self-Regulation Questionnaire-A (Ryan & Connell, 1989) are freely available research tools. The research was conducted under the academic supervision of the School of Education, CHRIST (Deemed to be University), Bengaluru, and received institutional research support only, with no external funding or commercial sponsorship. School examination data were obtained with written authorization from school authorities in Sangareddy district, Telangana, India, following institutional ethical review board approval. All participants provided written parental informed consent and student consent in accordance with institutional ethical protocols. The author affirms that the data reported in this chapter are authentic, derived from the actual study dataset, and have not been fabricated, falsified, selectively reported, or manipulated in any way.

11. CONCLUSION

Improvements were observed in sustained attention, academic self-regulation, and academic performance. Evidence gathered in this study is practically significant, which confirms the intervention as a genuine program to implement in educational settings. The intervention remains accessible, particularly within the socioeconomically disadvantaged school context. Anapana relies only on the guided instructions and the student's own breath. This mindfulness meditation intervention requires no additional resources once introduced.

These results matter as they are theoretically rational. The empirical findings align with the attention regulatory theory (Posner & Petersen, 1990; Y. Y. Tang et al., 2007) and self-regulated learning theory (Zimmerman, 2000). The results of this research indicate that the mindfulness meditation intervention is not only philosophically meaningful but also practically effective in classroom settings.

The conceptual understanding gained from this research indicated that artificial intelligence (AI) offers a powerful context for supporting and extending mindfulness practices in education without altering their core, essential nature. What remains is to extend this research to larger studies with increased sample sizes, longer durations, and more rigorous experimental designs integrated with AI-driven tools to strengthen the evidence base to support wider adoption across various educational settings.

A practical next step is pilot implementation in three or more schools with pre-registered analyses and AI-enabled measurement.

REFERENCES

Act, R. T. E. (2009). The Right of Children to Free and Compulsory Education Act 2009. *The Gazette of India*.

Aggarwal, J. C., & Agrawal, S. P. (1989). *National Policy on Education: Agenda for India 2001*. ERIC.

Arns, M., Clark, C. R., Trullinger, M., DeBeus, R., Mack, M., & Aniftos, M. (2020). Neurofeedback and attention-deficit/hyperactivity-disorder (ADHD) in children: Rating the evidence and proposed guidelines. *Applied Psychophysiology and Biofeedback*, *45*(2), 39–48. DOI: 10.1007/s10484-020-09455-2 PMID: 32206963

Baer, R. A. (2003). Mindfulness training as a clinical intervention: A conceptual and empirical review. *Clinical Psychology : a Publication of the Division of Clinical Psychology of the American Psychological Association*, *10*(2), 125–143. DOI: 10.1093/clipsy.bpg015

Bhatt, A., Watanabe, K., Santhosh, J., Dengel, A., & Ishimaru, S. (2025). ABCDE: Appearance-Based Confidence Detection by Evaluating Gaze Behavior Using Deep Learning. *International Journal of Activity and Behavior Computing*, *2025*(1), 1–24.

Boekaerts, M., Zeidner, M., & Pintrich, P. R. (1999). *Handbook of Self-Regulation*. Elsevier.

Bosch, B., DeJesus, M. A., Poulton, N. C., Zhang, W., Engelhart, C. A., Zaveri, A., Lavalette, S., Ruecker, N., Trujillo, C., Wallach, J. B., Li, S., Ehrt, S., Chait, B. T., Schnappinger, D., & Rock, J. M. (2021). Genome-wide gene expression tuning reveals diverse vulnerabilities of M. tuberculosis. *Cell*, *184*(17), 4579–4592. DOI: 10.1016/j.cell.2021.06.033 PMID: 34297925

Brown, K. W., & Ryan, R. M. (2003). The benefits of being present: Mindfulness and its role in psychological well-being. *Journal of Personality and Social Psychology*, *84*(4), 822–848. DOI: 10.1037/0022-3514.84.4.822 PMID: 12703651

Buddhaghosa, B. (2020). *The path of purification: Visuddhimagga*. Pariyatti.

Bussalb, A., Collin, S., Barthélemy, Q., Ojeda, D., Bioulac, S., Blasco-Fontecilla, H., Brandeis, D., Ouakil, D. P., Ros, T., & Mayaud, L. (2019). Is there a cluster of high theta-beta ratio patients in attention deficit hyperactivity disorder? *Clinical Neurophysiology : Official Journal of the International Federation of Clinical Neurophysiology*, *130*(8), 1387–1396. DOI: 10.1016/j.clinph.2019.02.021 PMID: 31176621

Carmody, J., & Baer, R. A. (2009). How long does a mindfulness-based stress reduction program need to be? A review of class contact hours and effect sizes for psychological distress. *Journal of Clinical Psychology*, *65*(6), 627–638. DOI: 10.1002/jclp.20555 PMID: 19309694

Chambers, R., Gullone, E., & Allen, N. B. (2009). Mindful emotion regulation: An integrative review. *Clinical Psychology Review*, *29*(6), 560–572. https://doi.org/https://doi.org/10.1016/j.cpr.2009.06.005. DOI: 10.1016/j.cpr.2009.06.005 PMID: 19632752

Creswell, J. D. (2017). Mindfulness interventions. *Annual Review of Psychology*, *68*(1), 491–516. DOI: 10.1146/annurev-psych-042716-051139 PMID: 27687118

Creswell, J. D., Myers, H. F., Cole, S. W., & Irwin, M. R. (2009). Mindfulness meditation training effects on CD4+ T lymphocytes in HIV-1 infected adults: A small randomized controlled trial. *Brain, Behavior, and Immunity*, *23*(2), 184–188. DOI: 10.1016/j.bbi.2008.07.004 PMID: 18678242

Denkova, E., Tardibuono, T. K., Zanesco, A. P., Sanchez Montenegro, C., Rooks, J. D., Rogers, S. L., & Jha, A. P. (2026). Evaluating Mindfulness Training as a Cognitive Performance Enhancement Tool: Insights from Two Pragmatic Cluster-Randomized Trials in an Elite Military Educational Setting. *Mindfulness*, *17*(4), 1–20. DOI: 10.1007/s12671-026-02786-x

Dhar, P. L. (2006). Insights from Modern Science into the Practice of "Insight Meditation." *Science and Spirituality in Modern India*, 230.

Dhiman, S. K. (2020). Doing Vipassana the Buddha's way: A seeker's immersion in mindfulness in life and leadership. In *The routledge companion to mindfulness at work* (pp. 585–603). Routledge.

Dunning, D. L., Griffiths, K., Kuyken, W., Crane, C., Foulkes, L., Parker, J., & Dalgleish, T. (2019a). Research Review: The effects of mindfulness-based interventions on cognition and mental health in children and adolescents–a meta-analysis of randomized controlled trials. *Journal of Child Psychology and Psychiatry, and Allied Disciplines*, *60*(3), 244–258. DOI: 10.1111/jcpp.12980 PMID: 30345511

Dunning, D. L., Griffiths, K., Kuyken, W., Crane, C., Foulkes, L., Parker, J., & Dalgleish, T. (2019b). Research Review: The effects of mindfulness-based interventions on cognition and mental health in children and adolescents–a meta-analysis of randomized controlled trials. *Journal of Child Psychology and Psychiatry, and Allied Disciplines*, *60*(3), 244–258. DOI: 10.1111/jcpp.12980 PMID: 30345511

Dutt, V. (n.d.). Organized by the Indian Knowledge System and Mental Health Applications (IKSMHA) Centre, IIT Mandi. *Workshop Page*, (469), 472.

Firth, A. M., Cavallini, I., Sütterlin, S., & Lugo, R. G. (2019). Mindfulness and self-efficacy in pain perception, stress and academic performance. The influence of mindfulness on cognitive processes. *Psychology Research and Behavior Management*, *12*, 565–574. DOI: 10.2147/PRBM.S206666 PMID: 31413648

Flook, L., Smalley, S. L., Kitil, M. J., Galla, B. M., Kaiser-Greenland, S., Locke, J., Ishijima, E., & Kasari, C. (2010). Effects of mindful awareness practices on executive functions in elementary school children. *Journal of Applied School Psychology*, *26*(1), 70–95. DOI: 10.1080/15377900903379125

Galindo-Aldana, G., Montoya-Rivera, L. A., Esqueda-Elizondo, J. J., Inzunza-Gonzalez, E., Garcia-Guerrero, E. E., Padilla-Lopez, A., Bautista, T. G., & Torres-González, C. (2025). Mindfulness-based intervention effects on EEG and executive functions: A systematic review. *Brain Sciences*, *15*(3), 324. DOI: 10.3390/brainsci15030324 PMID: 40149845

Gera, P. (2024). *Integrating Mindfulness: Enhancing Art and Design Student Well-being through AI Voice Assistants and Wearable Technology*. OCAD University.

Goenka, S. N. (2012a). *Discourse summaries*. Pariyatti Publishing.

Goenka, S. N. (2012b). *Meditation now: Inner peace through inner wisdom*. Pariyatti Publishing.

Grossman, P., Niemann, L., Schmidt, S., & Walach, H. (2004). Mindfulness-based stress reduction and health benefits: A meta-analysis. *Journal of Psychosomatic Research*, *57*(1), 35–43. https://doi.org/https://doi.org/10.1016/S0022-3999(03)00573-7. DOI: 10.1016/S0022-3999(03)00573-7 PMID: 15256293

Hart, W. (2011). *The art of living: Vipassana meditation as taught by SN Goenka*. Pariyatti.

Hofmann, S. G., Sawyer, A. T., Witt, A. A., & Oh, D. (2010). The effect of mindfulness-based therapy on anxiety and depression: A meta-analytic review. *Journal of Consulting and Clinical Psychology*, *78*(2), 169–183. DOI: 10.1037/a0018555 PMID: 20350028

Holmes, W. (2020). Artificial intelligence in education. In *Encyclopedia of education and information technologies* (pp. 88–103). Springer. DOI: 10.1007/978-3-030-10576-1_107

Hölzel, B. K., Carmody, J., Vangel, M., Congleton, C., Yerramsetti, S. M., Gard, T., & Lazar, S. W. (2011). Mindfulness practice leads to increases in regional brain gray matter density. *Psychiatry Research. Neuroimaging*, *191*(1), 36–43. https://doi .org/https://doi.org/10.1016/j.pscychresns.2010.08.006. DOI: 10.1016/j.pscychres-ns.2010.08.006 PMID: 21071182

Hölzel, B. K., Lazar, S. W., Gard, T., Schuman-Olivier, Z., Vago, D. R., & Ott, U. (2011). How Does Mindfulness Meditation Work? Proposing Mechanisms of Action From a Conceptual and Neural Perspective. *Perspectives on Psychological Science : A Journal of the Association for Psychological Science*, *6*(6), 537–559. DOI: 10.1177/1745691611419671 PMID: 26168376

Hosseini, M., Arefi, M., & Sajjadian, I. (2019). Effectiveness of Time-Perspective Training on Time-Balancing and Self-Regulation among Female Students. *International Journal of Behavioral Sciences*, *13*(3), 118–122.

Hwang, J., Castelli, D. M., & Gonzalez-Lima, F. (2016). Cognitive enhancement by transcranial laser stimulation and acute aerobic exercise. *Lasers in Medical Science*, *31*(6), 1151–1160. DOI: 10.1007/s10103-016-1962-3 PMID: 27220529

Jha, A. P., Krompinger, J., & Baime, M. J. (2007). Mindfulness training modifies subsystems of attention. *Cognitive, Affective & Behavioral Neuroscience*, *7*(2), 109–119. DOI: 10.3758/CABN.7.2.109 PMID: 17672382

Jon Kabat-Zin. (2003). *Mindfulness-Based Interventions in Context Past Present and Future -Clin Psych Sci Pract - 2006 - Kabat-Zinn -.pdf*.

Kabat-Zinn, J. (1982). An outpatient program in behavioral medicine for chronic pain patients based on the practice of mindfulness meditation: Theoretical considerations and preliminary results. *General Hospital Psychiatry*, *4*(1), 33–47. DOI: 10.1016/0163-8343(82)90026-3 PMID: 7042457

Kabat-Zinn, J. (2009). *Wherever you go, there you are: Mindfulness meditation in everyday life*. Hachette UK.

Kabat-Zinn, J. (2015). Mindfulness. *Mindfulness*, *6*(6), 1481–1483. DOI: 10.1007/s12671-015-0456-x

Kim, E., Moon, C. W., Kim, S., Ozkan, E., & Lomas, T. (2022). Mindfulness Intervention Courses in STEM Education: A Qualitative Assessment. In *Lecture Notes in Networks and Systems: 349 LNNS*. DOI: 10.1007/978-3-030-90677-1_16

Kuh, G. D., Kinzie, J. L., Buckley, J. A., Bridges, B. K., & Hayek, J. C. (2006). *What matters to student success: A review of the literature* (Vol. 8). National Post-secondary Education Cooperative Washington.

Lalanza, J. F., Lorente, S., Bullich, R., García, C., Losilla, J.-M., & Capdevila, L. (2023). Methods for heart rate variability biofeedback (HRVB): A systematic review and guidelines. *Applied Psychophysiology and Biofeedback*, *48*(3), 275–297. DOI: 10.1007/s10484-023-09582-6 PMID: 36917418

Lay, U. K. (2008). *Manual of Vipassana Meditation* (Third). Vipassana Research Institute, Dhamma Giri. https://www.vridhamma.org/

Lehrer, P. M., & Gevirtz, R. (2014). Heart rate variability biofeedback: How and why does it work? *Frontiers in Psychology*, *5*, 756. DOI: 10.3389/fpsyg.2014.00756 PMID: 25101026

Liew, J., Morris, A. S., & Kerr, K. L. (2023). *Emotion regulation processes as transdiagnostic in adolescence and early adulthood: A neurobioecological systems framework.*

Luckin, R., Holmes, W., & Forcier, L. B. (2018). *An argument for AI in education*. UCL Knowledge Lab. [Google Scholar]

Luxton, D. D. (2016). An introduction to artificial intelligence in behavioral and mental health care. In *Artificial intelligence in behavioral and mental health care* (pp. 1–26). Elsevier. DOI: 10.1016/B978-0-12-420248-1.00001-5

Mandinach, E. B., & Schildkamp, K. (2021). Misconceptions about data-based decision making in education: An exploration of the literature. *Studies in Educational Evaluation*, *69*, 100842. DOI: 10.1016/j.stueduc.2020.100842

Maynard, B. R., Solis, M. R., Miller, V. L., & Brendel, K. E. (2017). Mindfulness-based interventions for improving cognition, academic achievement, behavior, and socioemotional functioning of primary and secondary school students. *Campbell Systematic Reviews*, *13*(1), 1–144. DOI: 10.4073/CSR.2017.5

Meditation, T. W. (n.d.). *The Anapanasati Sutta: Sutta.*

Meiklejohn, J., Phillips, C., Freedman, M. L., Griffin, M. L., Biegel, G., Roach, A., Frank, J., Burke, C., Pinger, L., & Soloway, G. (2012). Integrating mindfulness training into K-12 education: Fostering the resilience of teachers and students. *Mindfulness*, *3*(4), 291–307.

Miller, J. J., Fletcher, K., & Kabat-Zinn, J. (1995). Three-year follow-up and clinical implications of a mindfulness meditation-based stress reduction intervention in the treatment of anxiety disorders. *General Hospital Psychiatry*, *17*(3), 192–200. DOI: 10.1016/0163-8343(95)00025-M PMID: 7649463

Misra, G. (2017). Effects of Mindfulness Meditation on Self-Compassion and Self-Construal among Adolescents. *Journal of Child and Family Studies*, *26*(7), 1984–1994. DOI: 10.1007/s10826-017-0736-5

Mitsea, E., Drigas, A., & Skianis, C. (2024). Artificial intelligence, immersive technologies, and neurotechnologies in breathing interventions for mental and emotional health: A systematic review. *Electronics (Basel)*, *13*(12), 2253. DOI: 10.3390/electronics13122253

Montessori, M. (n.d.). *The Absorbent Mind: i* (Number May 1949).

Mrazek, M. D., Zedelius, C. M., Gross, M. E., Mrazek, A. J., Phillips, D. T., & Schooler, J. W. (2017). Mindfulness in education: Enhancing academic achievement and student well-being by reducing mind-wandering. In *Mindfulness in social psychology* (pp. 139–152). Routledge. DOI: 10.4324/9781315627700-10

Mueller, S. T., & Piper, B. J. (2014). The Psychology Experiment Building Language (PEBL) and PEBL Test Battery. *Journal of Neuroscience Methods*, *222*, 250–259. https://doi.org/https://doi.org/10.1016/j.jneumeth.2013.10.024. DOI: 10.1016/j.jneumeth.2013.10.024 PMID: 24269254

Napoli, M., Krech, P. R., & Holley, L. C. (2005). Mindfulness Training for Elementary School Students. *Journal of Applied School Psychology*, *21*(1), 99–125. DOI: 10.1300/J370v21n01_05

NCERT, T. (2007). *National curriculum framework 2005*.

Nota, L., Soresi, S., & Zimmerman, B. J. (2004). Self-regulation and academic achievement and resilience: A longitudinal study. *International Journal of Educational Research*, *41*(3), 198–215. DOI: 10.1016/j.ijer.2005.07.001

Patarathipakorn, O., Pawa, K. K., Sritipsukho, P., Tansuhaj, K., Bhamarapravatana, K., & Suwannarurk, K. (2025). Aanapanasati Meditation and Stress Reduction Among Health Science University Students. *The Open Public Health Journal*, *18*(1), e18749445380247. DOI: 10.2174/0118749445380247250225075656

Posner, M. I., & Petersen, S. E. (1990). The attention system of the human brain. *Annual Review of Neuroscience*, *13*(1), 25–42. DOI: 10.1146/annurev.ne.13.030190.000325 PMID: 2183676

Pradhan, S., & Bhutia, Y. (2025). Impact of Anapanasati meditation on well-being of secondary school students in Teesta, Kalimpong District, West Bengal. *Int J Psychiatr Res*, *8*(4), 1–10. DOI: 10.33425/2641-4317.1225

Rosen, L. D., Lim, A. F., Felt, J., Carrier, L. M., Cheever, N. A., Lara-Ruiz, J. M., Mendoza, J. S., & Rokkum, J. (2014). Media and technology use predicts ill-being among children, preteens and teenagers independent of the negative health impacts of exercise and eating habits. *Computers in Human Behavior*, *35*, 364–375. DOI: 10.1016/j.chb.2014.01.036 PMID: 25717216

Ryan, R., & Connell, J. (1989). Academic Self-Regulation Questionnaire (SRQ-A). *Journal of Personality and Social Psychology*, *4*(1), 88–100.

Schunk, D. H., & Greene, J. A. (2017). Historical, contemporary, and future perspectives on self-regulated learning and performance. In *Handbook of self-regulation of learning and performance* (pp. 1–15). Routledge. DOI: 10.4324/9781315697048-1

SDG. U. N. (2018). Sustainable development goals. *United Nations*.

Segal, Z. V., Teasdale, J. D., Williams, J. M., & Gemar, M. C. (2002). The mindfulness-based cognitive therapy adherence scale: Inter-rater reliability, adherence to protocol and treatment distinctiveness. *Clinical Psychology & Psychotherapy*, *9*(2), 131–138. DOI: 10.1002/cpp.320

Siegel, R. D., & Germer, C. K. O. A. (2009). Mindfulness: What Is It? Where Did It Come From? In *Clinical Handbook of Mindfulness*.

Siemens, G. (2013). Learning analytics: The emergence of a discipline. *The American Behavioral Scientist*, *57*(10), 1380–1400. DOI: 10.1177/0002764213498851

Singhal, P. (2012). Continuous and comprehensive evaluation: A study of teachers' perception. *Delhi Business Review*, *13*(1), 81–99. DOI: 10.51768/dbr.v13i1.131201207

Suldo, S., Thalji, A., & Ferron, J. (2011). Longitudinal academic outcomes predicted by early adolescents' subjective well-being, psychopathology, and mental health status yielded from a dual factor model. *The Journal of Positive Psychology*, *6*(1), 17–30. DOI: 10.1080/17439760.2010.536774

Tang, Y.-Y., Hölzel, B. K., & Posner, M. I. (2015). The neuroscience of mindfulness meditation. *Nature Reviews. Neuroscience*, *16*(4), 213–225. DOI: 10.1038/nrn3916 PMID: 25783612

Tang, Y. Y., Ma, Y., Wang, J., Fan, Y., Feng, S., Lu, Q., Yu, Q., Sui, D., Rothbart, M. K., Fan, M., & Posner, M. I. (2007). Short-term meditation training improves attention and self-regulation. *Proceedings of the National Academy of Sciences of the United States of America*, *104*(43), 17152–17156. DOI: 10.1073/pnas.0707678104 PMID: 17940025

Teper, R., Segal, Z. V., & Inzlicht, M. (2013). Inside the Mindful Mind: How Mindfulness Enhances Emotion Regulation Through Improvements in Executive Control. *Current Directions in Psychological Science*, *22*(6), 449–454. DOI: 10.1177/0963721413495869

Thera, N. (1962). *The Heart of Buddhist Meditation (pp. 7Y113)*. Samuel Weiser.

VanLehn, K. (2011). The relative effectiveness of human tutoring, intelligent tutoring systems, and other tutoring systems. *Educational Psychologist*, *46*(4), 197–221. DOI: 10.1080/00461520.2011.611369

Vyas, M. V. (1975). *The Bhagavad Gita*. Maharshi Ved vyas.

Winne, P. H., & Hadwin, A. F. (2013). nStudy: Tracing and supporting self-regulated learning in the Internet. In *International handbook of metacognition and learning technologies* (pp. 293–308). Springer.

Xie, Y., Zhao, B., Dai, M., Zhou, J.-P., Sun, Y., Tan, T., Xie, W., Shen, L., & Yu, Z. (2025). Physllm: Harnessing large language models for cross-modal remote physiological sensing. *ArXiv Preprint ArXiv:2505.03621*.

Zawacki-Richter, O., Marín, V. I., Bond, M., & Gouverneur, F. (2019). Systematic review of research on artificial intelligence applications in higher education–where are the educators? *International Journal of Educational Technology in Higher Education*, *16*(1), 39. DOI: 10.1186/s41239-019-0171-0

Zenner, C., Herrnleben-Kurz, S., & Walach, H. (2014). Mindfulness-based interventions in schools-A systematic review and meta-analysis. *Frontiers in Psychology*, *5*(JUN). DOI: 10.3389/fpsyg.2014.00603 PMID: 25071620

Zimmerman, B. J. (1994). Dimensions of academic self-regulation: A conceptual framework for education. *Self-Regulation of Learning and Performance: Issues and Educational Applications*, *1*, 21–33.

Zimmerman, B. J. (2000). Attaining self-regulation: A social cognitive perspective. In *Handbook of self-regulation* (pp. 13–39). Elsevier. DOI: 10.1016/B978-012109890-2/50031-7

Zimmerman, B. J. (2002). Becoming a self-regulated learner: An overview. *Theory into Practice*, *41*(2), 64–70. DOI: 10.1207/s15430421tip4102_2

Zoefel, B., Huster, R. J., & Herrmann, C. S. (2011). Neurofeedback training of the upper alpha frequency band in EEG improves cognitive performance. *NeuroImage*, *54*(2), 1427–1431. DOI: 10.1016/j.neuroimage.2010.08.078 PMID: 20850552

Compilation of References

Abadi, M., Chu, A., Goodfellow, I., McMahan, H. B., Mironov, I., Talwar, K., & Zhang, L. (2016). Deep learning with differential privacy. *Proceedings of the 2016 ACM SIGSAC Conference on Computer and Communications Security* (pp. 308-318). ACM.

Act, R. T. E. (2009). The Right of Children to Free and Compulsory Education Act 2009. *The Gazette of India*.

Adeyemi, J. O. (2024). *Enhancing Elderly Wellness through AI-Powered Yoga and Exercise Support Systems*. https://www.researchsquare.com/article/rs-3809481/latest

Agarwal, V., Sharma, K., & Rajpoot, A. K. (2022). AI based Yoga Trainer-Simplifying home yoga using mediapipe and video streaming. *2022 3rd International Conference for Emerging Technology (INCET)*, 1–5. https://ieeexplore.ieee.org/abstract/document/9824332/

Aggarwal, J. C., & Agrawal, S. P. (1989). *National Policy on Education: Agenda for India 2001*. ERIC.

Agrawal, Y., Shah, Y., & Sharma, A. (2020, April 1). Implementation of Machine Learning Technique for Identification of Yoga Poses. DOI: 10.1109/CSNT48778.2020.9115758

Aksan, S. M. (2025). Ethics and morality from the perspective of eastern philosophy and theirimplications for modern life. *Kamara Journal*, *2*(2), 21–35. DOI: 10.62872/kj.v2i2.474

Alanezi, F. (2024). Assessing the Effectiveness of ChatGPT in Delivering Mental Health Support: A Qualitative Study. *Journal of Multidisciplinary Healthcare*, *17*, 461–471. DOI: 10.2147/JMDH.S447368

Al-Romeedy, B. S., & Singh, A. (2025). Reimagining Customer Relations Through AI Innovation. In Darwish, D., & Kumar, S. (Eds.), *Utilizing AI and Machine Learning in Financial Analysis* (pp. 351–368). IGI Global Scientific Publishing., DOI: 10.4018/979-8-3693-8507-4.ch019

Anderson, T., Thompson, L., & Davis, M. (2021). Digital competencies for yoga teachers: Training needs in the technology age. *Journal of Yoga Education, 15*(2), 87–103.

Ansari, A. I., & Singh, A. (2024). Growth and Opportunity of Medical Tourism in the Indian Healthcare Sector: A Critical Review. In Hassan, V., Albattat, A., & Basheer, S. (Eds.), *Impact of AI and Robotics on the Medical Tourism Industry* (pp. 290–301). IGI Global Scientific Publishing., DOI: 10.4018/979-8-3693-2248-2.ch013

Araujo, D., Couceiro, M., Seifert, L., Sarmento, H., & Davids, K. (2021). Artificial Intelligence in Sport Performance Analysis. New York: Routledge, 2020.: Routledge. DOI: 10.4324/9781003163589

Arin, H. (2023). *AI and the Human Experience: Embracing the Age of Intelligent Machines*. Holly Arin. https://books.google.com/books?hl=en&lr=&id=3QzkEAAAQBAJ&oi=fnd&pg=PA7&dq=AI+for+Community+Building+and+Human%E2%80%93AI+Collaboration+in+Yoga&ots=1XfC3ds9wG&sig=BEIWYVCuxhqpm8UCWUDC-OUOlBk

Arns, M., Clark, C. R., Trullinger, M., DeBeus, R., Mack, M., & Aniftos, M. (2020). Neurofeedback and attention-deficit/hyperactivity-disorder (ADHD) in children: Rating the evidence and proposed guidelines. *Applied Psychophysiology and Biofeedback, 45*(2), 39–48. DOI: 10.1007/s10484-020-09455-2 PMID: 32206963

Ashok, B. (2025). *Surendiran, and S. Babu, "Yoga pose estimation using MoveNet deep learning models* (Vol. 50). Sādhanā.

Askegaard, S., & Eckhardt, G. M. (2012). Glocal yoga: Re-appropriation in the Indian consumptionscape. *Marketing Theory, 12*(1), 45–60. DOI: 10.1177/1470593111424180

Atkinson, N. L., & Permuth-Levine, R. (2009). Benefits, barriers, and cues to action of yoga practice: A focus group approach. *American Journal of Health Behavior, 33*(1), 3–14. DOI: 10.5993/AJHB.33.1.1

Attila Biró, Antonio Ignacio Cuesta-Vargas, & László Szilágyi. (2024). AI-controlled training method for performance hardening or injury recovery in sports. DOI: 10.1109/SAMI60510.2024.10432911

Aturi, N. R. (2021). Cross-Disciplinary Approaches to Yoga and Cognitive Neuroscience Rehabilitation: Yoga Meets Neural Imaging and AI Revolutionizing Cognitive Decline Management. [IJIRMPS]. *Int. J. Innov. Res. Mod. Prob. Sol.*, *9*(6), 1–5.

Baer, R. A. (2003). Mindfulness training as a clinical intervention: A conceptual and empirical review. *Clinical Psychology : a Publication of the Division of Clinical Psychology of the American Psychological Association*, *10*(2), 125–143. DOI: 10.1093/clipsy.bpg015

Balpande, M., Sharma, J., Nair, A., Khandelwal, M., & Dhanray, S. (2023). AI Based Gym Trainer and Diet Recommendation System. *2023 IEEE 4th Annual Flagship India Council International Subsections Conference (INDISCON)*, 1–7. https://ieeexplore.ieee.org/abstract/document/10270066/

Banerjee, P., & Banerjee, S. (2025). Integrating Indian knowledge systems with artificial intelligence: A pathway to culturally rooted innovation. *Indian Knowledge System through the Ages: From Vedas to Modern Science*, 168.

Barbhuiya, S. (2025). Indian knowledge system (iks): Its implications in social life. DOI: 10.71097/IJSAT.v16.i3.8082

Basireddy, R., Reddy, K. R. S., & Pakkiraiah, Y. (2023). Complimentary and Supplementary Yoga in Sports. *International Journal for Multidisciplinary Research*, *5*(4), 5928. Advance online publication. DOI: 10.36948/ijfmr.2023.v05i04.5928

Becker, R. O. (1990). *Cross Currents*. Penguin Books.

Beirne, K., Rozanowska, M., & Votruba, M. (2017). Photostimulation of Mitochondria as a Treatment for Retinal Neurodegeneration. *Mitochondrion*, *36*, 85–95. DOI: 10.1016/j.mito.2017.05.002 PMID: 28499983

Belkhir, L., & Elmeligi, A. (2018). Assessing ICT global emissions footprint: Trends to 2040 & recommendations. *Journal of Cleaner Production*, *177*, 448–463. DOI: 10.1016/j.jclepro.2017.12.239

Bennett, J. P. (2019). Medical Hypothesis: Neurodegenerative Diseases Arise from Oxidative Damage to Electron Tunneling Proteins in Mitochondria. *Medical Hypotheses*, *127*, 1–4. DOI: 10.1016/j.mehy.2019.03.034 PMID: 31088629

Bharathi, S. T., Raj, F., Krishnan, R. S., Rajalakshmi, V., Kumar, V. V., & Anchitaalagammai, J. V. (2024). MentalHealthAI: Utilizing Deep Learning for Accurate Stress Level Prediction. 1705–1712. DOI: 10.1109/ICACRS62842.2024.10841747

Bhatt, A., Watanabe, K., Santhosh, J., Dengel, A., & Ishimaru, S. (2025). ABCDE: Appearance-Based Confidence Detection by Evaluating Gaze Behavior Using Deep Learning. *International Journal of Activity and Behavior Computing, 2025*(1), 1–24.

Bobade, P., & Vani, M. (2020). Stress Detection with Machine Learning and Deep Learning using Multimodal Physiological Data. *2020 Second International Conference on Inventive Research in Computing Applications (ICIRCA)*, 51–57. DOI: 10.1109/ICIRCA48905.2020.9183244

Boekaerts, M., Zeidner, M., & Pintrich, P. R. (1999). *Handbook of Self-Regulation*. Elsevier.

Bosch, B., DeJesus, M. A., Poulton, N. C., Zhang, W., Engelhart, C. A., Zaveri, A., Lavalette, S., Ruecker, N., Trujillo, C., Wallach, J. B., Li, S., Ehrt, S., Chait, B. T., Schnappinger, D., & Rock, J. M. (2021). Genome-wide gene expression tuning reveals diverse vulnerabilities of M. tuberculosis. *Cell, 184*(17), 4579–4592. DOI: 10.1016/j.cell.2021.06.033 PMID: 34297925

Braboszcz, C., Cahn, B. R., Levy, J., Fernandez, M., & Delorme, A. (2017). Increased Gamma Brainwave Amplitude Compared to Control in Three Different Meditation Traditions. *PLoS One, 12*(1), e0170647. DOI: 10.1371/journal.pone.0170647

Braveman, P. A., Kumanyika, S., Fielding, J., LaVeist, T., Borrell, L. N., Manderscheid, R., & Troutman, A. (2011). Health disparities and health equity: The issue is justice. *American Journal of Public Health, 101*(S1), S149–S155. DOI: 10.2105/AJPH.2010.300062

Brennan, B. A. (1988). *Hands of Light: A Guide to Healing Through the Human Energy Field*. Bantam.

Brennan, B. A. (1993). *Light Emerging: The Journey of Personal Healing*. Bantam.

Brown, K. W., & Ryan, R. M. (2003). The benefits of being present: Mindfulness and its role in psychological well-being. *Journal of Personality and Social Psychology, 84*(4), 822–848. DOI: 10.1037/0022-3514.84.4.822 PMID: 12703651

Brown, K., & Richards, P. (2022). The digital yoga instructor: Career transformations in wellness technology. *International Journal of Sport and Exercise Psychology, 18*(3), 234–251.

Brulle, R. J., & Pellow, D. N. (2006). Environmental justice: Human health and environmental inequalities. *Annual Review of Public Health, 27*(1), 103–124. DOI: 10.1146/annurev.publhealth.27.021405.102124

Bryant, E. F. (2009). *The Yoga Sutras of Patanjali: A new edition, translation, and commentary*. North Point Press.

Buçinca, Z., Swaroop, S., Paluch, A. E., Murphy, S. A., & Gajos, K. Z. (2024). *Towards Optimizing Human-Centric Objectives in AI-Assisted Decision-Making With Offline Reinforcement Learning* (arXiv:2403.05911). arXiv. https://doi.org// arXiv.2403.05911DOI: 10.48550

Buddhaghosa, B. (2020). *The path of purification: Visuddhimagga*. Pariyatti.

Bussalb, A., Collin, S., Barthélemy, Q., Ojeda, D., Bioulac, S., Blasco-Fontecilla, H., Brandeis, D., Ouakil, D. P., Ros, T., & Mayaud, L. (2019). Is there a cluster of high theta-beta ratio patients in attention deficit hyperactivity disorder? *Clinical Neurophysiology : Official Journal of the International Federation of Clinical Neurophysiology*, *130*(8), 1387–1396. DOI: 10.1016/j.clinph.2019.02.021 PMID: 31176621

Büssing, A., Michalsen, A., Khalsa, S. B. S., Telles, S., & Sherman, K. J. (2012). Effects of yoga on mental and physical health: A short summary of reviews. *Evidence-Based Complementary and Alternative Medicine : eCAM*, *2012*, 165410. DOI: 10.1155/2012/165410

Cahn, B. R., & Polich, J. (2006). States of meditation and traits of the meditator: EEG, ERP and neuroimaging studies. *Psychological Bulletin*, *132*(2), 180–211. DOI: 10.1037/0033-2909.132.2.180 PMID: 16536641

Campanelli, S., Tort, A. B. L., & Lobão-Soares, B. (2020). Pranayamas and Their Neurophysiological Effects. *International Journal of Yoga*, *13*(3), 183–192. DOI: 10.4103/ijoy.IJOY_91_19

Cao, Z., Hidalgo, G., Simon, T., Wei, S. E., & Sheikh, Y. (2021). OpenPose: Real-time multi-person 2D pose estimation using part affinity fields. *IEEE Transactions on Pattern Analysis and Machine Intelligence*, *43*(1), 172–186. DOI: 10.1109/ TPAMI.2019.2929257 PMID: 31331883

Cardone, D., & Merla, A. (2017). New Frontiers for Applications of Thermal Infrared Imaging Devices: Computational Psychopshysiology in the Neurosciences. *Sensors (Basel)*, *17*(5), 1042. DOI: 10.3390/s17051042

Carmody, J., & Baer, R. A. (2009). How long does a mindfulness-based stress reduction program need to be? A review of class contact hours and effect sizes for psychological distress. *Journal of Clinical Psychology*, *65*(6), 627–638. DOI: 10.1002/jclp.20555 PMID: 19309694

Cervellin, G., & Lippi, G. (2011). From Music-Beat to Heart-Beat: A Journey in the Complex Interactions Between Music, Brain and Heart. *European Journal of Internal Medicine*, *22*(4), 371–374. DOI: 10.1016/j.ejim.2011.02.019 PMID: 21767754

Chambers, R., Gullone, E., & Allen, N. B. (2009). Mindful emotion regulation: An integrative review. *Clinical Psychology Review*, *29*(6), 560–572. https://doi.org/https://doi.org/10.1016/j.cpr.2009.06.005. DOI: 10.1016/j.cpr.2009.06.005 PMID: 19632752

Chamola, V., Gummana, E. P., Madan, A., Rout, B. K., & Coelho Rodrigues, J. J. P. (2024). Advancements in yoga pose estimation using artificial intelligence: A survey. *Current Bioinformatics*, *19*(3), 264–280. DOI: 10.2174/1574893618666230508105440

Chanda, A. (2025). Religion and technology: Ethical implications of integrating artificial intelligence into religious practice and experience. *Indonesian Journal of Religion, Spirituality, and Humanity*, *4*(1), 25–54. DOI: 10.18326/ijoresh.v4i1.25-54

Chaturvedi, S. (2024). Human values from Indian philosophy to solve AI alignment problem. *International Journal for Multidisciplinary Research*, *6*(3), 22099. Advance online publication. DOI: 10.36948/ijfmr.2024.v06i03.22099

Chelishcheva, E. (2023). *Innovation in the Yoga and Ayurveda Industry: Exploring the role of technology and entrepreneurship*. https://www.theseus.fi/handle/10024/811266

Chen, I. Y., Joshi, S., Ghassemi, M., & Ranganath, R. (2023). "Probabilistic machine learning for healthcare," *npj Digital Medicine*, vol. 6.

Chen, K., & Chan, A. H. (2019). Gerontechnology acceptance by elderly: A systematic review. *Interdisciplinary Journal of Information, Knowledge, and Management*, *14*, 29–55.

Chen, R., Liu, Q., & Chen, Z. (2024). Research on Wearable Sensors Data Collection and Health Assessment based on Machine Learning. *Proceedings of the 2024 International Conference on Smart Healthcare and Wearable Intelligent Devices*, 227–231. DOI: 10.1145/3703847.3703885

Chen, Y., & Lin, C. (2020). Sustainability practices in digital wellness platforms: An exploratory study. *Journal of Sustainable Business*, *28*(4), 112–129.

Chhabra, G., Narayanan, A., Samantha, S., & Samanta, S. (2013). "Human Aura: A New Vedic Approach." *International Conference on Mechanical and Industrial Engineering*, 26 May 2013, New Delhi. ISBN 978-93-82208-95-2.

Chittineni, A., Kotagiri, Y. S., Kolli, M., Kollipara, T., Modepalli, J. R., & Namburi, S. K. (2023). A Real-Time Virtual Yoga Assistant Using Machine Learning. *2023 3rd International Conference on Smart Data Intelligence (ICSMDI)*, 316–321. https://ieeexplore.ieee.org/abstract/document/10127894/

Choudhury, K., ... (2025). "Steganography in the digital age: An in-depth review of techniques," in *ASCIS 2024*, CCIS, vol. 2424, Springer, Cham, DOI: 10.1007/978-3-031-86290-8_24

Conde, J., & Svantesson, D. J. B. (2024). The five generations of facial recognition usage and the Australian privacy law. *International Data Privacy Law*, *14*(3), 247–258. DOI: 10.1093/idpl/ipae007

Coroama, V. C., Hilty, L. M., & Birtel, M. (2013). Effects of Internet-based multiple-site conferences on greenhouse gas emissions. *Telematics and Informatics*, *30*(4), 362–374. DOI: 10.1016/j.tele.2011.11.006

Cramer, H. (2023). Artificial Intelligence, Complementary and Integrative Medicine: A Paradigm Shift in Health Care Delivery and Research? *Journal of Integrative and Complementary Medicine*, *29*(3), 131–133. DOI: 10.1089/jicm.2023.0040

Cramer, H., Lauche, R., Klose, P., Lange, S., Langhorst, J., & Dobos, G. J. (2017). Yoga for improving health-related quality of life, mental health and cancer-related symptoms in women diagnosed with breast cancer. *The Cochrane Library*, *2017*(1), CD010802. DOI: 10.1002/14651858.CD010802.pub2

Cramer, H., Lauche, R., Langhorst, J., & Dobos, G. (2013). Yoga for depression: A systematic review and meta-analysis. *Depression and Anxiety*, *30*(11), 1068–1083. DOI: 10.1002/da.22166

Cramer, H., Lauche, R., Langhorst, J., & Dobos, G. (2016). Is one yoga style better than another? A systematic review of associations of yoga style and conclusions in randomized yoga trials. *Complementary Therapies in Medicine*, *25*, 178–187. DOI: 10.1016/j.ctim.2016.02.015

Creswell, J. D. (2017). Mindfulness interventions. *Annual Review of Psychology*, *68*(1), 491–516. DOI: 10.1146/annurev-psych-042716-051139 PMID: 27687118

Creswell, J. D., Myers, H. F., Cole, S. W., & Irwin, M. R. (2009). Mindfulness meditation training effects on CD4+ T lymphocytes in HIV-1 infected adults: A small randomized controlled trial. *Brain, Behavior, and Immunity*, *23*(2), 184–188. DOI: 10.1016/j.bbi.2008.07.004 PMID: 18678242

Davies, R., & Mitchell, S. (2021). Content creation in the digital wellness economy: Skills, compensation, and career pathways. *Media Industries Journal*, *8*(2), 45–67.

Davis, F. D. (1989). Perceived usefulness, perceived ease of use, and user acceptance of information technology. *Management Information Systems Quarterly, 13*(3), 319–340. DOI: 10.2307/249008

de Carvalho-Guimarães, F. B., Correa, K. L., de Souza, T. P., Rodríguez Amado, J. R., Ribeiro-Costa, R. M., & Silva-Júnior, J. O. C. (2022). A Review of Pickering Emulsions: Perspectives and Applications. *Pharmaceuticals (Basel, Switzerland), 15*(11), 1413. DOI: 10.3390/ph15111413

de Goede, P., Wefers, J., Brombacher, E. C., Schrauwen, P., & Kalsbeek, A. (2018). Circadian Rhythms in Mitochondrial Respiration. *Journal of Molecular Endocrinology, 60*(3), R115–R130. DOI: 10.1530/JME-17-0196 PMID: 29378772

De Michelis, E. (2004). A history of modern yoga: Patanjali and Western esotericism. *Continuum.*

de Sousa, M. C., Caldas, I. L., Rizzato, F. B., Pakter, R., & Steffens, F. M. (2012). Controlling Chaos in Wave-Particle Interactions. *Physical Review E: Statistical, Nonlinear, and Soft Matter Physics, 86*(1 Pt 2), 016217. DOI: 10.1103/PhysRevE.86.016217 PMID: 23005517

Denkova, E., Tardibuono, T. K., Zanesco, A. P., Sanchez Montenegro, C., Rooks, J. D., Rogers, S. L., & Jha, A. P. (2026). Evaluating Mindfulness Training as a Cognitive Performance Enhancement Tool: Insights from Two Pragmatic Cluster-Randomized Trials in an Elite Military Educational Setting. *Mindfulness, 17*(4), 1–20. DOI: 10.1007/s12671-026-02786-x

Dey, D. N. C. (2024). Harmonizing The Threads of Well-Being: Ai (Artificial Intelligence), Spirituality, Healthcare, And Management. *Spirituality, Healthcare, And Management (April 24, 2024).* https://papers.ssrn.com/sol3/papers.cfm?abstract_id=5002655

Dhakate, H., Anasane, S., Shah, S., Thakare, R., & Rawat, S. G. (2024). Enhancing Yoga Practice: Real-time Pose Analysis and Personalized Feedback. *2024 International Conference on Emerging Systems and Intelligent Computing (ESIC)*, 35–40. https://ieeexplore.ieee.org/abstract/document/10481659/

Dhankhar, A., & Sharma, R. (2023). Evolution of Yoga. *International Journal of Physiology Nutrition and Physical Education, 8*(2), 510–513. DOI: 10.22271/journalofsport.2023.v8.i2g.2846

Dhar, P. L. (2006). Insights from Modern Science into the Practice of "Insight Meditation." *Science and Spirituality in Modern India*, 230.

Dhiman, S. K. (2020). Doing Vipassana the Buddha's way: A seeker's immersion in mindfulness in life and leadership. In *The routledge companion to mindfulness at work* (pp. 585–603). Routledge.

Dhinakaran, D., Raja, S. E., Jasmine, J. J., Kumar, P. V., & Ramani, R. (2025). The Future of Well-Being: AI-Powered Health Management with Privacy at its Core. In B. Bhushan, A. Khanday, K. Aurangzeb, S. K. Sharma, & P. Nand (Eds.)

Ding, D., Lawson, K. D., Kolbe-Alexander, T. L., Finkelstein, E. A., Katzmarzyk, P. T., Van Mechelen, W., & Pratt, M. (2017). The economic burden of physical inactivity: A global analysis of major non-communicable diseases. *The Lancet*, 388(10051), 1311-1324. Duffy, B. E., Pinch, A., Sannon, S., & Sawey, M. (2021). The nested precarities of creative labor on social media. *Social Media + Society*, *7*(2), 20563051211021370.

Dirlich, G., Vogl, L., Plaschke, M., & Strian, F. (1997). Cardiac Field Effects on the EEG. *Electroencephalography and Clinical Neurophysiology*, *102*(4), 307–315. DOI: 10.1016/S0013-4694(96)96506-2 PMID: 9146492

Dittakavi, B., Bavikadi, D., Desai, S. V., Chakraborty, S., Reddy, N., Balasubramanian, V. N., Callepalli, B., & Sharma, A. (2022). Pose tutor: An explainable system for pose correction in the wild. *Proceedings of the IEEE/CVF Conference on Computer Vision and Pattern Recognition*, 3540–3549. DOI: 10.1109/CVPRW56347.2022.00398

Doshi, M. (2023). "A comparison of data mining approaches for forecasting sales of FMCG food products," in *Proc. ICCCNT*, Delhi, India, pp. 1–7, DOI: 10.1109/ICCCNT56998.2023.10307432

Doshi, M., Hirapara, J., Ranpara, R., Khachariya, H., Patel, A. K., Jhanwar, K., & Choudhury, K. (2025). Enhancing FMCG sales prediction using recurrent neural networks and economic indicators. *IET Conference Proceedings,* 2025(7), 1223–1230. https://doi.org/DOI: 10.1049/icp.2025.1574

Duan, J., Xiong, J., Li, Y., & Ding, W. (2024). Deep learning based multimodal biomedical data fusion: An overview and comparative review. *Information Fusion*, *112*, 102536. DOI: 10.1016/j.inffus.2024.102536

Duda, A. T., Clarke, A. R., & Barry, R. J. (2024). Mindfulness meditation alters neural oscillations independently of arousal. *International Journal of Psychophysiology : Official Journal of the International Organization of Psychophysiology*, *205*, 112439. DOI: 10.1016/j.ijpsycho.2024.112439

Dunning, D. L., Griffiths, K., Kuyken, W., Crane, C., Foulkes, L., Parker, J., & Dalgleish, T. (2019a). Research Review: The effects of mindfulness-based interventions on cognition and mental health in children and adolescents–a meta-analysis of randomized controlled trials. *Journal of Child Psychology and Psychiatry, and Allied Disciplines*, *60*(3), 244–258. DOI: 10.1111/jcpp.12980 PMID: 30345511

Duppala, V. R., Marepalli, H. Y., Jain, K., Anusha, K., Thangavel, S. K., Kumar, B. S., Bindu, A., Satish, L., & Sekar, J. (2024). Aatma yoga: Automation of yoga pose recognition and recommendation using deep learning. *2024 International Conference on Inventive Computation Technologies (ICICT)*, 1315–1322. https://ieeexplore.ieee.org/abstract/document/10544761/

Dutt, V. (n.d.). Organized by the Indian Knowledge System and Mental Health Applications (IKSMHA) Centre, IIT Mandi. *Workshop Page*, (469), 472.

Eden, D. (1998). *Energy Medicine*. Penguin Putnam.

Einstein, A. (1955). *The Meaning of Relativity* (5th ed.). Princeton University Press.

Ercikan, K., & McCaffrey, D. F. (2022). Optimizing Implementation of Artificial-Intelligence-Based Automated Scoring: An Evidence Centered Design Approach for Designing Assessments for AI-based Scoring. *Journal of Educational Measurement*, *59*(3), 272–287. Advance online publication. DOI: 10.1111/jedm.12332

Eysenbach, G. (2001). What is e-health? *Journal of Medical Internet Research*, *3*(2), e20. DOI: 10.2196/jmir.3.2.e20

Ferrández, R. (2024). *From yogic powers to technological powers. Contemporary yoga and transhumanist spirituality*. https://philpapers.org/rec/FORFYP

Ferrarelli, F., Smith, R., Dentico, D., Riedner, B. A., Zennig, C., Benca, R. M., Lutz, A., Davidson, R. J., & Tononi, G. (2013). Experienced mindfulness meditators exhibit higher parietal-occipital EEG gamma activity during NREM sleep. *PLoS One*, *8*(8), e73417. DOI: 10.1371/journal.pone.0073417

Fialoke, S., Tripathi, V., Thakral, S., Dhawan, A., Majahan, V., & Garg, R. (2024). Functional connectivity changes in meditators and novices during yoga nidra practice. *Scientific Reports*, *14*(1), 12957. DOI: 10.1038/s41598-024-63765-7

Firth, A. M., Cavallini, I., Sütterlin, S., & Lugo, R. G. (2019). Mindfulness and self-efficacy in pain perception, stress and academic performance. The influence of mindfulness on cognitive processes. *Psychology Research and Behavior Management*, *12*, 565–574. DOI: 10.2147/PRBM.S206666 PMID: 31413648

Flook, L., Smalley, S. L., Kitil, M. J., Galla, B. M., Kaiser-Greenland, S., Locke, J., Ishijima, E., & Kasari, C. (2010). Effects of mindful awareness practices on executive functions in elementary school children. *Journal of Applied School Psychology*, *26*(1), 70–95. DOI: 10.1080/15377900903379125

Frawley, D. (1999). *Yoga & Ayurveda: Self-Healing and Self-Realization*. Lotus Pr.

Fuadi, A., Nuwairah, N., Rani, S., Ilham, I., & Herlita, J. (2025). Culturally responsive AI: Designing emotion recognition systems that account for diverse non-verbal communication styles. *International Journal of Research in Counseling.*, *4*(1), 12–22. DOI: 10.70363/ijrc.v4i1.274

Galindo-Aldana, G., Montoya-Rivera, L. A., Esqueda-Elizondo, J. J., Inzunza-Gonzalez, E., Garcia-Guerrero, E. E., Padilla-Lopez, A., Bautista, T. G., & Torres-González, C. (2025). Mindfulness-based intervention effects on EEG and executive functions: A systematic review. *Brain Sciences*, *15*(3), 324. DOI: 10.3390/brainsci15030324 PMID: 40149845

Ganesh, K., & Ramudhin, A. (2024). Leveraging AI to Mitigate Risks in Yoga Practice: A Real-Time Posture Correction Application. *Proceedings of the 12th International Conference on Sport Sciences Research and Technology Support*, 241–250. DOI: 10.5220/0013063300003828

Gao, J., Sun, R., Leung, H. K., Roberts, A., Wu, B. W. Y., Tsang, E. W., Tang, A. C. W., & Sik, H. H. (2023). Increased neurocardiological interplay after mindfulness meditation: A brain oscillation-based approach. *Frontiers in Human Neuroscience*, *17*, 1008490. Advance online publication. DOI: 10.3389/fnhum.2023.1008490

Garbett, A., Degutyte, Z., Hodge, J., & Astell, A. (2021). Towards Understanding People's Experiences of AI Computer Vision Fitness Instructor Apps. *Designing Interactive Systems Conference 2021*, 1619–1637. DOI: 10.1145/3461778.3462094

Garg, M. (2025). *Spiritual Artificial Intelligence (SAI): Towards a New Horizon*. Springer Nature Switzerland., DOI: 10.1007/978-3-031-73719-0

Garrison, K., Thomas, R., & Williams, P. (2020). Healthcare cost implications of digital wellness interventions: A systematic review. *Health Economics Review*, *10*(1), 1–18.

Gera, P. (2024). *Integrating Mindfulness: Enhancing Art and Design Student Well-being through AI Voice Assistants and Wearable Technology*. OCAD University.

Ghiya, S. (2017). Alternate nostril breathing: A systematic review of clinical trials. *International Journal of Research in Medical Sciences*, *5*(8), 3273. DOI: 10.18203/2320-6012.ijrms20173523

Ghosh, K. (n.d.). *Chatur-Varna in the AI Era: Integrating Bhagavad Gita's*. Retrieved January 11, 2026, from https://www.researchgate.net/profile/Debi-Prasad-Ghosh/publication/389634950_Chatur-Varna_in_the_AI_Era_Integrating_Bhagavad_Gita's_Ethical_and_Spiritual_Philosophy_for_Human-AI_Symbiosis/links/67ca8c35cc055043ce6ec4e8/Chatur-Varna-in-the-AI-Era-Integrating-Bhagavad-Gitas-Ethical-and-Spiritual-Philosophy-for-Human-AI-Symbiosis.pdf

Global Wellness Institute. (2022). *Global wellness economy monitor 2022*. Global Wellness Institute.

Godrej, F. (2017). The neoliberal yogi and the politics of yoga. *Political Theory, 45*(6), 772–800. DOI: 10.1177/0090591716643604

Goenka, S. N. (2012a). *Discourse summaries*. Pariyatti Publishing.

Goenka, S. N. (2012b). *Discourse Summaries*. Pariyatti Publishing.

Goenka, S. N. (2012d). *Meditation now: Inner peace through inner wisdom*. Pariyatti Publishing.

González, M. J., Olalde, J., Ward, T. D., & Miranda-Massari, J. R. (2019). Physiological Modulation: The Orthomolecular Explanation of Phytotherapy Based on the Systemic Medicine Approach. *Journal of Orthomolecular Medicine, 34*(1).

González, M. J., Seyfried, T., Nicolson, G. L., Barclay, B. J., Matta, J., Vasquez, A., D'Agostino, D., Olalde, J., Duconge, J., Hunninghake, R., Berdiel, M. J., & Cintrón, A. (2018). Mitochondrial Correction: A New Therapeutic Paradigm for Cancer and Degenerative Diseases. *Journal of Orthomolecular Medicine, 33*(4).

González, M. J., Sutherland, E., & Olalde, J. (2019). Quantum Functional Energy Medicine: The Next Frontier of Restorative Medicine. *Journal of Restorative Medicine, 8*(1), 1–7. DOI: 10.14200/jrm.2019.0114

Gosalia, M., Dedhia, R., Doshi, S., Sharma, R., & Mangla, M. (2024). Individualized Guidance in Yoga Practice: A Comparative Analysis of Technology Solutions. *2024 International Conference on Electrical Electronics and Computing Technologies (ICEECT), 1*, 1–6. https://ieeexplore.ieee.org/abstract/document/10739307/

Gosalia, M., Dedhia, R., Doshi, S., Sharma, R., & Mangla, M. (2024). Individualized Guidance in Yoga Practice: A Comparative Analysis of Technology Solutions. *2024 International Conference on Electrical Electronics and Computing Technologies (ICEECT)*, 1, 1–6. DOI: 10.1109/ICEECT61758.2024.10739307

Govinda, K. (2002). *A Handbook of Chakra Healing: Spiritual Practice for Health, Harmony and Inner Peace*. Konecky & Konecky.

Graham, M., Hjorth, I., & Lehdonvirta, V. (2017). Digital labour and development: Impacts of global digital labour platforms and the gig economy on worker livelihoods. *Transfer: European Review of Labour and Research, 23*(2), 135–162. DOI: 10.1177/1024258916687250

Graham, M., & Woodcock, J. (2018). Towards a fairer platform economy: Introducing the Fairwork Foundation. *Alternate Routes, 29*, 242–253.

Grand View Research. (2023). *Mindfulness meditation apps market size, share & trends analysis report by platform, by subscription, by end-use*. Grand View Research.

Grimes, J. A. (1996). *A Concise Dictionary of Indian Philosophy: Sanskrit Terms Defined in English*. State University of New York Press.

Grossman, P., Niemann, L., Schmidt, S., & Walach, H. (2004). Mindfulness-based stress reduction and health benefits: A meta-analysis. *Journal of Psychosomatic Research, 57*(1), 35–43. https://doi.org/https://doi.org/10.1016/S0022-3999(03)00573 -7. DOI: 10.1016/S0022-3999(03)00573-7 PMID: 15256293

Gupta, N., Arora, Y., Yadav, S., Aggarwal, N., GUPTA, S., GUPTA, M., PRIYADARSHI, P., & KAUR, S. (2025). Enhancing wellness through AI-powered yoga assistant: A human activity recognition application. *JOURNAL OF INFORMATION AND OPTIMIZATION SCIENCES, 46*(1), 143–155.

Hamblin, M. R. (2018). Photobiomodulation for Traumatic Brain Injury and Stroke. *Journal of Neuroscience Research, 96*(4), 731–743. DOI: 10.1002/jnr.24190 PMID: 29131369

Hammerschlag, R., Levin, M., McCraty, R., Bat, N., Ives, J. A., Lutgendorf, S. K., & Oschman, J. L. (2015). Biofield Physiology: A Framework for an Emerging Discipline. *Global Advances in Health and Medicine : Improving Healthcare Outcomes Worldwide, 4*(1_suppl, Suppl), 35–41. DOI: 10.7453/gahmj.2015.015.suppl PMID: 26665040

Hampton, K. N., & Wellman, B. (2018). Lost and saved... again: The moral panic about the loss of community takes hold of social media. *Contemporary Sociology, 47*(6), 643–651. DOI: 10.1177/0094306118805415

Hanwari, E., Kanani, J., Bhavsar, Y., & Shah, N. (2024). AI Based Personal Yoga Assistant. *2024 IEEE International Conference on Interdisciplinary Approaches in Technology and Management for Social Innovation (IATMSI), 2*, 1–5. https://ieeexplore.ieee.org/abstract/document/10502646/

Hanwari, E., Kanani, J., Bhavsar, Y., & Shah, N. (2024). AI Based Personal Yoga Assistant. *2024 IEEE International Conference on Interdisciplinary Approaches in Technology and Management for Social Innovation (IATMSI)*, 2, 1–5.

Haridasan, J. T., & Raj, E. D. (2023). Deep learning system for paddy plant disease detection and classification. *Environmental Monitoring and Assessment*, *195*(1), 120. DOI: 10.1007/s10661-022-10656-x PMID: 36399232

Harishbhai Tilala, M., Kumar Chenchala, P., Choppadandi, A., Kaur, J., Naguri, S., Saoji, R., & Devaguptapu, B. (2024). Ethical Considerations in the Use of Artificial Intelligence and Machine Learning in Health Care: A Comprehensive Review. *Cureus*, *16*(6), e62443. DOI: 10.7759/cureus.62443

Hart, W. (2011). *The art of living: Vipassana meditation as taught by SN Goenka.* Pariyatti.

Haryanto, C. Y., Vu, M. H., Nguyen, T. D., Lomempow, E., Nurliana, Y., & Taheri, S. (2024). SecGenAI: Enhancing Security of Cloud-based Generative AI Applications within Australian Critical Technologies of National Interest (arXiv:2407.01110). arXiv.

Hasan, M. M., Islam, M. U., Murad, M. A. H., & Uddin, M. J. (2025). A comprehensive survey on data augmentation for time-series classification of medical wearable sensor data. *Artificial Intelligence in Medicine*, *158*, 102985.

Hasanzadeh, F., Josephson, C. B., Waters, G., Adedinsewo, D., Azizi, Z., & White, J. A. (2025). "Bias recognition and mitigation strategies in artificial intelligence healthcare applications," *npj. Digital Medicine*, *8*(1), 154. Advance online publication. DOI: 10.1038/s41746-025-01503-7 PMID: 40069303

Hirpara, J., Doshi, M., Patel, A., & Choudhury, K. (2025). A Study on Machine Learning Algorithms: Forecasting Crop Prices. In Rajagopal, S., Popat, K., Meva, D., Bajeja, S., & Mudholkar, P. (Eds.), *Artificial Intelligence Based Smart and Secured Applications. ASCIS 2024. Communications in Computer and Information Science* (Vol. 2427). Springer., DOI: 10.1007/978-3-031-86299-1_4

Hofmann, S. G., Sawyer, A. T., Witt, A. A., & Oh, D. (2010). The effect of mindfulness-based therapy on anxiety and depression: A meta-analytic review. *Journal of Consulting and Clinical Psychology*, *78*(2), 169–183. DOI: 10.1037/a0018555 PMID: 20350028

Holmes, W. (2020). Artificial intelligence in education. In *Encyclopedia of education and information technologies* (pp. 88–103). Springer. DOI: 10.1007/978-3-030-10576-1_107

Hölzel, B. K., Carmody, J., Vangel, M., Congleton, C., Yerramsetti, S. M., Gard, T., & Lazar, S. W. (2011). Mindfulness practice leads to increases in regional brain gray matter density. *Psychiatry Research. Neuroimaging*, *191*(1), 36–43. https://doi.org/https://doi.org/10.1016/j.pscychresns.2010.08.006. DOI: 10.1016/j.pscychresns.2010.08.006 PMID: 21071182

Hölzel, B. K., Lazar, S. W., Gard, T., Schuman-Olivier, Z., Vago, D. R., & Ott, U. (2011). How Does Mindfulness Meditation Work? Proposing Mechanisms of Action From a Conceptual and Neural Perspective. *Perspectives on Psychological Science : A Journal of the Association for Psychological Science*, *6*(6), 537–559. DOI: 10.1177/1745691611419671 PMID: 26168376

Hosseini, M., Arefi, M., & Sajjadian, I. (2019). Effectiveness of Time-Perspective Training on Time-Balancing and Self-Regulation among Female Students. *International Journal of Behavioral Sciences*, *13*(3), 118–122.

Hwang, J., Castelli, D. M., & Gonzalez-Lima, F. (2016). Cognitive enhancement by transcranial laser stimulation and acute aerobic exercise. *Lasers in Medical Science*, *31*(6), 1151–1160. DOI: 10.1007/s10103-016-1962-3 PMID: 27220529

Ieger-Raittz, R., De Pierri, C. R., Perico, C. P., Costa, F. de F., Bana, E. G., Vicenzi, L., Machado, D. J. S., Marchaukoski, J. N., & Raittz, R. T. (2025). What are we learning with Yoga? Mapping the scientific literature on Yoga using a vector-text-mining approach. *PLoS One*, *20*(5), e0322791. DOI: 10.1371/journal.pone.0322791 PMID: 40440353

Insights, C. B. (2023). *Wellness tech funding report: AI-powered fitness and meditation platforms*. CB Insights Research.

International Telecommunication Union (ITU). (2023). *Measuring digital development: Facts and figures 2023*. ITU Publications.

Irfan, M., Ali, A., & Rehman, A. U. (2025). Integrating artificial intelligence with naturopathy and yoga for chronic disease management: A systematic review. *Journal of Integrative and Complementary Medicine*, *31*(2), 115–134.

Irfan, N., Zafar, S., Shakil, K. A., Wani, M. A., Kumar, S. N., Jaiganesh, A., & Abubeker, K. M. (2025). Integrating AI predictive analytics with naturopathic and yoga-based interventions in a data-driven preventive model to improve maternal mental health and pregnancy outcomes. *Scientific Reports*, *15*(1), 23878. DOI: 10.1038/s41598-025-07885-8

Ismail Fawaz, H., Forestier, G., Weber, J., Idoumghar, L., & Muller, P. A. (2019). Deep learning for time series classification: A review. *Data Mining and Knowledge Discovery*, *33*(4), 917–963. DOI: 10.1007/s10618-019-00619-1

Iyengar, B. K. S. (2010). *Light on Pranayama*. The Crossroad Publishing Company. Chapter 5: Nadis and Chakras.

Jahnavi, G. (2025). Smart yoga asana recommender: Leveraging nlp for health-driven suggestions. *International Journal for Research in Applied Science and Engineering Technology*, *13*(7), 2167–2174. DOI: 10.22214/ijraset.2025.73331

Jain, A. R. (2014). *Selling yoga: From counterculture to pop culture*. Oxford University Press. DOI: 10.1093/acprof:oso/9780199390236.001.0001

Jain, A. R. (2020). Who is saving whom? Colonial missionizing and yoga. *International Journal of Hindu Studies*, *24*(1), 39–66.

Jain, I., Srivastava, R., Srivastava, V., Sinha, V., & Juneja, A. (2025). Ethical Decision-Making in Yoga Posture Detection through AI: Fostering Responsible Technology Integration. In Juneja, S., Dhanaraj, R. K., Juneja, A., Sathyamoorthy, M., & Shaikh, A. (Eds.), *Ethical Decision-Making Using Artificial Intelligence* (1st ed., pp. 99–123). Wiley., DOI: 10.1002/9781394275311.ch5

Javed, H., Muqeet, H. A., Javed, T., Rehman, A. U., & Sadiq, R. (2024). Ethical frameworks for machine learning in sensitive healthcare applications. *IEEE Access : Practical Innovations, Open Solutions*, *12*, 16233–16254. DOI: 10.1109/ACCESS.2023.3340884

Jebamikyous, H., Li, M., Suhas, Y., & Kashef, R. (2023). Leveraging machine learning and blockchain in E-commerce and beyond: Benefits, models, and application. *Discover Artificial Intelligence*, *3*(1), 3. DOI: 10.1007/s44163-022-00046-0

Jha, A. P., Krompinger, J., & Baime, M. J. (2007). Mindfulness training modifies subsystems of attention. *Cognitive, Affective & Behavioral Neuroscience*, *7*(2), 109–119. DOI: 10.3758/CABN.7.2.109 PMID: 17672382

Jon Kabat-Zin. (2003). *Mindfulness-Based Interventions in Context Past Present and Future -Clin Psych Sci Pract - 2006 - Kabat-Zinn -.pdf.*

Jose, J., & Shailesh, S. (2021). Yoga Asana Identification: A Deep Learning Approach. *IOP Conference Series. Materials Science and Engineering*, *1110*(1), 012002. DOI: 10.1088/1757-899X/1110/1/012002

Joshi, R. R. (2004). Biostatistical approach to Ayurveda: Tridosha quantification. *Journal of Alternative and Complementary Medicine (New York, N.Y.), 10*(5), 879–889. DOI: 10.1089/acm.2004.10.879 PMID: 15650478

Jugran, S. (2024). Yogasanas and Their Importance in Stree Rog. *International Journal of Advanced Research, 12*(04), 877–890. DOI: 10.21474/IJAR01/18627

Kabat-Zinn, J. (2009). *Wherever you go, there you are: Mindfulness meditation in everyday life*. Hachette UK.

Kabat-Zinn, J. (1982). An outpatient program in behavioral medicine for chronic pain patients based on the practice of mindfulness meditation: Theoretical considerations and preliminary results. *General Hospital Psychiatry, 4*(1), 33–47. DOI: 10.1016/0163-8343(82)90026-3 PMID: 7042457

Kabat-Zinn, J. (2015). Mindfulness. *Mindfulness, 6*(6), 1481–1483. DOI: 10.1007/s12671-015-0456-x

Kaplan, A. M., & Haenlein, M. (2010). Users of the world, unite! The challenges and opportunities of social media. *Business Horizons, 53*(1), 59–68. DOI: 10.1016/j.bushor.2009.09.003

Kaur, C., & Singh, P. (2015). EEG Derived Neuronal Dynamics during Meditation: Progress and Challenges. *Advances in Preventive Medicine, 614723*, 1–10. Advance online publication. DOI: 10.1155/2015/614723

Kavitha, N., Pal, P., Pal, G. K., Bharadwaj, B., & Nanda, N. (2024). Effects of Slow Breathing Exercises on Cardiac Autonomic Functions in Anxiety Disorder-A Randomised Control Trial. *Annals of Neurosciences, 09727531241266094*, 09727531241266094. Advance online publication. DOI: 10.1177/09727531241266094

Keny, V. (2025). Can artificial intelligence experience spirituality?. *Journal of advances in science and technology, 22* (2). DOI: 10.29070/3t5w4a12

Kher, D., & Patel, D. M. (2021). A Comprehensive Review on Wearable Health Monitoring Systems. *The Open Biomedical Engineering Journal, 15*(1), 213–225. DOI: 10.2174/1874120702115010213

Kim, E., Moon, C. W., Kim, S., Ozkan, E., & Lomas, T. (2022). Mindfulness Intervention Courses in STEM Education: A Qualitative Assessment. In *Lecture Notes in Networks and Systems: 349 LNNS*. DOI: 10.1007/978-3-030-90677-1_16

Kim, H. G., Cheon, E. J., Bai, D. S., Lee, Y. H., & Koo, B. H. (2018). Heart rate variability and stress: A meta-analysis and review of the literature. *Psychiatry Investigation, 15*(3), 235–245. DOI: 10.30773/pi.2017.08.17 PMID: 29486547

Kim, K. K., & Backonja, U. (2025). Digital health equity frameworks and key concepts: A scoping review. *Journal of the American Medical Informatics Association : JAMIA*, *32*(5), 932–944. DOI: 10.1093/jamia/ocaf017 PMID: 39936843

Kontos, E., Blake, K. D., Chou, W. Y. S., & Prestin, A. (2014). Predictors of eHealth usage: Insights on the digital divide from the Health Information National Trends Survey 2012. *Journal of Medical Internet Research*, *16*(7), e172. DOI: 10.2196/jmir.3117

Kuh, G. D., Kinzie, J. L., Buckley, J. A., Bridges, B. K., & Hayek, J. C. (2006). *What matters to student success: A review of the literature* (Vol. 8). National Postsecondary Education Cooperative Washington.

Kumar, S., & Singh, R. (2021). Digital divide in health technology adoption: Urban-rural disparities in India. *The Journal of Rural Health : Official Journal of the American Rural Health Association and the National Rural Health Care Association*, *37*(2), 312–325.

Kuruvilla, S., & Gopalakrishna, G. K. Pillai, null, Kim, S., McDougall, L., Soon, G. C., Matsabisa, M., & Briand, S. (2025). Traditional medicine and its contributions to science, health equity and sustainability. Bulletin of the World Health Organization, *103*(11), 642-642A. DOI: 10.2471/BLT.25.295061

Lad, V. (2002). *Textbook of Ayurveda: Fundamental principles*. The Ayurvedic Press.

Lagopoulos, J., Xu, J., Rasmussen, I., Vik, A., Malhi, G. S., Eliassen, C. F., Arntsen, I. E., Saether, J. G., Hollup, S., Holen, A., Davanger, S., & Ellingsen, Ø. (2009). Increased theta and alpha EEG activity during nondirective meditation. *Journal of Alternative and Complementary Medicine (New York, N.Y.)*, *15*(11), 1187–1192. DOI: 10.1089/acm.2009.0113

Lalanza, J. F., Lorente, S., Bullich, R., García, C., Losilla, J.-M., & Capdevila, L. (2023). Methods for heart rate variability biofeedback (HRVB): A systematic review and guidelines. *Applied Psychophysiology and Biofeedback*, *48*(3), 275–297. DOI: 10.1007/s10484-023-09582-6 PMID: 36917418

Lavanya, V., Premkumar K, & Rohith R. (2024). AI Enhanced Yoga Pose Detection And Alignment Using Deep Learning. DOI: 10.1109/INOCON60754.2024.10512108

Lay, U. K. (2008). *Manual of Vipassana Meditation* (Third). Vipassana Research Institute, Dhamma Giri. https://www.vridhamma.org/

Lazarou, I., Oikonomou, V. P., Mpaltadoros, L., Grammatikopoulou, M., Alepopoulos, V., Stavropoulos, T. G., Bezerianos, A., Nikolopoulos, S., Kompatsiaris, I., & Tsolaki, M.RADAR-AD Consortium. (2023). Eliciting brain waves of people with cognitive impairment during meditation exercises using portable electroencephalography in a smart-home environment: A pilot study. *Frontiers in Aging Neuroscience*, *15*, 1167410. DOI: 10.3389/fnagi.2023.1167410

Lehrer, P. M., & Gevirtz, R. (2014). How and why does biofeedback on heart rate variability work? *Frontiers in Psychology*, *5*, 756. DOI: 10.3389/fpsyg.2014.00756 PMID: 25101026

Leslie, D. (2023). *Understanding Artificial Intelligence Ethics and Safety*. The Alan Turing Institute.

Liew, J., Morris, A. S., & Kerr, K. L. (2023). *Emotion regulation processes as transdiagnostic in adolescence and early adulthood: A neurobioecological systems framework*.

Liu, M., Ning, Y., Teixayavong, S., Liu, X., Mertens, M., Shang, Y., Li, X., Miao, D., Liao, J., Xu, J., Ting, D. S. W., Cheng, L. T.-E., Ong, J. C. L., Teo, Z. L., Tan, T. F., RaviChandran, N., Wang, F., Celi, L. A., Ong, M. E. H., & Liu, N. (2025). "A scoping review and evidence gap analysis of clinical AI fairness," *npj. Digital Medicine*, *8*(1), 360. Advance online publication. DOI: 10.1038/s41746-025-01667-2 PMID: 40517148

Liu, S., & Guo, L. R. (2024). Data ownership in the AI-powered integrative health care landscape. *JMIR Medical Informatics*, *12*, e57754. DOI: 10.2196/57754

Lochtefeld, J. G. (2002). *The Illustrated Encyclopedia of Hinduism: A–M*. The Rosen Publishing Group.

Lomas, T., Ivtzan, I., & Fu, C. H. Y. (2015). Mindfulness' neurophysiology: A systematic review on EEG oscillations. *Neuroscience and Biobehavioral Reviews*, *57*, 401–410. DOI: 10.1016/j.neubiorev.2015.09.018 PMID: 26441373

Luckin, R., Holmes, W., & Forcier, L. B. (2018). *An argument for AI in education*. UCL Knowledge Lab. [Google Scholar]

Luxton, D. D. (2016). An introduction to artificial intelligence in behavioral and mental health care. In *Artificial intelligence in behavioral and mental health care* (pp. 1–26). Elsevier. DOI: 10.1016/B978-0-12-420248-1.00001-5

Mahajan, P. (2025). *The Soul of the AI: Governance, Ethics, and the Future of Human–AI Integration*. Zenodo. https://hal.science/hal-05140138/ DOI: 10.14293/PR2199.001783.v1

Mallinson, J., & Singleton, M. (2017). *Roots of Yoga*. Penguin Books.

Mandinach, E. B., & Schildkamp, K. (2021). Misconceptions about data-based decision making in education: An exploration of the literature. *Studies in Educational Evaluation*, *69*, 100842. DOI: 10.1016/j.stueduc.2020.100842

Manikumar, T., Kankanala, J., Kishore, K., & Sriram, L. (2024). Real Time Yoga Posture Location and Assessment Utilizing Deep Learning. *2024 International Conference on Sustainable Communication Networks and Application (ICSCNA)*, 751–756. https://ieeexplore.ieee.org/abstract/document/10863926/

Mani, P., Thangavelu, A., Sharma, A., & Chaudhari, N. (2017). A Real Time Monitoring System for Yoga Practitioners. *International Journal of Intelligent Engineering and Systems*, *10*(3), 85–93. DOI: 10.22266/ijies2017.0630.10

Marade, A., Suvarna, K., Chaudhari, P., & Bhandiwad, P. V. (2025). Spiritual.ai: An ai-driven platform for enhancing mental, emotional, and spiritual well-being. *International Journal for Research in Applied Science and Engineering Technology*, *13*(4), 4211–4216. DOI: 10.22214/ijraset.2025.64703

Martinez, L., Chen, M., & Rodriguez, A. (2020). Quality stratification in digital health platforms: Access and equity implications. *Journal of Medical Internet Research*, *22*(8), e18234.

Mateus, N., Abade, E., Coutinho, D., Ángel Gómez, M., Peñas, C. L., & Sampaio, J. (2024). Empowering the Sports Scientist with Artificial Intelligence in Training, Performance, and Health Management. *Sensors (Basel)*, *25*(1), 139–139. DOI: 10.3390/s25010139 PMID: 39796930

Matsuyama, H., Kawaguchi, N., & Lim, B. Y. (2023). *IRIS: Interpretable Rubric-Informed Segmentation for Action Quality Assessment. ArXiv*. Cornell University., DOI: 10.1145/3581641.3584048

Maynard, B. R., Solis, M. R., Miller, V. L., & Brendel, K. E. (2017). Mindfulness-based interventions for improving cognition, academic achievement, behavior, and socioemotional functioning of primary and secondary school students. *Campbell Systematic Reviews*, *13*(1), 1–144. DOI: 10.4073/CSR.2017.5

Mazurova, E., Standaert, W., Penttinen, E., & Tan, F. T. C. (2021). Paradoxical Tensions Related to AI-Powered Evaluation Systems in Competitive Sports. *Information Systems Frontiers*, *24*(3), 897–922. Advance online publication. DOI: 10.1007/s10796-021-10215-8 PMID: 34867076

Meditation, T. W. (n.d.). *The Anapanasati Sutta : Sutta :* Meiklejohn, J., Phillips, C., Freedman, M. L., Griffin, M. L., Biegel, G., Roach, A., Frank, J., Burke, C., Pinger, L., & Soloway, G. (2012). Integrating mindfulness training into K-12 education: Fostering the resilience of teachers and students. *Mindfulness*, *3*(4), 291–307.

Mehra, R., ... (2026). AI-Driven Yoga Therapy Validation with Blockchain Health Records. Patent No. 202511656788 / 202511030786. Indian Patent Office.

Meskó, B., Drobni, Z., Bényei, É., Gergely, B., & Győrffy, Z. (2017). Digital health is a cultural transformation of traditional healthcare. *mHealth*, *3*, 38. DOI: 10.21037/mhealth.2017.08.07

Miao, Z., Wang, J., & Yu, C. (2024). FairPose: Toward fairness-aware human pose estimation. *IEEE Transactions on Pattern Analysis and Machine Intelligence*.

Miller, J. J., Fletcher, K., & Kabat-Zinn, J. (1995). Three-year follow-up and clinical implications of a mindfulness meditation-based stress reduction intervention in the treatment of anxiety disorders. *General Hospital Psychiatry*, *17*(3), 192–200. DOI: 10.1016/0163-8343(95)00025-M PMID: 7649463

Misra, G. (2017). Effects of Mindfulness Meditation on Self-Compassion and Self-Construal among Adolescents. *Journal of Child and Family Studies*, *26*(7), 1984–1994. DOI: 10.1007/s10826-017-0736-5

Mitchell, M.. "Model cards for model reporting," in *Proc. ACM Conf. on Fairness, Accountability, and Transparency (FAccT)*, 2023, pp. 220–229.

Mitsea, E., Drigas, A., & Skianis, C. (2024a). Artificial intelligence, immersive technologies, and neurotechnologies in breathing interventions for mental and emotional health: A systematic review. *Electronics (Basel)*, *13*(12), 2253. DOI: 10.3390/electronics13122253

Mittelstadt, B. D., & Floridi, L. (2016). The ethics of big data: Current and foreseeable issues in biomedical contexts. *Science and Engineering Ethics*, *22*(2), 303–341. DOI: 10.1007/s11948-015-9652-2

Moga, M., & Bengston, W. (2010). Moga, M.M., W.F. Bengston (2010) Anomalous magnetic field activity during a bioenergy healing experiment. J. Sci. Exploration 24(3): 397-410. *Journal of Scientific Exploration*, *24*, 397–410.

Mondal, S. (2024). Proposed physiological mechanisms of pranayama: A discussion. *Journal of Ayurveda and Integrative Medicine*, *15*(1), 100877. DOI: 10.1016/j.jaim.2023.100877

Montessori, M. (n.d.). *The Absorbent Mind: i* (Number May 1949).

Mrazek, M. D., Zedelius, C. M., Gross, M. E., Mrazek, A. J., Phillips, D. T., & Schooler, J. W. (2017). Mindfulness in education: Enhancing academic achievement and student well-being by reducing mind-wandering. In *Mindfulness in social psychology* (pp. 139–152). Routledge. DOI: 10.4324/9781315627700-10

Mueller, S. T., & Piper, B. J. (2014). The Psychology Experiment Building Language (PEBL) and PEBL Test Battery. *Journal of Neuroscience Methods*, *222*, 250–259. https://doi.org/https://doi.org/10.1016/j.jneumeth.2013.10.024. DOI: 10.1016/j.jneumeth.2013.10.024 PMID: 24269254

Muktibodhananda, S. (1998). *Hatha Yoga Pradipika*. https://www.amazon.com/Hatha-Yoga-Pradipika-Swami-Muktibodhananda/dp/8185787387

Muktibodhananda, S. (2012). *Hatha Yoga Pradipika*. https://www.amazon.in/Hatha-Yoga-Pradipika-Swami-Muktibodhananda-ebook/dp/B01BRF5MFO

Mundargi, B. V., Mutalikdesai, V., & Balakrishnan, A. (2024). A Bird's Eye View on the Integration of Artificial Intelligence (AI) In Ayurveda. *Journal of Ayurveda and Integrated Medical Sciences*, *9*(8), 167–172. DOI: 10.21760/jaims.9.8.25

Murphy, A., Bowen, K., Naqa, I. M. E., Yoga, B., & Green, B. L. (2025). Bridging Health Disparities in the Data-Driven World of Artificial Intelligence: A Narrative Review. *Journal of Racial and Ethnic Health Disparities*, *12*(4), 2367–2379. DOI: 10.1007/s40615-024-02057-2

Mütze, C., Mitzinger, D., & Haller, H. (2025). Effectiveness of pranayama for mental disorders: A systematic review and meta-analysis of randomized controlled trials. *Frontiers in Psychiatry*, *16*, 1616996. Advance online publication. DOI: 10.3389/fpsyt.2025.1616996

Nair, M. (2020). Commodification, appropriation, and representation: Yoga in the United States. In *Handbook of Research on the Global Impacts and Roles of Immersive Media* (pp. 290–312). IGI Global.

Nandram, S. S., Bindlish, P. K., Sukhada, & Shrestha, A. K. (2022). Spirituality led ethical decision making with yogic yamas and niyamas. DOI: 10.51327/EHZW1674

Napoli, M., Krech, P. R., & Holley, L. C. (2005). Mindfulness Training for Elementary School Students. *Journal of Applied School Psychology*, *21*(1), 99–125. DOI: 10.1300/J370v21n01_05

Narine, A., Moazzamipeiro, F., Mangal, G., & Moazzamipeiro, M. (2025). Transforming ayurveda research through the synergy of AI technology and traditional wisdom. *Annals of Ayurvedic Medicine*, *14*(2), 156–156. DOI: 10.5455/AAM.219889

Nazari, G., Kaur, P., MacDermid, J. C., & Edwards, C. (2021). Wearable smartwatches during yoga practice: Considerations for HRV-based monitoring. *Sensors (Basel)*, *21*(4), 1257. DOI: 10.3390/s21041257 PMID: 33578794

NCERT, T. (2007). *National curriculum framework 2005.*

Nesin, J., & Sathyamoorthy, G. (2025). Psychoneuroimmunology of yoga and meditation: Mechanisms and clinical applications. In Sharma, S., & Gupta, R. (Eds.), *Indian Knowledge Systems in Modern Healthcare* (pp. 112–145). IGI Global.

Neufeld, D., & Dellaert, B. (2020). Consumer response to subscription-based wellness platforms: Price, value, and utilization patterns. *Journal of Service Research*, *23*(4), 412–428.

Ng, J. Y., Cramer, H., Lee, M. S., & Moher, D. (2024). Traditional, complementary, and integrative medicine and artificial intelligence: Novel opportunities in healthcare. *Integrative Medicine Research*, *13*(1), 101024. DOI: 10.1016/j.imr.2024.101024

Norori, N., Hu, Q., Aellen, F. M., Faraci, F. D., & Tzovara, A. (2023). Addressing bias in big data and AI for health care: A call for open science. *Patterns (New York, N.Y.)*, *2*(10), 100347. DOI: 10.1016/j.patter.2021.100347 PMID: 34693373

Nota, L., Soresi, S., & Zimmerman, B. J. (2004). Self-regulation and academic achievement and resilience: A longitudinal study. *International Journal of Educational Research*, *41*(3), 198–215. DOI: 10.1016/j.ijer.2005.07.001

Novrianto, A., Gustion, D., & Rahmawati, E. (2025). AI-Powered Performance Appraisal: Balancing Automation with Human Judgment in Performance Management Systems. Journal of Economics and Management Scienties, 389–396. DOI: 10.37034/jems.v7i3.163

Nuong Deri, M. ., Singh, A., Zaazie, P. ., & Anandene, D. . (2024). Leveraging Artificial Intelligence in Higher Educational Institutions: A Comprehensive Overview. Revista De Educación Y Derecho, (30). DOI: 10.1344/REYD2024.30.45777

Özsezer, G., & Mermer, G. (2025). Real-Time Prediction of Correct Yoga Asanas in Healthy Individuals With Artificial Intelligence Techniques: A Systematic Review for Nursing. *Nursing Open*, *12*(8), e70278. DOI: 10.1002/nop2.70278

Padhi, M. M. (2016). Evolution of Yoga and Physiotherapy. *Journal of Yoga and Physiotherapy*, *1*(2). Advance online publication. DOI: 10.19080/JYP.2016.01.555556

Pallathadka, H., & Roy, P. (2025). Commandments in hinduism and sanatana dharma: A comprehensive scholarly review of ethical imperatives and their contemporary relevance. *Integrated Journal for Research in Arts and Humanities*, *5*(3), 380–393. DOI: 10.55544/ijrah.5.3.46

Pallathadka, H., & Roy, P. D. (2025). Hindu Responses to Artificial Intelligence: Theological and Ethical Frameworks for Human Technology Relationships. *International Journal for Research Trends in Social Science & Humanities*, *3*(2), 868–890. DOI: 10.61463/ijrtssh.vol.3.issue2.147

Pal, R., Adhikari, D., Heyat, M. B. B., Ullah, I., & You, Z. (2023). Yoga meets intelligent internet of things: Recent challenges and future directions. *Bioengineering (Basel, Switzerland)*, *10*(4), 459. DOI: 10.3390/bioengineering10040459

Pandi-Perumal, S. R., Spence, D. W., Srivastava, N., Kanchibhotla, D., Kumar, K., Sharma, G. S., Gupta, R., & Batmanabane, G. (2022). The Origin and Clinical Relevance of Yoga Nidra. *Sleep and Vigilance*, *6*(1), 61–84. DOI: 10.1007/s41782-022-00202-7

Park, C. L., Elwy, A. R., Maiya, M., Sarkin, A. J., Riley, K. E., Eisen, S. V., Gutierrez, I., Finkelstein-Fox, L., Lee, S. Y., Casteel, D., Braun, T., & Groessl, E. J. (2020). The essential properties of yoga questionnaire (EPYQ): Psychometric properties. *International Journal of Yoga Therapy*, *30*(1), 23–38. DOI: 10.17761/2018-00016R2

Park, C. L., Finkelstein-Fox, L., Sacco, S. J., Braun, T. D., & Lazar, S. (2018). How does yoga reduce stress? A clinical trial examining psychological mechanisms. *Stress and Health : Journal of the International Society for the Investigation of Stress*, *34*(2), 245–256.

Patarathipakorn, O., Pawa, K. K., Sritipsukho, P., Tansuhaj, K., Bhamarapravatana, K., & Suwannarurk, K. (2025). Aanapanasati Meditation and Stress Reduction Among Health Science University Students. *The Open Public Health Journal*, *18*(1), e18749445380247. DOI: 10.2174/0118749445380247250225075656

Patel, M. S., Asch, D. A., & Volpp, K. G. (2020). Wearable devices as facilitators, not drivers, of health behavior change. *Journal of the American Medical Association*, *313*(5), 459–460. DOI: 10.1001/jama.2014.14781

Pavithra, S., Dhanya, R., Dharshana, M., Fathima, I. N., & Soundariya, S. (2025). Tech yoga: The smart mat revolution. *I-Manager's Journal on Embedded Systems*, *13*(2), 46. DOI: 10.26634/jes.13.2.21490

Pavlopoulos, A., Rachiotis, T., & Maglogiannis, I. (2024). An Overview of Tools and Technologies for Anxiety and Depression Management Using AI. *Applied Sciences (Basel, Switzerland)*, *14*(19), 9068–9068. DOI: 10.3390/app14199068

Pisaniello, A. (2024). The Game Changer: How Artificial Intelligence is Transforming Sports Performance and Strategy. Geopolitical. *Social Security and Freedom Journal*, *7*(1), 75–84. DOI: 10.2478/gssfj-2024-0006

Popkova, E. G. (2024). Spirituality in the realities of digitalization of society in the era of intelligent machines development. *Journal of Economics*, *32*(1), 170–186. Advance online publication. DOI: 10.22363/2313-2329-2024-32-1-170-186

Posner, M. I., & Petersen, S. E. (1990). The attention system of the human brain. *Annual Review of Neuroscience*, *13*(1), 25–42. DOI: 10.1146/annurev.ne.13.030190.000325 PMID: 2183676

Pradhan, B. (2014). *Yoga and Mindfulness-Based Cognitive Therapy: A Clinical Guide*. Springer.

Pradhan, S., & Bhutia, Y. (2025). Impact of Anapanasati meditation on well-being of secondary school students in Teesta, Kalimpong District, West Bengal. *Int J Psychiatr Res*, *8*(4), 1–10. DOI: 10.33425/2641-4317.1225

Pramanik, D., & Singh, V. (2023).. . *PHILOSOPHY OF THE BODY ACCORDING TO THE ANCIENT TEXTS OF HATHA YOGA.*, *13*, 156–162.

Prasanna, M., Arunkumar, T., & Arunkumar, S. (2017). A Mobile Application Based Smart System for Supporting Yoga Activities and Health Monitoring. *Research Journal of Pharmacy and Technology*, *10*(11), 3863. DOI: 10.5958/0974-360X.2017.00701.6

Prasher, B., Negi, S., Aggarwal, S., Mandal, A. K., Sethi, T. P., Deshmukh, S. R., & Mukerji, M. (2008). Biochemical and whole genome correlates of extreme constitutional types defined in Ayurveda. *Journal of Translational Medicine*, *6*(1), 48. DOI: 10.1186/1479-5876-6-48 PMID: 18782426

Prathomwong, P., & Singsuriya, P. (2022). Ethical Framework of Digital Technology, Artificial Intelligence, and Health Equity. *Asia Social Issues*, *15*(5), 252136. DOI: 10.48048/asi.2022.252136

Rachakonda, L., Bapatla, A. K., Mohanty, S. P., & Kougianos, E. (2020a). SaYoPillow: A Blockchain-Enabled, Privacy-Assured Framework for Stress Detection, Prediction and Control Considering Sleeping Habits in the IoMT (arXiv:2007.07377). arXiv.

Radha, M., Fonseca, P., Moreau, A., Ross, M., Cerny, A., Anderer, P., & Aarts, R. M. (2019). A machine learning approach to predict sleep stages using data from multiple wearable sensors. *Frontiers in Neuroscience*, *13*, 1032.

Rahul, M. (2023). Fitness and Yoga in Sports. *International Journal for Multidisciplinary Research*, *5*(6). Advance online publication. DOI: 10.36948/ijfmr.2023.v05i06.9428

Rai, D., Kumar, A., & Baghel, A. (2024). Pose Detection Using OpenCV and Media Pipe. 1–6. DOI: 10.1109/ICIC3S61846.2024.10603040

Rajendran, A. K., & Sethuraman, S. C. (2023). A survey on yogic posture recognition. *IEEE Access : Practical Innovations, Open Solutions*, *11*, 11183–11223. DOI: 10.1109/ACCESS.2023.3240769

Ranpara, R., Hirpara, J., Doshi, M., & Shah, D. (2025). A novel Bayesian-inspired framework for proactive detection and mitigation of zero-day attacks in distributed network architectures. *IET Conference Proceedings,* 2025(7), 1168–1175. https://doi.org/DOI: 10.1049/icp.2025.1567

Raval, H. Y., Parikh, S. M., & Patel, H. R. (2022). Self-maintained health surveillance artificial intelligence assistant. In Handbook of Research on Lifestyle Sustainability and Management Solutions Using AI, Big Data Analytics, and Visualization (pp. 168–184). IGI Global Scientific Publishing. DOI: 10.4018/978-1-7998-8786-7.ch010

Raveena, N. M., & Rathod, L. L. (2024). ROLE OF AI IN TALENT IDENTIFICATION AND PERFORMANCE PREDICTION IN TRACK AND FIELD. *ShodhKosh Journal of Visual and Performing Arts*, *5*(7SE). Advance online publication. DOI: 10.29121/shodhkosh.v5.i7SE.2024.5878

Rawat, K., Chandravanshi, D., Sahu, V., & Pedhekar, S. R. (2025). The perspectives of yoga in maintaining psycho-social health and overall well-being. *Journal of Neonatal Surgery*, *14*(6), 291–295. DOI: 10.63682/jns.v14i6.3259

Ray, A. (2025a). AI Agent Engineering: Building LLM-COT-Powered Intelligent AI Agents (Total Guide). *Compassionate AI*, *2*(4), 87–89.

Ray, A. (2025b). AI Agents and Robots in Peacekeeping Force and Social Care: Compassionate AI Technologies. *Compassionate AI*, *3*(9), 75–77.

Ray, S. (2025). Consciousness in transformers? A critical philosophical analysis of emergent AI capabilities. *AI & Society*, *40*(1), 55–78.

Rosen, L. D., Lim, A. F., Felt, J., Carrier, L. M., Cheever, N. A., Lara-Ruiz, J. M., Mendoza, J. S., & Rokkum, J. (2014). Media and technology use predicts ill-being among children, preteens and teenagers independent of the negative health impacts of exercise and eating habits. *Computers in Human Behavior, 35*, 364–375. DOI: 10.1016/j.chb.2014.01.036 PMID: 25717216

ROy, S., & DESHPANDE, Sanja. H. (n.d.). Coupling Technology with Traditional Knowledge for Health and Wellbeing: Harnessing AI. *Science for Sustainability and Wellbeing in the Anthropocene Opportunities, Challenges, and AI*, 263.

Rubik, B., Muehsam, D., Hammerschlag, R., & Jain, S. (2015). Biofield Science and Healing: History, Terminology, and Concepts. *Global Advances in Health and Medicine : Improving Healthcare Outcomes Worldwide*, *4*(1_suppl, Suppl), 8–14. DOI: 10.7453/gahmj.2015.038.suppl

Ryan, R., & Connell, J. (1989). Academic Self-Regulation Questionnaire (SRQ-A). *Journal of Personality and Social Psychology*, *4*(1), 88–100.

Sabry, F., Eltaras, T., Labda, W., Alzoubi, K., & Malluhi, Q. (2022). Machine Learning for Healthcare Wearable Devices: The Big Picture. *Journal of Healthcare Engineering*, *2022*(1), 4653923. DOI: 10.1155/2022/4653923

Sadaria, D., Khachariya, H., & Hirpara, J. (2023). Priti, Dr. Haresh Khachariya, and Dr. Jignesh Hirpara. "Exploring the Diverse Applications of Deep Learning Across Multiple Domains.". *Recent Research Reviews Journal*, *2*(1), 183–200. DOI: 10.36548/rrrj.2023.1.16

Schmidt, P., Reiss, A., Duerichen, R., Marberger, C., & Van Laerhoven, K. (2018). Introducing WESAD, a multimodal dataset for wearable stress and affect detection. *Proceedings of the 20th ACM International Conference on Multimodal Interaction* (pp. 400-408). DOI: 10.1145/3242969.3242985

Schunk, D. H., & Greene, J. A. (2017). Historical, contemporary, and future perspectives on self-regulated learning and performance. In *Handbook of self-regulation of learning and performance* (pp. 1–15). Routledge. DOI: 10.4324/9781315697048-1

SDG. U. N. (2018). Sustainable development goals. *United Nations.*

Segal, Z. V., Teasdale, J. D., Williams, J. M., & Gemar, M. C. (2002). The mindfulness-based cognitive therapy adherence scale: Inter-rater reliability, adherence to protocol and treatment distinctiveness. *Clinical Psychology & Psychotherapy*, *9*(2), 131–138. DOI: 10.1002/cpp.320

Selvaraj, K., & Priya, S. (2025). Adaptive Yoga Intervention System for Remote Workers: A Computer Vision and AI-Based Framework. *International Journal of Yoga, Sports and Health Sciences*. https://ijyshs.melangepublications.com/index.php/ijyshs/article/view/2

Setiawati, D., Hakim, H. A., & Yoga, F. A. H. (2020). Optimizing personal data protection in Indonesia: Lesson learned from China, South Korea, and Singapore. *Indonesian Comparative Law Review*, *2*(2), 95–109. DOI: 10.18196/iclr.2219

Shaffer, F., & Ginsberg, J. P. (2017). Heart rate variability measures and norms. *Frontiers in Public Health*, *5*, 258. DOI: 10.3389/fpubh.2017.00258 PMID: 29034226

Shah, M., Gandhi, K., Pandhi, B. M., Padhiyar, P., & Degadwala, S. (2023). Computer Vision & Deep Learning based Realtime and Pre-Recorded Human Pose Estimation. DOI: 10.1109/ICAAIC56838.2023.10141279

Shaik, T., Tao, X., Li, L., Xie, H., & Velásquez, J. D. (2024). A survey of multimodal information fusion for smart healthcare: Mapping the journey from data to wisdom. *Information Fusion*, *102*, 102040. DOI: 10.1016/j.inffus.2023.102040

Shajari, S., Kuruvinashetti, K., Komeili, A., & Sundararaj, U. (2023). The Emergence of AI-Based Wearable Sensors for Digital Health Technology: A Review. *Sensors (Basel)*, *23*(23), 9498. DOI: 10.3390/s23239498

Shao, R., Man, I. S. C., & Lee, T. M. C. (2024). The Effect of Slow-Paced Breathing on Cardiovascular and Emotion Functions: A Meta-Analysis and Systematic Review. *Mindfulness*, *15*(1), 1–18. DOI: 10.1007/s12671-023-02294-2

Sharma, D., & Tiwari, R. (2024). Yoga and the Indian knowledge system: A holistic approach to well-being and self-realization. DOI: 10.69758/GIMRJ/2412IV-02V12P0002

Sharma, R.K. (1997). Fifth Edition. Chaukhambha Sanskrit Series Office, Varanasi. Chapter 30, Shloka 3–4.

Sharma, S., ... (2025). Effect of Yoga-based Interventions on Heart Rate Variability and Anxiety Among Students: A Systematic Review and Meta-Analysis. Journal of Ayurveda and Integrative Medicine (or similar). https://pmc.ncbi.nlm.nih.gov/articles/PMC12700775/

Sharma, A. K., & Sharma, R. (2024). Comparative Analysis of Data Protection Laws and ai Privacy Risks in brics Nations: A Comprehensive Examination. *Global Journal of Comparative Law*, *13*(1), 56–85.

Sharma, K., Anand, A., & Kumar, R. (2020). The role of Yoga in working from home during the COVID-19 global lockdown. *Work : A Journal of Prevention, Assessment, and Rehabilitation*, *66*(4), 731–737. DOI: 10.3233/WOR-203219 PMID: 32925134

Sharma, S. K., & Gaur, S. (2024). Optimizing Nutritional Outcomes: The Role of AI in Personalized Diet Planning. *International Journal for Research Publication and Seminar*, *15*(2), 107–116. DOI: 10.36676/jrps.v15.i2.15

Sharpe, E., Lacombe, A., Sadowski, A., Phipps, J., Heer, R., Rajurkar, S., Hanes, D., Jindal, R. D., & Bradley, R. (2021). Investigating Components of Pranayama for Effects on Heart Rate Variability. *Journal of Psychosomatic Research*, *148*, 110569. DOI: 10.1016/j.jpsychores.2021.110569

Sherlin, L. H., Arns, M., Lubar, J., Heinrich, H., Kerson, C., Strehl, U., & Sterman, M. B. (2011). Neurofeedback and basic learning theory. *Journal of Neurotherapy*, *15*(4), 292–304. DOI: 10.1080/10874208.2011.623089

Shih, C.-L., Liu, J.-Y., Anggraini, I. T., Xiao, Y., Funabiki, N., & Fan, C.-P. (2024). A yoga pose difficulty level estimation method using OpenPose for self-practice systems. *Information (Basel)*, *15*(12), 789. Advance online publication. DOI: 10.3390/info15120789

Shrivastava, D., Khilavdiya, Y., Gurele, S., & Mishra, D. (2024). Yoga Posture AI Assistant. *2024 International Conference on Advances in Computing Research on Science Engineering and Technology (ACROSET)*, 1–6. https://ieeexplore.ieee.org/abstract/document/10743779/

Siegel, R. D., & Germer, C. K. O. A. (2009). Mindfulness: What Is It? Where Did It Come From? In *Clinical Handbook of Mindfulness*.

Siemens, G. (2013). Learning analytics: The emergence of a discipline. *The American Behavioral Scientist*, *57*(10), 1380–1400. DOI: 10.1177/0002764213498851

Sikarwar, K., Venu, N., Dubey, A., & Bisen, D. (2025). AI-Based System for Real-Time Yoga Pose Detection and Correction. 2025 IEEE International Students' *Conference on Electrical, Electronics and Computer Science (SCEECS)*, 1–6.

Silas, N. (2024). AI in Chemistry: The Future of Scientific Discovery. *The Scientific Spectrum of AI Enhancing The Future*, 192.

Singh, B. (n.d.). *Integrating AI and Yogic Sciences: A Data-Driven Approach to Well-Being*. Retrieved January 11, 2026, from https://holisticyog.in/pdfs/Articles/1.pdf

Singh, L. (2024). *Revolutionizing Care: Developing an AI-Human Synergy Mental Health Application for Mental Health Worker's Well-Being* [PhD Thesis, Capella University]. https://search.proquest.com/openview/a3f04b7f88337706ce9bf96f23428956/1?pq-origsite=gscholar&cbl=18750&diss=y

Singh, R., Kumar, P., Ansari, M. H., & Dwivedi, M. (2024). Yoga Pose Detection Using Artificial Intelligence and Machine Learning. *2024 2nd International Conference on Disruptive Technologies (ICDT)*, 887–892. https://ieeexplore.ieee.org/abstract/document/10489410/

Singh, A., & Vats, A. (2025). Safe and Trusted Artificial Intelligence: Privacy as the cornerstone for digital transformation in Traditional Medicine. *International Journal of Ayurveda Research*, *6*(4), 286–292. DOI: 10.4103/ijar.ijar_340_25

Singhal, P. (2012). Continuous and comprehensive evaluation: A study of teachers' perception. *Delhi Business Review*, *13*(1), 81–99. DOI: 10.51768/dbr.v13i1.131201207

Singh, J., Kumar, S., & Arora, A. S. (2018). Thermographic evaluation of mindfulness meditation using dynamic IR imaging. *Infrared Physics & Technology*, *95*, 81–87. DOI: 10.1016/j.infrared.2018.10.029

Singleton, M. (2013). Transnational Exchange and the Genesis of Modern Postural Yoga. Transcultural Research - Heidelberg Studies on Asia and Europe in a Global Context, 37–56. DOI: 10.1007/978-3-319-00315-3_2

Singleton, M. (2010). *Yoga body: The origins of modern posture practice*. Oxford University Press. DOI: 10.1093/acprof:oso/9780195395358.001.0001

Sinha, N., & Sinha, R. K. (2024). Harnessing the Potential of Artificial Intelligence in Yoga Therapy. *International Journal of Yoga*, *17*(3), 242–245. DOI: 10.4103/ijoy.ijoy_124_24 PMID: 39959510

Soumma, S. B., Mamun, A., & Ghasemzadeh, H. (2025). AI-powered wearable sensors for health monitoring and clinical decision making. *Current Opinion in Biomedical Engineering*, *36*, 100628. DOI: 10.1016/j.cobme.2025.100628

Sprengel, M., Teo, L., Allen, S., Ijssennagger, N., Hammerschlag, R., Dyer, N., & Crawford, C. (2025). Biofield Therapies Clinical Research Landscape: A Scoping Review and Interactive Evidence Map. *Journal of Integrative and Complementary Medicine*, *31*(5), 406–430. Advance online publication. DOI: 10.1089/jicm.2024.0773

Srivastava, R., Khanna, P., & Anand, A. (2020). Digital Yoga Interventions in Social Distancing Era. *Annals of Neurosciences*, *097275312094516*. Advance online publication. DOI: 10.1177/0972753120945165 PMID: 34733049

Stahlschmidt, S. R., Ulfenborg, B., & Synnergren, J. (2022). Multimodal deep learning for biomedical data fusion: A review. *Briefings in Bioinformatics*, *23*(2), bbab569. Advance online publication. DOI: 10.1093/bib/bbab569

Stapleton, P. B., Buchan, C., Mitchell, I., McGrath, Y., Gorton, P., & Carter, B. (2019). An initial investigation of neural changes in overweight adults with food cravings after emotional freedom techniques. *OBM Integrative and Complimentary Medicine*, *4*(1), 1–12. Advance online publication. DOI: 10.21926/obm.icm.1901010

Suldo, S., Thalji, A., & Ferron, J. (2011). Longitudinal academic outcomes predicted by early adolescents' subjective well-being, psychopathology, and mental health status yielded from a dual factor model. *The Journal of Positive Psychology*, *6*(1), 17–30. DOI: 10.1080/17439760.2010.536774

Sulong, G. B., & Randles, N. M. (2023). Computer Vision Using Pose Estimation. *Wasit Journal of Computer and Mathematics Science (Print)*, *2*(1), 54–58. DOI: 10.31185/wjcm.111

Sundararajan, A. (2016). *The sharing economy: The end of employment and the rise of crowd-based capitalism*. MIT Press.

Tang, Y. Y., Ma, Y., Wang, J., Fan, Y., Feng, S., Lu, Q., Yu, Q., Sui, D., Rothbart, M. K., Fan, M., & Posner, M. I. (2007). Short-term meditation training improves attention and self-regulation. *Proceedings of the National Academy of Sciences of the United States of America*, *104*(43), 17152–17156. DOI: 10.1073/pnas.0707678104 PMID: 17940025

Tang, Y.-Y., Hölzel, B. K., & Posner, M. I. (2015a). The neuroscience of mindfulness meditation. *Nature Reviews. Neuroscience*, *16*(4), 213–225. DOI: 10.1038/nrn3916 PMID: 25783612

Teper, R., Segal, Z. V., & Inzlicht, M. (2013). Inside the Mindful Mind: How Mindfulness Enhances Emotion Regulation Through Improvements in Executive Control. *Current Directions in Psychological Science*, *22*(6), 449–454. DOI: 10.1177/0963721413495869

Thatte, D. G. (2016). *Elements of Shaarira Rachana* (1st ed.). Chaukhambha Orientalia.

Thayer, J. F., Ahs, F., Fredrikson, M., Sollers, J. J.III, & Wager, T. D. (2012). A meta-analysis of heart rate variability and neuroimaging studies: Implications for heart rate variability as a marker of stress and health. *Neuroscience and Biobehavioral Reviews*, *36*(2), 747–756. DOI: 10.1016/j.neubiorev.2011.11.009 PMID: 22178086

Thera, N. (1962). *The Heart of Buddhist Meditation (pp. 7Y113)*. Samuel Weiser.

Thompson, R., & Larson, P. (2020). Hybrid wellness models: Integrating technology and human instruction. *The Journal of Business Strategy*, *41*(4), 23–31.

Townsend, B. (2025). Multiculturalism and AI value alignment. DOI: 10.1093/9780198945215.003.0178

Tripathi, R. L. (2025). AI Meets Mindfulness: Redefining Spirituality and Meditation in the Digital Age. *The Voice of Creative Research*, *7*(1), 17–26. DOI: 10.53032/tvcr/2025.v7n1.03

Tripathi, S. M. (2021). Yogic theory of consciousness and its neuroscientific correlates: Chitta, Vritti, and the default mode network. *Journal of Consciousness Studies*, *28*(5-6), 112–145.

Trisia, R. (2025). Maintaining spiritual and balance technology in the AI era. *JKP: Jurnal Konseling dan Pendidikan, 13* (2), 150-155. DOI: 10.29210/1150800

Tyagi, R., Yadav, R., & Mishra, D. (2024). Technological Insights into Yoga Posture Recognition: A State-of-the-Art Review. *2024 International Conference on Communication, Computer Sciences and Engineering (IC3SE)*, 1–7. https://ieeexplore.ieee.org/abstract/document/10593008/

Upadhyay, A., Basha, N. K., & Ananthakrishnan, B. (2023). Deep learning-based yoga posture recognition using the Y_PN-MSSD model. *Healthcare (Basel)*, *11*(4), 609. DOI: 10.3390/healthcare11040609 PMID: 36833142

Vallabhaneni, N., & Prabhavathy, P. (2021). The analysis of the impact of yoga on healthcare and conventional strategies for human pose recognition. *Turkish Journal of Computer and Mathematics Education*, *12*(6), 1772–1783. DOI: 10.17762/turcomat.v12i6.4032

Van Dijk, J. A. (2005). *The deepening divide: Inequality in the information society*. Sage Publications.

VanLehn, K. (2011). The relative effectiveness of human tutoring, intelligent tutoring systems, and other tutoring systems. *Educational Psychologist*, *46*(4), 197–221. DOI: 10.1080/00461520.2011.611369

Venkatasubramanian, A. (2023). A digital health trust framework guided by values from the science of yoga. *Oxford Open Digital Health*, *1*, oqad007. DOI: 10.1093/oodh/oqad007

Venkatesh, V., Thong, J. Y., & Xu, X. (2012). Consumer acceptance and use of information technology: Extending the unified theory of acceptance and use of technology. *Management Information Systems Quarterly*, *36*(1), 157–178. DOI: 10.2307/41410412

Verma, P., Sharma, R., & Rajput, N. S. (2023). Enhancing yoga practice through real-time posture detection and correction using artificial intelligence: A comprehensive review. *NeuroQuantology : An Interdisciplinary Journal of Neuroscience and Quantum Physics*, *21*(6), 1053.

Vijayalakshmi, P. S., & A, D. D. (2025). The Personalized Fitness and Nutrition Coach. *International Journal of Research Publication and Reviews*, *6*(4), 6822–6826. DOI: 10.55248/gengpi.6.0425.14155

Vyas, M. V. (1975). *The Bhagavad Gita*. Maharshi Ved vyas.

Vyshnivskyi, D., Liashenko, O., & Yeromina, N. (2023). HUMAN POSE ESTIMATION SYSTEM USING DEEP LEARNING ALGORITHMS. *Navigation and Communication Control Systems Collection of Scientific Papers*, *2*(72), 75–79. DOI: 10.26906/SUNZ.2023.2.075

Waghmode, P., Shitole, A., Telrandhe, M., & Bide, P. J. (2023, May 1). Real-time Yoga Pose Classification and Correction: YogaAI. DOI: 10.1109/INCET57972.2023.10170599

Walter, M., Lovett, R., Maher, B., Williamson, B., Prehn, J., Bodkin-Andrews, G., & Lee, V. (2021). Indigenous Data Sovereignty in the Era of Big Data and Open Data. *The Australian Journal of Social Issues*, *56*(2), 143–156. DOI: 10.1002/ajs4.141

Wang, Y.-C., Lu, Y., Grunwald, S., Chu, S. L., Kamble, P., & Kumar, J. (2024). An AI Approach to Support Student Mental Health: Case of Developing an AI-Powered Web-Platform with Nature-Based Mindfulness. *Journal of Hospitality & Tourism Education*, *36*(3), 267–280. DOI: 10.1080/10963758.2024.2369128

Warden, P., & Situnayake, D. (2019). *TinyML: Machine learning with TensorFlow Lite on Arduino and other ultra low-power microcontrollers*. O'Reilly Media.

White, D. G. (2012). *Yoga in Practice*. Princeton University Press. DOI: 10.1515/9781400839933

Williams, D., Thompson, K., & Martinez, S. (2021). Adherence and outcomes in digital versus in-person yoga interventions: A comparative effectiveness study. *Complementary Therapies in Medicine*, *58*, 102693.

Wilson, S., et al. (2025). Feasibility and Effectiveness of Portable/Remote Heart Rate Variability (HRV) Biofeedback Training in Treating Stress and Mental Health Difficulties: A Systematic Review. Applied Psychophysiology and Biofeedback. https://doi.org/doi:10.1007/s10484-025-09751-9

Winne, P. H., & Hadwin, A. F. (2013). nStudy: Tracing and supporting self-regulated learning in the Internet. In *International handbook of metacognition and learning technologies* (pp. 293–308). Springer.

Woodroffe, J. (1974). *The Serpent Power*. Dover Publications.

World Health Organization. (2022). *World mental health report: Transforming mental health for all*. WHO.

World Health Organization. Ethics and Governance of Artificial Intelligence for Health: Guidance on Large Multi-Modal Models, Geneva, Switzerland, 2025.

Xiang, , Andrews, J. T. A., Bourke, R. L., Thong, W., LaChance, J. M., Georgievski, T., Modas, A., Rahmattalabbi, A., Ba, Y., Nagpal, S., Papakyriakopoulos, O., Zhao, D., Xue, J., Matthews, V., Gong, L., Hoag, A. T., Cimpoi, M., Sankaranarayanan, S., Hutiri, W., & Spranger, M. (2025). Fair human-centric image dataset for ethical AI benchmarking. *Nature*, *648*(8092), 97–108. DOI: 10.1038/s41586-025-09716-2 PMID: 41193813

Xie, Y., Zhao, B., Dai, M., Zhou, J.-P., Sun, Y., Tan, T., Xie, W., Shen, L., & Yu, Z. (2025). Physllm: Harnessing large language models for cross-modal remote physiological sensing. *ArXiv Preprint ArXiv:2505.03621*.

Xi, Y., Huang, T., & Yang, Z. (2026). Multimodal human action recognition and personalized sports health promotion: A deep learning framework integrating wearable sensor fusion. *Frontiers in Neurorobotics*, *20*, 1785114. Advance online publication. DOI: 10.3389/fnbot.2026.1785114 PMID: 42037737

Xu, Y., Zhang, Z., & Wang, Y. (2024). *Cross-cultural generalization in vision-based human activity recognition* (Vol. 149). Pattern Recognition.

Xu, Z.. (2024). “Addressing fairness issues in deep learning-based medical image analysis: A systematic review,” *npj. Digital Medicine*, *7*, 286. PMID: 39420149

Yenishettil, S., Karajkhede, G., & Panat, L. (2024). Virtual yoga teacher with AI model for yoga posture correction for good health. DOI: 10.23919/ITUK62727.2024.10772930

Ying, J.. "LDPose: Towards inclusive human pose estimation for limb-deficient individuals in the wild," in *Proc. IEEE/CVF Int. Conf. on Computer Vision (ICCV)*, 2025. DOI: 10.1109/ICCV51701.2025.00920

Yoga Alliance & Yoga Journal. (2021). *2021 yoga in America study*. Yoga Alliance.

Yoga Ratnam, K. K. (2025). Generative artificial intelligence in public health research and scientific communication: A narrative review of real applications and future directions. *Digital Health, 11*, 20552076251362070. DOI: 10.1177/20552076251362070 PMID: 40842935

Yoon, J., Jarrett, D., & Van der Schaar, M. (2019). Time-series generative adversarial networks. Advances in Neural Information Processing Systems (NeurIPS), 32, 5508-5518.

Yuan, Y., Liu, B., Li, H., Li, M., Song, Y., Wang, R., Wang, T., & Zhang, H. (2022). Flexible Wearable Sensors in Medical Monitoring. *Biosensors (Basel), 12*(12), 1069. DOI: 10.3390/bios12121069

Zaccaro, A., Piarulli, A., Laurino, M., Garbella, E., Menicucci, D., Neri, B., & Gemignani, A. (2018). How Breath-Control Can Change Your Life: A Systematic Review on Psycho-Physiological Correlates of Slow Breathing. *Frontiers in Human Neuroscience, 12*, 353. DOI: 10.3389/fnhum.2018.00353

Zaheer, S. (n.d.). Designing Emotion-Aware UX: Leveraging Sentiment Analysis to Adapt Digital Experiences. Retrieved January 13, 2026

Zawacki-Richter, O., Marín, V. I., Bond, M., & Gouverneur, F. (2019). Systematic review of research on artificial intelligence applications in higher education–where are the educators? *International Journal of Educational Technology in Higher Education, 16*(1), 39. DOI: 10.1186/s41239-019-0171-0

Zenner, C., Herrnleben-Kurz, S., & Walach, H. (2014a). Mindfulness-based interventions in schools-A systematic review and meta-analysis. *Frontiers in Psychology, 5*(JUN). Advance online publication. DOI: 10.3389/fpsyg.2014.00603 PMID: 25071620

Zhao, X., Zheng, H., & Zhang, Q. (2025). Modern Advances in Artificial Intelligence Across the Athletic Domain. *Concurrency and Computation, 37*(9-11), e70068. Advance online publication. DOI: 10.1002/cpe.70068

Zhao, Y., Ni, Q., & Zhou, R. (2018). What factors influence the mobile health service adoption? A meta-analysis and the moderating role of age. *International Journal of Information Management, 43*, 342–350. DOI: 10.1016/j.ijinfomgt.2017.08.006

Zhou, H., Li, Y., & Huang, K. (2024). AI-assisted physical activity monitoring for personalized wellness. *Sensors (Basel), 24*(2).

Zhu, L., Spachos, P., Ng, P. C., Yu, Y., Wang, Y., Plataniotis, K., & Hatzinakos, D. (2023). Stress Detection Through Wrist-Based Electrodermal Activity Monitoring and Machine Learning. *IEEE Journal of Biomedical and Health Informatics, 27*(5), 2155–2165. DOI: 10.1109/JBHI.2023.3239305

Zickerick, B., Thönes, S., Kobald, S. O., Wascher, E., Schneider, D., & Küper, K. (2020a). Differential Effects of Interruptions and Distractions on Working Memory Processes in an ERP Study. *Frontiers in Human Neuroscience, 14*, 84. DOI: 10.3389/fnhum.2020.00084

Zimmerman, B. J. (1994). Dimensions of academic self-regulation: A conceptual framework for education. *Self-Regulation of Learning and Performance: Issues and Educational Applications, 1*, 21–33.

Zimmerman, B. J. (2000). Attaining self-regulation: A social cognitive perspective. In *Handbook of self-regulation* (pp. 13–39). Elsevier. DOI: 10.1016/B978-012109890-2/50031-7

Zimmerman, B. J. (2002). Becoming a self-regulated learner: An overview. *Theory into Practice, 41*(2), 64–70. DOI: 10.1207/s15430421tip4102_2

Zoefel, B., Huster, R. J., & Herrmann, C. S. (2011). Neurofeedback training of the upper alpha frequency band in EEG improves cognitive performance. *NeuroImage, 54*(2), 1427–1431. DOI: 10.1016/j.neuroimage.2010.08.078 PMID: 20850552

About the Contributors

Ayoub Khan(Senior member IEEE) received his Ph. D (Electrical Engg.) from Jamia Millia Islamia, New Delhi, India, and Master of Technology (Computer Science and Engineering) from Guru Gobind Singh Indraprastha, New Delhi, India. Presently, he is working as Deputy Director, Smart Cyber-Physical System (CPS) Research Centre, University of Bisha, Saudi Arabia with interests in Internet of Things, RFID, Wireless Sensors Networks, Ad Hoc Network, Smart Cities, Industrial IoT, and signal processing, NFC, Routing in Network-on-Chip, Real Time and Embedded Systems. He is a certified Chief Information Security Officer (CISO) and Certified Information Security Manager (CISM). He has more than 14 years of experience in his research and consultancy area.

Raghav Mehra is a Professor and Program Leader of AIML at Chandigarh University with over 21 years of academic and research experience. He has served as HOD, Dean of Academics, and Assistant Director in reputed AICTE and UGC-approved institutions, leading them to achieve ISO, NBA, and NAAC accreditations.

S. Kanaga Suba Raja is a Professor and Associate Dean at the School of Computing, SRM Institute of Science and Technology, Tiruchirappalli, with over 20 years of teaching and research experience in Computer Science and Engineering. He has supervised 13 Ph.D. scholars, published more than 120 international journal papers, including 23 in SCI/WoS-indexed journals, and authored 9 book chapters.

Pushkar Praveen is an Assistant Professor in the Department of Electronics and Communication Engineering at G.B. Pant Institute of Engineering and Technology, Pauri Garhwal, Uttarakhand, India. He received his Ph.D. in Electronics and Communication Engineering from Uttarakhand Technical University and M.Tech. in VLSI Design from CDAC Noida. He has over 13 years of academic and industry experience. His research interests include electronic device and circuit design, VLSI systems, embedded systems, Internet of Things (IoT). Dr. Praveen has published several research articles in reputed SCI/SCIE and Scopus-indexed journals and conferences. He has also contributed to multiple edited books and book chapters. He is actively involved in organizing faculty development programs, conferences, and research projects funded by national and international agencies. Dr. Praveen is a member of professional organizations including IEEE, IAENG, and ISTE.

Rijwan Khan is currently working as Professor & Dean FoCA at Marwadi University, India . He also worked as Dean Emerging Technologies and Training at ABES Institute of Technology, Ghaziabad. He completed his PhD in 2017 from Jamia Millia Islamia University, New Delhi, India. He has more than 20 years' experience of teaching. He served as Head of Department-CSE in ABESIT and also Dean Research in ABESIT. He is editor in chief of Journal of Engineering, Science and Mathematics (JESM). He is guest editor of more than 15 journals. He edited 10 books in Elsevier, IGI Global, CRC and Bentham Science. He published 12 SCI Indexed Journal Papers, 21 Scopus Indexed Journal Papers and 21 Conference papers and 19 book chapters. He was keynote speaker in an international conference in Muscat, Oman conducted by Ministry of Agriculture, Oman. He has H index 25 and I index 40 and number of citations are more than 2500. He is member of ACM, ISTE, IETE.

***

Yagnik Dave is a dedicated physiotherapist and currently serves as an assistant professor at Marwadi University, Rajkot. He is guiding PG and PhD scholars. With over 7.5 years of academic, clinical, and research experience, he has established himself as an emerging contributor to the field of physiotherapy education and practice. Dr. Dave has an extensive research portfolio, with more than 40 publications, many of which are indexed in Scopus and Web of Science, reflecting the quality and impact of his scholarly work. He has actively participated in academic forums, presenting over 6 papers at various national and international conferences, contributing to knowledge exchange and professional development within the physiotherapy community. In addition to his research contributions, Dr. Yagnik Dave has authored one book and has published five patents, showcasing his commitment to innovation and advancement in healthcare sciences. Through his academic leadership, clinical expertise, and research-driven approach, Dr. Yagnik Dave continues to significantly contribute to the growth of physiotherapy as a health science profession. He has also conducted various expert sessions on topics like CPR, yoga integration with physiotherapy, advancements in cardiac rehabilitation, and strategic exercise planning for obesity.

Ashwin R. Dobariya is an academic and researcher with over 22+ years of experience in computer science and information technology. Currently working as an Associate Professor at Marwadi University, Rajkot, he holds a Ph.D. with his research specialization in image processing, machine vision, artificial intelligence, machine learning, and deep learning. As a dedicated Ph.D. supervisor, Dr. Dobariya is actively guiding research scholars at Marwadi University. His academic contributions include numerous publications in national and international journals and conferences, along with many patents. A prolific author, he has written five books on C programming. He has also contributed to the scholarly community as a session chair and reviewer at many reputed international conferences. In recognition of his outstanding academic and institutional contributions, Dr. Dobariya received the "Best Outstanding Performer" award from Marwadi University in year 2015 and 2016.

Jaypalsinh A. Gohil is an academician and researcher with over 20 years of experience in higher education and research. He holds a Ph.D. in Computer Science from MK Bhavnagar University and has published extensively in reputed international journals and conferences, including Springer-indexed publications. His research interests include blockchain technology, database systems, concurrency control, machine learning, and emerging applications in real estate and IoT. He is an Oracle Academy Certified Professional and serves as a Ph.D. supervisor for multiple research scholars. Dr. Gohil is also a co-author of three patent publications focused on IoT-based smart systems, waste disposal management, and agricultural water supply optimization, reflecting his commitment to translating research into practical solutions. He has authored textbooks on system analysis, design, and development, and actively contributes to curriculum design and faculty development initiatives.

Hemang Jani is a Professor and In-charge Principal at the Institute of Physiotherapy, Ganpat University (Mehsana, Gujarat), with more than 15 years of academic, clinical, and research experience in physiotherapy. He has made significant contributions in the areas of cardiopulmonary rehabilitation, exercise prescription, musculoskeletal physiotherapy, and community health. Dr. Jani is an editorial board member of Nature's Scientific Reports and the Physiotherapy and Occupational Therapy Journal and serves as a reviewer for more than 14 national and international journals, including the European Respiratory Journal and the American Journal of Sports Medicine. His Ph.D. research focuses on yogic and breathing interventions for sedentary smokers, aligning with his interest in integrative rehabilitation and public health.

Ashish Kakkad (PT) Professor & Principal, Faculty of Physiotherapy, Marwadi University, Rajkot, Gujarat, India He passed his BPT and MPT from the Government

Physiotherapy College, Gujarat University, Ahmedabad. He has a PhD in the topic of stroke prognosis. He has a total of 15+ years of teaching experience. He has published one book, "Fundamentals of Electrotherapy and Biomedical Physics," under Jaypee International Publication. He has also launched a mobile application in the Google Play store named "Stroke recovery predictor" for the prognosis of stroke recovery. He is a member of the Professional Physiotherapy Council, National Commission for Allied & Healthcare Professionals. He has been awarded twice by the Indian Association for his significant contribution to the field. He has published 40+ research papers and 18 IPR (Design/Patent/Copyright). His area of interest is electrodiagnosis. He is a recognised PhD guide.

Harmanpreet Kaur is an eminent academician, researcher, and sportsperson, currently serving as an Associate Professor and Former Head, Department of Physical Education, Lovely Professional University, Punjab. She has made exceptional contributions to the fields of Physical Education, Sports Sciences, and Research Innovation through her academic leadership, research excellence, and athletic achievements. Dr. Kaur has published over 80 research papers in reputed national and international journals, authored 4 books, and contributed to 7 book chapters. With extensive research guidance experience, she has mentored 40 M.P.Ed, 20 M.Phil, and 7 Ph.D. scholars to successful completion. She has also participated in 50+ national and international conferences, workshops, and faculty development programmes (FDPs) and holds 10+ copyrights and patents, including one recognized under Artificial Intelligence Innovation by Lovely Professional University. In recognition of her remarkable achievements, Dr. Harmanpreet Kaur has received several prestigious awards, including: • Mother Teresa Award by Human Growth and Development Society • Young Researcher Award by INSC – Institute of Scholars, under the Ministry of MSME, Government of India • Innotek Award on Patent in Artificial Intelligence by Lovely Professional University Beyond academia, Dr. Kaur is actively engaged in sports administration and development. She serves as the Joint Secretary of Punjab Women Hockey Association and Hockey Punjab, and is the President of Floorball Association of Punjab as well as a Member of the Floorball Federation of India. She is also affiliated with professional bodies such as AIAER (All India Association for Educational Research) and INSC (Institute of Scholars). An accomplished hockey player, Dr. Kaur has brought laurels to her name and the nation by securing four Gold Medals in All India Inter-University Championships, two Silver Medals in Senior National Championships, and two Bronze Medals in National Games. Her outstanding performance earned her the title of Best Player of India at the Senior National Competition.

Swasti Mehra is an undergraduate student of Instrumentation and Control Engineering at Sant Longowal Institute of Engineering and Technology (SLIET), India. Her academic interests lie in Internet of Things (IoT), biomedical instrumentation, and emerging applications of Artificial Intelligence in healthcare. She is actively involved in developing smart monitoring systems, including a non-contact sleep monitoring project using thermal sensing and embedded platforms. She is particularly interested in the integration of IoT with yoga-based wellness systems and contributes to research in the area of YogAI, focusing on technology-driven preventive healthcare and personalized wellness solutions.

Ratnesh Kumar Namdeo is an accomplished academician with over 15 years of teaching experience in Computer Science and Applications. He is currently serving as an Assistant Professor in the Faculty of Computer Applications at Marwadi University, Rajkot (Gujarat), where he contributes to undergraduate and postgraduate teaching, curriculum enhancement and academic mentoing. His research expertise spans Neural Networks, Machine Learning, Cloud Computing, and Neuro-Fuzzy Systems. He has published multiple research papers in UGC CARE and peer-reviewed journals and holds two published patents in the domains of cloud security and machine-learning-based data classification. Dr. Ratnesh Namdeo has also edited a book on Data Science and actively participates in conferences, workshops, and faculty development programs. Throughout his career, he has held significant roles such as Head of Department, Online Examination Cell In-Charge, Career Guidance Cell Coordinator, and Examination Superintendent for MPPSC, UPSC, CUET, and NIELIT examinations. His academic contributions also include serving as a Board of Studies member at Govt. M.H. College, Jabalpur. Dr. Ratnesh Namdeo holds a Ph.D. in Computer Science and Applications, with his research focused on neuro-fuzzy models for non-linear climatological time series data. He is passionate about innovative teaching, research excellence, and advancing technology-driven education.

Prakasha G S is an Associate Professor at School of Education, Christ University Central campus, Bangalore, India. He has 21+ years of teaching and research experiences in Education. His research interest areas are Teacher-education, Educational-technology, Teaching-learning, Assessment-evaluation, and Higher education. He has published research articles in peer-reviewed journals indexed in Scopus and web of science. He conducts Quantitative data-analysis workshops and delivers lectures on Research and Publication. He is an active editorial board member for Sage Open, Springer Nature, Tylor & Francis, and IGI Global. He is actively involved in research activities, which have national and international importance.

N. Rajkumar is a Research Scholar at the School of Education, Christ (Deemed to be) University, Central Campus, Bengaluru, India. His research is situated within the interdisciplinary field of mindfulness in education. He is committed to advancing research that bridges traditional contemplative practices with contemporary educational psychology. Email: n.rajkumar@res.christuniversity.in

Amrik Singh is working as Professor and HOD in the School of Hotel Management and Tourism at Lovely Professional University, Punjab, India. He obtained his Ph.D. degree in Hotel Management from Kurukshetra University, Haryana, India. He has published 115 Scopus-indexed publications. He has published 12 patents, and 01 patent has been granted in the inter-disciplinary domain. Dr. Amrik Singh participated and acted as a resource person in various national and international conferences, seminars, research workshops, and industry talks. He has published 20 books with IGI Global Publication, Emerald Publication, Bentham Publication, Nova Publication etc., on trending areas such as Food waste, Artificial Intelligence, Mountain Tourism, Virtual tourism, Healthcare Tourism, Guest behavior in tourism and hospitality. His area of research interest are Accommodation management, sustainability, Green practices, Human Resource Management in Hospitality, Artificial Intelligence, AR VR in hospitality, Hotel pricing, Employee Disability, Work life balance, women empowerment etc. He is currently guiding 8 Ph.D. scholars, and 5 Ph.D. scholars have been awarded Ph.D.

Sandeep Kumar Singh is a faculty in the area of Information Systems and Analytics at Jindal Global Business School, O.P. Jindal Global University, Sonipat. Prior to joining Jindal Global Business School, he worked as an Assistant Professor at JKLU Jaipur for two years. He has earned his Ph.D. in computational physics from Antwerpen University, Belgium. His PhD work focused on mathematical modeling and simulation of two-dimensional materials. Post to his PhD, he worked as a research scientist in Sweden for four years in energy storage systems, bioelectronics. He also did MTech in industrial mathematics and scientific computing from IIT Madras, Chennai. His current research interests are to apply complex mathematical modeling in the business and financial world.

Dimple Thakar is an Assistant Professor in the Department of Computer Applications at Marwadi University, Rajkot, India, with over 21 years of academic and industry experience. She holds a Ph.D. in Computer Science with a specialization in Image Processing. Her research interests span Artificial Intelligence, Machine Learning, medical image analysis, image steganography, data hiding techniques, and cyber security applications. She is an active member of professional bodies such as IEEE and ACM and contributes to the scholarly community through peer review, editorial responsibilities, and international conference organization. Dr. Thakar has published research articles, book chapters, and conference papers with reputed publishers including CRC Press and Springer. She also serves as Editor-in-Chief and editorial board member of international journals. Dr. Thakar is a recognized keynote speaker and delivered a keynote address on AI-Enhanced Air and Water Quality Monitoring at the international conference "Sustainable AI 2025: AI for a Greener Planet." Her academic work reflects a strong interdisciplinary and application-driven research approach.

Index

N

P

Q

R

S

T

W

Y

www.ingramcontent.com/pod-product-compliance
Lightning Source LLC
LaVergne TN
LVHW060005031026
849161LV00025B/1427
* 9 7 9 8 2 6 0 0 2 4 6 3 8 *